DENTAL SECRETS

DENTAL
SECRETS

STEPHEN T. SONIS, D.M.D., D.M.Sc.

Professor and Chairman
Department of Oral Medicine and
  Diagnostic Sciences
Harvard School of Dental Medicine
Chief, Division of Oral Medicine and Dentistry
Brigham and Women's Hospital
Boston, Massachusetts

HANLEY & BELFUS, INC./ Philadelphia
MOSBY/ St. Louis • Baltimore • Boston • Chicago • London
  Philadelphia • Sydney • Toronto

Publisher: HANLEY & BELFUS, INC.
                210 S. 13th Street
                Philadelphia, PA 19107
                (215) 546-7293

North American and worldwide sales and distribution:

                MOSBY
                11830 Westline Industrial Drive
                St. Louis, MO 63146

In Canada: Times Mirror Professional Publishing, Ltd.
                130 Flaska Drive
                Markham, Ontario L6G 1B8
                Canada

Library of Congress Cataloging-in-Publication Data

Dental secrets / edited by Stephen T. Sonis.
    p.   cm.
    Includes bibliographical references and index.
    ISBN 1-56053-063-4
    1. Dentistry—Examinations, questions, etc.   I. Sonis, Stephen T.
    |DNLM: 1. Dental Care—examination questions.   WU 18 D4165 1994|
    RK57.D48   1994
    617.6'0076—dc20
    DNLM/DLC
    for Library of Congress   94-14804
                                                                  CIP

DENTAL SECRETS   ISBN 1-56053-063-4

Library of Congress catalog card number   94-14804

Last digit is the print number: 9   8   7   6   5   4   3   2   1

DEDICATION

To my father, H. Richard Sonis, D.D.S.

with admiration and gratitude.

CONTENTS

CONTRIBUTORS

Helene S. Bednarsh, B.S., R.D.H., M.P.H.
Program Manager, HIV Dental Ombudsperson Program, Community Dental Programs, Boston Department of Public Health, Boston, Massachusetts

Kathy J. Eklund, B.S., R.D.H., M.H.P.
Clinical Associate Professor of Dental Hygiene, Forsyth Dental Center, School for Dental Hygienists, Boston, Massachusetts

Elliot V. Feldbau, D.M.D.
Instructor in Operative Dentistry, Harvard School of Dental Medicine; Surgeon, Division of Oral Medicine and Dentistry, Brigham and Women's Hospital, Boston, Massachusetts

Steven P. Levine, D.M.D.
Assistant Clinical Professor, Department of Endodontics, Tufts University School of Dental Medicine, Boston, Massachusetts

Steven Migliorini, D.M.D.
Instructor, Department of Oral Medicine and Diagnostic Sciences, Harvard School of Dental Medicine; Surgeon, Division of Oral Medicine and Dentistry, Brigham and Women's Hospital, Boston, Massachusetts

John A. Molinari, Ph.D.
Professor and Chairman, Department of Biomedical Sciences, University of Detroit Mercy School of Dentistry, Detroit, Michigan

Mark S. Obernesser, D.D.S., M.M.Sc.
Instructor in Periodontology, Harvard School of Dental Medicine; Associate Surgeon, Brigham and Women's Hospital, Boston, Massachusetts

Edward S. Peters, D.M.D., M.S.
Instructor in Oral Medicine and Diagnostic Sciences, Harvard School of Dental Medicine; Associate Surgeon, Division of Oral Medicine and Dentistry, Brigham and Women's Hospital, Boston, Massachusetts

Dale Potter, D.D.S., M.P.H.
Instructor in Oral Medicine and Diagnostic Sciences, Harvard School of Dental Medicine; Director, Harvard-Brigham Residency Program in General Dentistry; Surgeon, Division of Oral Medicine and Dentistry, Brigham and Women's Hospital, Boston, Massachusetts

Andrew L. Sonis, D.M.D.
Associate Clinical Professor of Pediatric Dentistry, Harvard School of Dental Medicine; Associate in Dentistry, Department of Dentistry, Children's Hospital Medical Center; Surgeon, Division of Oral Medicine and Dentistry, Brigham and Women's Hospital, Boston, Massachusetts

Stephen T. Sonis, D.M.D., D.M.Sc.
Professor and Chairman, Department of Oral Medicine and Diagnostic Sciences, Harvard School of Dental Medicine; Chief, Division of Oral Medicine and Dentistry, Brigham and Women's Hospital, Boston, Massachusetts

Ralph B. Sozio, D.M.D.
Lecturer in Prosthetic Dentistry, Harvard School of Dental Medicine; Consultant, Division
of Oral Medicine and Dentistry, Brigham and Women's Hospital, Boston,
Massachusetts

Willie L. Stephens, D.D.S.
Instructor in Oral and Maxillofacial Surgery, Harvard School of Dental Medicine; Surgeon,
Division of Oral Medicine and Dentistry, Brigham and Women's Hospital, Boston,
Massachusetts

Richard W. Valachovic, D.M.D., M.Sc.
Associate Professor and Head, Division of Oral and Maxillofacial Radiology, Harvard
School of Dental Medicine; Attending Dentist, Department of Dentistry, Children's Hospital
Medical Center, Boston, Massachusetts

Sook-Bin Woo, D.M.D., M.M.Sc.
Instructor in Oral Medicine and Diagnostic Sciences, Harvard School of Dental Medicine;
Surgeon, Division of Oral Medicine and Dentistry, Brigham and Women's Hospital, Boston,
Massachusetts

PREFACE

This book was written by people who like to teach for people who like to learn. Its format of questions and short answers lends itself to the dissemination of information as the kinds of "pearls" that teachers are always trying to provide and for which students yearn. The format also permits a lack of formality not available in a standard text. Consequently, the reader will note smatterings of humor throughout the book. Our goal has been to provide a work that readers will enjoy and find useful and stimulating.

This book is not a substitute for the many excellent textbooks available in dentistry. It is our hope that readers will pursue additional readings in areas which they find stimulating. While short answers provide the passage of succinct information, they do not allow for much discussion in the way of background or rationale. We have tried to provide sufficient breadth in the sophistication of questions in each chapter to meet the needs of dental students, residents, and practitioners.

It has been a pleasure working with my colleagues who have contributed to this book. I would like to thank Mike Bokulich for initiating this project. Finally, I am grateful to Linda Belfus, our publisher and editor, for her assistance, attention to detail, and patience.

Stephen T. Sonis, D.M.D., D.M.Sc.
Boston, Massachusetts

THE FAR SIDE

By GARY LARSON

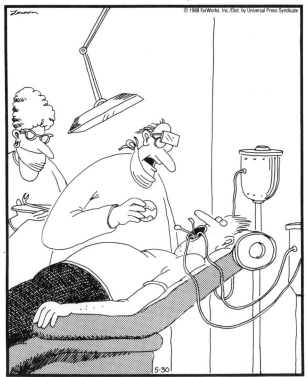

"Now open even wider, Mr. Stevens. ...
Just out of curiosity, we're going to see
if we can also cram in this tennis ball."

1. PATIENT MANAGEMENT: THE DENTIST–PATIENT RELATIONSHIP

Elliot V. Feldbau, D.M.D.

After you seat the patient, a 42-year-old woman, she turns to you and glibly says, "Doctor, I don't like dentists." How should you respond?

As you prepare to do a root canal on tooth number 9, a 58-year-old man responds, "The last time I had that dam on, I couldn't catch my breath. . . . It was horrible." How would you proceed? What may be the significance of his statement?

A 36-year-old woman who has not been to the dentist for almost 10 years tells you, "My last dentist said I was allergic to a local anesthetic. I passed out in the dental chair after the injection." How do you interpret this information? How do you proceed?

A 55-year-old man is referred for periodontal surgery. During the medical history, he states that he had his tonsils out at age 10 years and that since then any work on his mouth frightens him. He feels like gagging. How do you respond? What line of questioning do you pursue?

With each of the above patients, the dentist should be alerted that something is not routine. Each expresses deep concern and anxiety. This is clearly the time for the dentist to remove the gloves, lower the mask, and begin a comprehensive interview. Although responses to such situations may vary according to individual style, each clinician should proceed methodically and carefully to gather specific information based on the cues that the patient presents. By understanding each patient's comments and the feelings related to earlier experiences, the dentist can help the patient to see that change is possible and that coping with dental treatment is easily learned.

The following questions and answers are intended to provide a framework for conducting a therapeutic interview that increases patient compliance and reduces levels of anxiety.

1. What are two basic objectives of the initial patient interview?

1. A verbal exchange with the patient to discover all elements of the medical and personal history relevant to treating the patient's dental needs.

2. A nonverbal empathic exchange in which the following *feelings* are communicated to the patient: Attentiveness and concern for the patient

        Acceptance of the patient and his or her problem

        Support for the patient

        Involvement with the intent to help the patient

2. How may the preceding *feelings* be conveyed to a patient?

By listening attentively and giving your full attention, you demonstrate both a physical presence and a comprehension of what the patient relates. Appropriate physical attending skills enhance the process. Understanding what you hear allows you to respond to the content of a patient's remarks while clarifying and enlarging the issues discussed. The patient gains some insight into his or her problem, and rapport is further enhanced.

3. What useful physical attending skills comprise the nonverbal component of communication?

The adept use of face, voice, and body facilitates the classic bedside manner, including the following:

Eye contact: Looking at the patient without overt staring establishes rapport.

Facial expression: A smile or nod of the head to affirm shows warmth, concern, and interest.

Vocal characteristics: The voice is modulated to express meaning and to help the patient to understand important issues.

Body orientation: Facing patients as you stand or sit signals attentiveness. Turning away may seem like rejection.

Forward lean and proximity: Leaning forward tells a patient that you are interested and want to hear more, thus facilitating the patient's comments. Proximity infers intimacy, whereas distance signals less attentiveness. In general, 4–6 feet is considered a social, consultative zone.

A verbal message of low empathic value may be altered favorably by maintaining eye contact, forward trunk lean, and appropriate distance and body orientation. However, even a verbal message of high empathic content may be reduced to a lower value when the speaker does not have eye contact, turns away with backward lean, or maintains too far a distance. For example, do not tell the patient that you are concerned while washing your hands with your back to the dental chair!

4. During the interview, what cues alert the dentist to search for more information about a statement made by the patient?
Most people express information that they do not fully understand by using many generalizations, deletions, and distortions in their phrasing. For example, the comment, "I am a horrible patient," does not give much insight into the patient's intent. By probing further the dentist may discover specific fears or behaviors that the patient has deleted in the opening generalization. As a matter of routine, the dentist should be alert to such cues and use the interview to clarify and work through the patient's comments. As the interview proceeds, trust and rapport are built as a mutual understanding develops and levels of fear decrease.

5. Why is open-ended questioning useful as an interviewing format?
Questions that do not have specific yes or no answers give patients more latitude to express themselves. More information allows a better understanding of patients and their problems. The dentist is basically saying, "Tell me more about it." Throughout the interview the clinician listens to any cues that indicate the need to pursue further questioning for more information about expressed fears or concerns. Typical questions of the open-ended format include the following: "What brings you here today?," "Are you having any problems?," or "Please tell me more about it."

6. How can the dentist help the patient to relate more information or to talk about a certain issue in greater depth?
A communication technique called *facilitation by reflection* is helpful. One simply repeats the last word or phrase that was spoken in a questioning tone of voice. Thus when a patient says, "I am petrified of dentists," the dentist responds, "Petrified of dentists?" The patient usually elaborates.

The goal is to go from *generalization* to *specific fear* to the *origin* of the fear. The process is therapeutic and allows fears to be reduced or diminished as patients gain insight into their feelings.

7. How should one construct suggestions that help patients to alter their behavior or that influence the outcome of a command?
Negatives should be avoided in commands. Positive commands are more easily experienced, and compliance is usually greater. To experience a negation, the patient first creates the positive image and then somehow negates it. In experience only positive situations can be realized; language forms negation. For example, to experience the command "Do not run!" one may visualize (experience) oneself sitting, standing, or walking slowly. A more direct command is "Stop!" or "Walk!" Moreover, a negative command may create more resistance to compliance, whether voluntary or not. If you ask someone not to see elephants, he or she tends to see elephants first. Therefore, it may be best to ask patients to keep their mouth open widely rather than to say "Don't close"—or perhaps to suggest, "Rest open widely, please."

A permissive approach and indirect commands also create less resistance and enhance compliance. One may say, "If you stay open widely, I can do my procedure faster and better," or "By flossing daily, you will experience a fresher breath and a healthier smile." This style of suggestion is usually better received than a direct command.

Linking phrases—for example, "as," "while," or "when"—to join a suggestion with something that is happening in the patient's immediate experience provides an easier pathway for a patient to follow and further enhances compliance. Examples include the following: "As you lie in the chair, allow your mouth to rest open. While you take another deep breath, allow your body to relax further." In each example the patient easily identifies with the first experience and thus experiences the additional suggestion more readily.

Providing pathways to achieve a desired end may help patients to accomplish something that they do not know how to do on their own. Patients may not know how to relax on command; it may be more helpful to suggest that while they take in each breath slowly and see a drop of rain rolling off a leaf, they can let their whole body become loose and at ease. Indirect suggestions, positive images, linking pathways, and guided visualizations play a powerful role in helping patients to achieve desired goals.

8. How do the senses influence communication style?

Most people record experience in either the auditory, visual, or kinesthetic modes. They hear, they see, or they feel. Some individuals use a dominant mode to process information. Language can be chosen to match the modality that best fits the patient. If patients relate their problem in terms of feelings, responses related to how they feel may enhance communication. Similarly, a patient may say, "Doctor, that sounds like a good treatment plan," or "I see that this disorder is relatively common. Things look less frightening now." These comments suggest an auditory mode and a visual mode, respectively. Responding in similar terms enhances communication.

9. When is reassurance most valuable in the clinical session?

Positive supportive statements to the patient that he or she is going to do well or be all right are an important part of treatment. Everyone at some point may have doubts or fears about the outcome. Reassurance given too early, such as before a thorough examination of the presenting symptoms, may be interpreted by some patients as insincerity or as trivializing their problem. The best time for reassurance is after the examination, when a tentative diagnosis is reached. The support is best received by the patient at this point.

10. What type of language or phrasing is best avoided in patient communications?

Certain words or descriptions that are routine in the technical terminology of dentistry may be offensive or frightening to patients. Cutting, drilling, bleeding, injecting, or clamping may be anxiety-provoking terms to some patients. Furthermore, being too technical in conversations with patients may result in poor communication and provoke rather than reduce anxiety. It is beneficial to choose terms that are neutral yet informative. One may prepare a tooth rather than cut it, or dry the area rather than suction all the blood. This approach may be especially important during a teaching session when procedural and technical instructions are given as the patient lies helpless, listening to conversation that seems to exclude his or her presence as a person.

11. What common dental-related fears do patients experience?

Common dental-related fears focus on the following:
Pain
Drills (e.g., slipping, noise, smell)
Needles (deep penetration, tissue injury, numbness)
Loss of teeth
Surgery

12. List four elements common to all fears.
    Fear of the unknown   Fear of loss of control
    Fear of physical harm or bodily injury   Fear of helplessness and dependency
    Understanding the above elements of fear allows effective planning for treatment of the fearful and anxious patient.

13. During the clinical interview, how may one address such fears?
According to the maxim that fear dissolves in a trusting relationship, establishing good rapport with patients is especially important. Secondly, preparatory explanations may deal effectively with fear of the unknown and thus give a sense of control. Allowing patients to signal when they wish to pause or speak further alleviates fears of loss of control. Finally, well-executed dental technique and clinical practices minimize any unpleasantness.

14. How are dental fears learned?
Most commonly dental-related fears are learned directly from a traumatic experience in a dental or medical setting. The experience may be real or perceived by the patient as a threat, but a single event may lead to a lifetime of fear when any element of the traumatic situation is reexperienced. The situation may have occurred many years before, but the intensity of the recalled fear may continue to persist. Associated with the incident is the behavior of the past doctor. Thus, in diffusing learned fear, the behavior of the present doctor is paramount.

    Fears also may be learned indirectly as a vicarious experience from family members, friends, or even the media. Cartoons and movies often portray the pain and fear of the dental setting. How many times have dentists seen the negative reaction of patients to the term "root canal," even though they may not have had one?

    Past fearful experiences often occur during childhood when perceptions are out of proportion to events, but memories and feelings persist into adulthood with the same distortions. Feelings of helplessness, dependency, and fear of the unknown are coupled with pain and a possible uncaring attitude on the part of the dentist to condition a response of fear when any element of the past event is reexperienced. Indeed, such events may not even be available to conscious awareness.

15. How are the terms *generalization* and *modeling* related to the conditioning aspect of dental fears?
As discussed in the preceding question, dental fears may be seen as similar to classic Pavlovian conditioning. Such conditioning may result in **generalization,** by which the effects of the original episode spread to situations with similar elements. For example, the trauma of an injury or the details of an emergency setting, such as sutures or injections, may be generalized to the dental setting. Many adults who had tonsillectomies under ether anesthesia may generalize the childhood experience to the dental setting, complaining of difficulty with breathing or airway maintenance, difficulty with gagging, or the inability to tolerate oral injections.

    Modeling is vicarious learning through indirect exposure to traumatic events through parents, siblings, or any other source that affects the patient.

16. Why is understanding the patient's perception of the dentist so important in the control of fear and stress?
According to studies, patients perceive the dentist as both the **controller** of what the patient perceives as dangerous and as the **protector** from that danger. Thus the dentist's behavior and communications assume increased significance. The patient's ability to tolerate stress and to cope with fears depends on the ability to develop and maintain a high level of trust and confidence in the dentist. To achieve this goal, patients must express all the issues that they perceive as threatening, and the dentist must explain what he or she can do to address patient concerns and protect them from the perceived dangers. This is the purpose of the clinical interview. The result of this exchange should be increased trust and rapport and a subsequent decline in fear and anxiety.

17. How can learned fears be eliminated or unlearned?
Because fears of dental treatment are learned, relearning or unlearning is possible. A comfortable experience without the associated fearful and painful elements may eliminate the conditioned fear response and replace it with an adaptive and more comfortable coping response. The secret is to uncover through the interview process which elements resulted in the maladaption and subsequent response of fear, to eliminate them from the present dental experience by reinterpreting them for the adult patient, and to create a more caring and protected experience. During the interview the exchange of information and the insight gained by the patient decrease levels of fear, increase rapport, and establish trust in the doctor-patient relationship. The clinician needs only to apply expert operative technique to treat the vast majority of fearful patients.

18. What remarks may be given to a patient before beginning a procedure that the patient perceives as threatening?
Opening comments by the dentist to inform the patient about what to expect during a procedure—e.g., pressure, noise, pain—may reduce the fear of the unknown and the sense of helplessness. Control through knowing is increased with such preparatory communications.

19. How may the dentist further address the issue of loss of control?
A simple instruction that allows patients to signal by raising a hand if they wish to stop or speak returns a sense of control.

20. Define dental phobia.
A phobia is an irrational fear of a situation or object. The reaction to the stimulus is often greatly exaggerated in relation to the reality of the threat. The fears are beyond voluntary control, and avoidance is the primary coping mechanism. Phobias may be so intense that severe physiological reactions interfere with daily functioning, and in the dental setting acute syncopal episodes may result.

Almost all phobias are learned. The process of dealing with true dental phobia may require a long period of individual psychotherapy and adjunctive pharmacological sedation. However, relearning is possible, and establishing a good doctor–patient relationship is paramount.

21. What strategies may be used with the patient who gags on the slightest provocation?
The gag reflex is a basic physiological protective mechanism that occurs when the posterior oropharynx is stimulated by a foreign object; normal swallowing does not trigger the reflex. When overlying anxiety is present, especially if anxiety is related to the fear of being unable to breath, the gag reflex may be exaggerated. A conceptual model is the analogy to being "tickled." Most people can stroke themselves on the sole of the foot or under the arm without a reaction, but when the same stimulus is done by someone else, the usual results are laughter and withdrawal. Hence, if patients can eat properly, put a spoon in their mouth, or suck on their own finger, then usually they are considered physiologically normal and may be taught to accept dental treatment and even dentures with appropriate behavioral therapy.

In dealing with such patients, desensitization becomes the process of relearning. A review of the past history to discover episodes of impaired or threatened breathing is important. Childhood general anesthesia, near drowning, choking, or asphyxiation may have been the initiating event that created increased anxiety about being touched in the oral cavity. Patients may fear the inability to breathe, and the gag becomes part of their protective coping. Thus, reduction of anxiety is the first step; an initial strategy is to give information that allows patients to understand better their own response.

Instruction in nasal breathing may offer confidence in the ability to maintain a constant and uninterrupted air flow, even with oral manipulation. Eye fixation on a singular object may dissociate and distract the patient's attention away from the oral cavity. This technique may be especially helpful for taking radiographs and for brief oral examinations. For severe gaggers, hypnosis and nitrous oxide may be helpful; others may find use of a rubber dam reassuring. For some patients longer-term behavioral therapy may be necessary.

22. What is meant by the term anxiety? How is it related to fear?

Anxiety is a subjective state commonly defined as an unpleasant feeling of apprehension or impending danger in the presence of a real or perceived stimulus that the individual has learned to associate with a threat to well-being. The feelings may be out of proportion to the real threat, and the response may be grossly exaggerated. Such feelings may be present before the encounter with the feared situation and may linger long after the event. Associated somatic feelings include sweating, tremors, palpations, nausea, difficulty with swallowing, and hyperventilation.

Fear is usually considered an appropriate defensive response to a real or active threat. Unlike anxiety, the response is brief, the danger is external and readily definable, and the unpleasant somatic feelings pass as the danger passes. Fear is the classic "fight-or-flight" response and may serve as an overall protective mechanism by sharpening the senses and the ability to respond to the danger.

Whereas the response of fear does not usually rely on unhealthy actions for resolution, the state of anxiety often relies on noncoping and avoidance behaviors to deal with the threat.

23. How is stress related to pain and anxiety? What are some parameters of the stress response?

When an individual is stimulated by pain or anxiety, the result is a series of physiological responses dominated by the autonomic nervous system, the skeletal muscles, and the endocrine system. These physiologic responses define stress. In what is termed adaptive responses, the sympathetic responses dominate (increases in pulse rate, blood pressure, respiratory rate, peripheral vasoconstriction, skeletal muscle tone, and blood sugar; decreases in sweating, gut motility, and salivation). In an acute maladaptive response the parasympathetic responses dominate and a syncopal episode may result (decreases in pulse rate, blood pressure, respiratory rate, muscle tone; increases in salivation, sweating, gut motility, and peripheral vasodilation, with overall confusion and agitation).

In chronic maladaptive situations, psychosomatic disorders may evolve. The accompanying figure illustrates the relationships of fear, pain, and stress. It is important to control anxiety and stress during dental treatment. The medically compromised patient necessitates appropriate control to avoid potentially life-threatening situations.

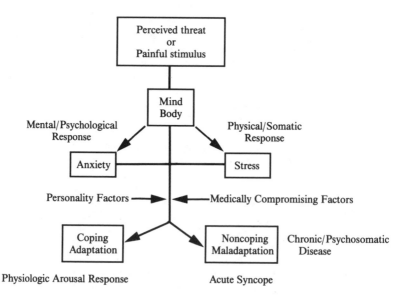

Relationships of pain, anxiety, stress, and reactions. (From Gregg JM: Psychosedation, Part 1. In McCarthy FM (ed): Emergencies in Dental Practice, 3rd ed. Philadelphia, W.B. Saunders, 1979, p 230, with permission.)

24. What is the relationship between pain and anxiety?

Many studies have shown the close relationship between pain and anxiety. The greater the anxiety of the individual, the more likely it is that he or she will interpret the response to a stimulus as painful. In addition, the pain threshold is lowered with increasing anxiety. Individuals who are debilitated, fatigued, or depressed respond to threats with a higher degree of undifferentiated anxiety and thus are more reactive to pain.

25. List four guidelines for the proper management of pain, anxiety and stress.

1. Make a careful assessment of the patient's anxiety and stress levels by a thoughtful interview. Uncontrolled anxiety and stress may lead to maladaptive situations that become life-threatening in the medically compromised individual. Prevention is the most important strategy.

2. From all information gathered, medical and personal, determine the correct methods for control of pain and anxiety. This assessment is critical to appropriate management. Monitoring the patient's responses to the chosen method is essential.

3. Use medications as adjuncts for positive reinforcement, not as methods of control. Drugs circumvent fear; they do not resolve conflicts. The need for good rapport and communication is always essential.

4. Adapt control techniques to fit the patient's needs. The use of a single modality for all patients may lead to failure; for example, the use of nitrous oxide sedation to moderate severe emotional problems.

26. Construct a model for the therapeutic interview of a self-identified fearful patient.

1. Recognize a patient's anxiety by acknowledgment of what the patient says or observation of the patient's demeanor. Recognition, which is both verbal and nonverbal, may be as simple as saying, "Are you nervous about being here?" This recognition indicates the dentist's concern, acceptance, supportiveness, and intent to help.

2. Facilitate patients' cues as they tell their story. Help them to go from generalizations to specifics, especially to past origins, if possible. Listen for generalizations, distortions, and deletions of information or misinterpretations of events as the patient talks.

3. Allow patients to speak freely. Their anxiety decreases as they tell their story, describing the nature of their fear and the attitude of previous doctors. Trust and rapport between doctor and patient also increase as the patient is allowed to speak to someone who cares and listens.

4. Give feedback to the patient. Interpretations of the information helps patients to learn new strategies for coping with their feelings and to adopt new behaviors by confronting past fears. Thus a new set of feelings and behaviors may replace maladaptive coping mechanisms.

5. Finally the dentist makes a commitment to protect the patient—a commitment that the patient may have perceived as absent in past dental experiences. Strategies include allowing the patient to stop a procedure by raising a hand or simply assuring a patient that you are ready to listen at any time.

27. Discuss behavioral methods that may help patients to cope with dental fears and related anxiety.

The first step for the dentist is to become knowledgeable of the patient and his or her presenting needs. Interviewing skills cannot be overemphasized. A trusting relationship is essential. As the clinical interview proceeds, fears are usually reduced to coping levels.

Because a patient cannot be anxious and relaxed at the same moment, teaching methods of relaxation may be helpful. Systematic relaxation allows the patient to cope with the dental situation. Guided visualizations may be helpful to achieve relaxation. Paced breathing also may be an aid to keeping patients relaxed. Guiding the rate of inspiration and expiration allows a hyperventilating patient to resume normal breathing, thus decreasing the anxiety level.

Hypnosis, a useful tool with a myriad of benefits, induces an altered state of awareness with heightened suggestibility for changes in behavior and physiologic responses. It is easily taught, and the benefits can be highly beneficial in the dental setting.

Informing patients of what they may experience during procedures addresses the specific fears of the unknown and loss of control. Sensory information, that is, what physical sensations may be expected—as well as procedural information is appropriate. Knowledge enhances a patient's coping skills.

Modeling, or observing a peer undergo successful dental treatment, may be beneficial. Videotapes are available for a variety of dental scenarios.

Methods of distraction may also improve coping responses. Audio or video programs have been reported to be useful for some patients.

28. Whom do dentists often consider their most "difficult" patient?

Surveys repeatedly show that dentists often view the anxious patient often as their most difficult challenge. Almost 80% of dentists report that they themselves become anxious with an anxious patient. The ability to assess carefully a patient's emotional needs helps the clinician to improve his or her ability to deal effectively with anxious patients.

29. What behaviors on the dentist's part do patients specify as reducing their anxiety?

Explain procedures before starting.
Give specific information during
  procedures.
Instruct the patient to be calm.
Forewarn about the possibility of pain.
Verbally support the patient:
  give reassurance.
Help patient to redefine the experience
  to minimize threat.

Give patient some control over
  procedures and pain.
Attempt to teach the patient to cope
  with distress.
Provide distraction and tension relief.
Attempt to build trust in the dentist.
Show personal warmth to the
  patient.

Source: Corah N: Dental anxiety: Assessment, reduction and increasing patient satisfaction. Dent Clin North Am 32:779–790, 1988.

30. What perceived behaviors on the dentist's part are associated with patient satisfaction?

The dentist

- assured me he would prevent pain
- was friendly
- worked quickly, but didn't rush
- had a calm manner
- gave me moral support

- reassured me that he would alleviate pain
- asked if I was concerned or nervous
- made sure that I was numb before starting to work.

Source: Corah N: Dental anxiety: Assessment, reduction and increasing patient satisfaction. Dent Clin North Am 32:779–790, 1988.

BIBLIOGRAPHY

1. Corah N: Dental anxiety: Assessment, reduction and increasing patient satisfaction. Dent Clin North Am 32:779–790, 1988.
2. Crasilneck HB, Hall JA: Clinical Hypnosis: Principles and Applications, 2nd ed. Orlando, FL, Grune & Stratton, 1985.
3. Dworkin SF, Ference TP, Giddon DB: Behavioral Science in Dental Practice. St. Louis, C.V. Mosby, 1978.
4. Friedman N, Cecchini JJ, Wexler M, et al: A dentist-oriented fear reduction technique: The iatrosedative process. Compend Cont Educ Dent 10:113–118, 1989.
5. Friedman N: Psychosedation. Part 2: Iatrosedation. In McCarthy FM (ed): Emergencies in Dental Practice, 3rd ed. Philadelphia, W.B. Saunders, 1979, pp 236–265.
6. Gregg JM: Psychosedation. Part 1: The nature and control of pain, anxiety, and stress. In McCarthy FM (ed): Emergencies in Dental Practice, 3rd ed. Philadelphia, W.B. Saunders, 1979, pp 220–235.
7. Jepsen CH: Behavioral foundations of dental practice. In Williams A (ed): Clark's Clinical Dentistry, Vol. 5. Philadelphia, J.B. Lippincott, 1993, pp 1–18.
8. Krochak M, Rubin JG: An overview of the treatment of anxious and phobic dental patients. Compend Cont Educ Dent 14:604–615, 1993.
9. Rubin JG, Kaplan A (eds): Dental Phobia and Anxiety. Dent Clin North Am 32, 1988.

2. TREATMENT PLANNING AND ORAL DIAGNOSIS

Stephen T. Sonis, D.M.D., D.M.Sc.

1. What are the objectives of pretreatment evaluation of a patient?

1. Establishment of a diagnosis
2. Determination of underlying medical conditions that may modify the oral condition or the patient's ability to tolerate treatment
3. Discovery of concomitant illnesses
4. Prevention of medical emergencies associated with dental treatment
5. Establishment of rapport with the patient

2. What are the essential elements of a patient history?

1. Chief complaint
2. History of the present illness (HPI)
3. Past medical history
4. Social history
5. Family history
6. Review of systems
7. Dental history

3. Define the chief complaint.

The chief complaint is the reason that the patient is seeking care, as described in the patient's own words.

4. What is the history of the present illness?

The HPI is a chronological description of the patient's symptoms and should include information relative to duration, location, character, and previous treatment.

5. What elements need to be included in the medical history?

Current status of the patient's general health
Hospitalizations
Medications
Allergies

6. What areas are routinely investigated in the social history?

Present and past occupations
Occupational hazards
Smoking, alcohol or drug use
Marital status

7. Why is the family history of interest to the dentist?

The family history often provides information relative to diseases of genetic origin or diseases that have a familial tendency. Examples include clotting disorders, atherosclerotic heart disease, psychiatric diseases, and diabetes mellitus.

8. How is the medical history most often obtained?

The medical history is obtained with a written health history questionnaire supplemented by a verbal history. The verbal history is imperative, because patients may leave out or misinterpret questions on the written form. For example, some patients may take daily aspirin and yet not consider it a "true" medication. The verbal history also allows the clinician to pursue positive answers on the written form and, in doing so, to establish rapport with the patient.

9. What techniques are used for physical examination of the patient? How are they used in dentistry?

Inspection, the most commonly used technique, is based on visual evaluation of the patient. **Palpation,** which involves touching and feeling the patient, is used to determine the consistency and shape of masses in the mouth or neck. **Percussion,** which involves differences in sound transmission of structures, has little application to the head and neck. **Auscultation,** the technique of listening to differences in the transmission of sound, is usually accomplished with a stethoscope. In dentistry it is most typically used to listen to changes in sounds emanating from the temporomandibular joint and in taking a patient's blood pressure.

10. What are the patient's vital signs?
Blood pressure
Pulse
Respiratory rate
Temperature

11. What are the normal values for the vital signs?
Blood pressure: 120 mmHg/80 mmHg
Pulse: 72 beats per minute
Respiratory rate: 16–20 respirations per minute
Temperature: 98.6°F or 37°C

12. What is a complete blood count (CBC)?
A CBC consists of a determination of the patient's hemoglobin, hematocrit, white blood cell count, and differential white blood cell count.

13. What are the normal ranges of a CBC?

Hemoglobin: men 14–18 g/dl
          women 12–16 g/dl
Hematocrit: men 40–54%
          women 37–47%
White blood count: 4,000–10,000
    cells/mm^3

Differential white blood count
    Neutrophils 50–70%
    Lymphocytes 30–40%
    Monocytes 3–7%
    Eosinophils 0–5%
    Basophils 0–1%

14. What is the most effective blood test to screen for diabetes mellitus?
The most effective screen for diabetes mellitus is fasting blood sugar.

15. What is the technique of choice for diagnosis of a soft-tissue lesion in the mouth?
With few exceptions, biopsy is the diagnostic technique of choice for virtually all soft-tissue lesions of the mouth.

16. Is there any alternative diagnostic technique to biopsy for the evaluation of suspected malignancies of the mouth?
Exfoliative cytology may be used as a screening technique for oral lesions. This technique is analogous to the Papanicolaou smear used to screen for cervical cancer. Unfortunately, a high rate of false negatives makes exfoliative cytology a dangerous practice in the screening of suspected oral cancers. It has value mainly in the diagnosis of certain viral, fungal and vesiculobullous diseases.

17. When is immunofluorescence of value in oral diagnosis?
Immunofluorescent techniques are of value in the diagnosis of a number of autoimmune diseases that affect the mouth, including pemphigus vulgaris and mucous membrane pemphigoid.

18. What elements should be included in the dental history?

1. Past dental visits, including frequency, reasons, previous treatment, and complications

2. Oral hygiene practices

3. Oral symptoms other than those associated with the chief complaint, including tooth pain or sensitivity, gingival bleeding or pain, tooth mobility, halitosis, and abscess formation

4. Past dental or maxillofacial trauma

5. Habits related to oral disease, such as bruxing, clenching, and nail biting

6. Dietary history

19. When is it appropriate to use microbiologic culturing in oral diagnosis?

1. **Bacterial infection.** Because the overwhelming number of oral infections are sensitive to treatment with penicillin, routine bacteriologic culture of primary dental infections is not generally indicated. However, cultures are indicated in patients who are immunocompromised or myelosuppressed for two reasons: (1) such patients are at significant risk for sepsis, and (2) the oral flora often change in such individuals. Cultures should be obtained for infections that are refractory to the initial course of antibiotics before changing antibiotics.

2. **Viral infection.** Immunocompromised patients who present with mucosal lesions may well be manifesting herpes simplex infection. A viral culture is warranted in these cases. Similarly, other viruses in the Herpes family, such as cytomegalovirus, can cause oral lesions in the immunocompromised patient and should be isolated, if possible. Routine culturing for primary or secondary herpes infections is not warranted in healthy patients.

3. **Fungal infection.** Candidiasis is the most common fungal infection affecting the oral mucosa. Because its appearance is often varied, especially in immunocompromised patients, fungal cultures are often of value. In addition, because candidal infection is a frequent cause of burning mouth, culture is often indicated in immunocompromised patients, even in the absence of visible lesions.

20. How do you obtain access to a clinical laboratory?

It is easy to obtain laboratory tests for your patients, even if you do not practice in a hospital. Community hospitals provide virtually all the laboratory services that your patients may require. Usually the laboratory provides order slips and culture tubes. Simply indicate the test needed and send the patient to the laboratory. Patients who need a test at night or on a weekend can generally be accommodated through the hospital's emergency department. Commercial laboratories also may be used. They, too, supply order forms. If you practice in a medical building with physicians, find out which laboratory they use. If they use a commercial laboratory, a pick-up service for specimens may well be provided. The most important issue is to ensure the quality of the laboratory. Adherence to the standards of the American College of Clinical Pathologists is a good indicator of laboratory quality.

21. What is the approximate cost of the following laboratory tests: complete blood count, platelet count, prothrombin time, fasting glucose, bacterial culture, and fungal culture?

CBC	$18	Fasting glucose	$13
Platelet count	$18	Bacterial culture	$32
Prothrombin time	$29	Fungal culture	$42

22. What are the causes of halitosis?

Halitosis may be caused by local factors in the mouth and by extraoral or systemic factors. Among the local factors are food retention, periodontal infection, caries, acute necrotizing gingivitis, and mucosal infection. Extraoral and systemic causes of halitosis include smoking, alcohol ingestion, pulmonary or bronchial disease, metabolic defects, diabetes mellitus, sinusitis, and tonsillitis.

23. What are the most commonly abused drugs in the United States?

Alcohol	Prescription medications
Marijuana	Tricyclic antidepressants
Cocaine	Sedative-hypnotics
Phencyclidine (PCP)	Narcotic analgesics
	Anxiolytic agents
	Diet aids
	Heroin

24. What are the common causes of lymphadenopathy?

1. **Infectious and inflammatory diseases** of all types. Common oral conditions causing lymphadenopathy are herpes infections, pericoronitis, aphthous or traumatic ulceration, and acute necrotizing ulcerative gingivitis.

2. **Immunologic diseases,** such as rheumatoid arthritis, systemic lupus erythematosus, and drug reactions.

3. **Malignant disease,** such as Hodgkin's disease, lymphoma, leukemia, and metastatic disease from solid tumors.

4. **Hyperthyroidism.**

5. **Lipid storage diseases,** such as Gaucher's and Niemann-Pick disease.

6. **Other conditions,** including sarcoidosis, amyloidosis, and granulomatosis.

25. How can one differentiate between lymphadenopathy associated with an inflammatory process and lymphadenopathy associated with tumor?

1. **Onset and duration.** Inflammatory nodes tend to have a more acute onset and course than nodes associated with tumor.

2. **Identification of an associated infected site.** An identifiable site of infection associated with an enlarged lymph node is probably the source of the lymphadenopathy. Effective treatment of the site should result in resolution of the lymphadenopathy.

3. **Symptoms.** Enlarged lymph nodes associated with an inflammatory process are usually tender to palpation. Nodes associated with tumor are not.

4. **Progression.** Continuous enlargement over time is associated with tumor.

5. **Fixation.** Inflammatory nodes are usually freely movable, whereas nodes associated with tumor are hard and fixed.

6. **Lack of response to antibiotic therapy.** Continued nodal enlargement in the face of appropriate antibiotic therapy should be viewed as suspicious.

7. **Distribution.** Unilateral nodal enlargement is a common presentation for malignant disease. In contrast, bilateral enlargement often is associated with systemic processes.

26. What is the most appropriate technique for lymph node diagnosis?

The most appropriate technique for lymph node diagnosis is biopsy or needle aspiration.

27. What are the most frequent causes of intraoral swelling?

The most frequent causes of intraoral swelling are infection and tumor.

28. Why does Polly get parrotitis?

Too many crackers.

29. Why do humans get parotitis?

Infection of viral or bacterial origin is the most common cause of parotitis in humans. Viruses causing parotitis are mumps, Coxsackie, and influenza. *Staphylococcus aureus,* the most common bacterial cause of parotitis, results in the production of pus within the gland. Other bacteria, such as actinomyces, streptococci, and gram-negative bacilli also may cause suppurative parotitis.

30. What are common causes of xerostomia?
Advanced age
Certain medications
Radiation therapy
Sjögren's syndrome

31. What is the presentation of a patient with a tumor of the parotid gland? How is the diagnosis made?
The typical patient with a parotid gland tumor presents with a firm, fixed mass in the region of the gland. Involvement of the facial nerve is common and results in facial palsy. Fine-needle biopsy is a commonly used technique for diagnosis. However, the small sample obtained by such technique may be limiting. CT and MRI are also often helpful in evaluating suspected tumors.

32. What are the major risk factors for oral cancer?
Tobacco and alcohol use are the major risk factors for the development of oral cancer.

33. What is the possible role of toluidine blue stain in oral diagnosis?
Because toluidine blue is a metachromatic nuclear stain, it has been reported to be preferentially absorbed by dysplastic and cancerous epithelium. Consequently, it has been used as a technique to screen oral lesions. The technique has a reported false-positive rate of 9% and a false-negative rate of 5%.

34. What are the common clinical presentations of oral cancers?
The two most common clinical presentations for oral cancer are a nonhealing ulcer and an area of leukoplakia.

35. What percent of keratotic white lesions in the mouth are dysplastic or cancerous?
Approximately 10% of such oral lesions are dysplastic or cancerous.

36. What is a simple way to differentiate clinically between necrotic and keratotic white lesions of the oral mucosa?
Necrotic lesions of the mucosa, such as those caused by burns or candidal infections, scrape off when gently rubbed with a moist tongue blade. On the other hand, because keratotic lesions result from epithelial changes, scrapping fails to dislodge them.

37. How long should one wait before obtaining a biopsy of an oral ulcer?
Virtually all ulcers caused by trauma or aphthous stomatitis heal within 14 days of presentation. Consequently, any ulcer that is present for 2 weeks or more should be biopsied.

38. What is the differential diagnosis of ulcers of the oral mucosa?

Traumatic ulcer	Chancre of syphilis
Aphthous stomatitis	Noma
Cancer	Necrotizing sialometaplasia
Tuberculosis	Deep fungal infection

39. Why is it a good idea to aspirate a pigmented lesion before obtaining a biopsy?
Because pigmented lesions may be vascular in nature, prebiopsy aspiration is prudent to prevent hemorrhage.

40. What are the major causes of pigmented oral and perioral lesions?
Pigmented lesions are due to either endogenous or exogenous sources. Among endogenous sources are melanoma, endocrine-related pigmentation (such as occurs in Addison's disease), and perioral pigmentation associated with intestinal polyposis or Peutz-Jehger's syndrome.

Exogenous sources of pigmentation include heavy metal poisoning (e.g., lead), amalgam tattoos, and changes caused by chemicals or medications. A common example of medication-related changes is black hairy tongue associated with antibiotics, particularly tetracycline, or bismuth-containing compounds, such as Pepto-Bismol.

41. Do any diseases of the oral cavity also present with lesions of the skin?
Numerous diseases can cause simultaneous lesions of the mouth and skin. Among the most common are lichen planus, erythema multiforme, lupus erythematosus, bullous pemphigoid, and pemphigus vulgaris.

42. What is the appearance of the skin lesion associated with erythema multiforme?
The skin lesion of erythema multiforme looks like an archery target with a central erythematous bullseye and a circular peripheral area. Hence, the lesions are called bullseye or target lesions.

43. A 25-year-old woman presents with the chief complaint of spontaneously bleeding gingiva. She also notes malaise. On oral examination you find that her hygiene is excellent. Would you suspect a local or systemic basis for her symptoms? What tests might you order to make a diagnosis?
Spontaneous bleeding, especially in the face of good oral hygiene, is most likely of systemic origin. Gingival bleeding is among the most common presenting signs of acute leukemia, which should be high on the differential diagnosis. A complete blood count and platelet count should provide data to help to establish a preliminary diagnosis. Definitive diagnosis most likely requires a bone marrow biopsy.

44. A 45-year-old, overweight man presents with suppurative periodontitis. As you review his history, he tells you that he is always hungry, drinks water almost every hour, and awakens four times each night to urinate. What systemic disease is most likely a cofactor in this man's periodontal disease? What test(s) might you order to help you with a diagnosis?
The complex of symptoms—polyuria, polyphagia, polydipsia, and suppurative periodontal disease—should raise a strong suspicion of diabetes mellitus. A fasting blood glucose test is the most efficacious way to screen for this disease.

45. A 60-year-old woman presents with the complaint of numbness of the left side of her mandible. Four years ago she had a mastectomy for treatment of breast cancer. What is the likely diagnosis? What is the first step you take to confirm it?
The mandible is not an infrequent site for metastatic breast cancer. As the metastatic lesion grows, it puts pressure on the inferior alveolar nerve and causes paresthesia. Radiographic evaluation of the jaw is a reasonable first step to make a diagnosis.

46. What endocrine disease may present with pigmented lesions of the oral mucosa?
Pigmented lesions of the oral mucosa may suggest Addison's disease.

47. What drugs cause gingival hyperplasia?
  Phenytoin
  Cyclosporine
  Nifedipine

48. What is the most typical presentation of the oral lesions of tuberculosis? How do you make a diagnosis?
The oral lesions of tuberculosis are thought to result from the presence of organisms brought into contact with the oral mucosa by sputum. A nonhealing ulcer, which is impossible to differentiate clinically from carcinoma, is the most common presentation in the mouth. Ulcers are most consistently present on the lateral borders of the tongue and may have a purulent

center. Lymphadenopathy also may be present. Diagnosis is made by histologic examination and demonstration of organisms in the tissue.

49. What are the typical oral manifestations of a patient with pernicious anemia?
The most common target site in the mouth is the tongue, which presents with a smooth, dorsal surface denuded of papillae. Angular cheilitis is a frequent accompanying finding.

50. What is the classic oral manifestation of Crohn's disease?
Mucosal lesions with a cobblestone appearance are associated with Crohn's disease.

51. List the oral changes that may occur in a patient who is receiving radiation therapy for treatment of a tumor on the base of the tongue.

Xerostomia	Osteoradionecrosis
Cervical and incisal edge caries	Mucositis

52. A patient presents for extraction of a carious tooth. In taking the history, you learn that the patient is receiving chemotherapy for treatment of a breast carcinoma. What information is critical before proceeding with the extraction?
Because cancer chemotherapy nonspecifically affects the bone marrow, the patient is likely to be myelosuppressed after treatment. Therefore, you need to know both the patient's white blood cell count and platelet count before initiating treatment.

53. What oral findings have been associated with the diuretic hydrochlorothiazide?
Lichen planus has been associated with hydrochlorothiazide.

54. Some patients believe that topical application of an aspirin to the mucosa next to a tooth will help odontogenic pain. How may you detect this form of therapy by looking in the patient's mouth?
Because of its acidity, topical application of aspirin to the mucosa frequently causes a chemical burn, which appears as a white, necrotic lesion in the area corresponding to aspirin placement.

BIBLIOGRAPHY

1. Atkinson JC, Fox PC: Sjögren's syndrome: Oral and dental considerations. J Am Dent Assoc 124:74, 1993.
2. Fenlon MR, McCartan BE: Validity of a patient self-completed health questionnaire in a primary dental care practice. Commun Dent Oral Epidemiol 20:130–132, 1992.
3. Harahap M: How to biopsy oral lesions. J Dermatol Surg Oncol 15:1077–1080, 1989.
4. Jones JH, Mason DK: Oral Manifestations of Systemic Disease, 2nd ed. Philadelphia, Bailliere Tindall/W.B. Saunders, 1990.
5. Laurin D, Brodeur JM, Leduc N, et al: Nutritional deficiencies and gastrointestinal disorders in the edentulous elderly: A literature review. J Can Dent Assoc 58:738–740, 1992.
6. McCarthy FM: Recognition, assessment and safe management of the medically compromised patient in dentistry. Anesth Prog 37:217–222, 1990.
7. O'Brien CJ, Seng-Jaw S, Herrera GA, et al: Malignant salivary tumors: Analysis of prognostic factors and survival. Head Neck Surg 9:82–92, 1986.
8. Redding SW, Olive JA: Relative value of screening tests of hemostasis prior to dental treatment. Oral Surg Oral Med Oral Pathol 59:34–36, 1985.
9. Rose LF, Steinberg BJ: Patient evaluation. Dent Clin North Am 31:53–73, 1987.
10. Sonis ST, Fazio RC, Fang L: Principles and Practice of Oral Medicine, 2nd ed. Philadelphia, W.B. Saunders, 1995.
11. Sonis ST, Woods PD, White BA: Oral complications of cancer therapies. NCI Monogr 9:29–32, 1990.
12. Williams AJ, Wray D, Ferguson A: The clinical entity of orofacial Crohn's disease. Q J Med 79:451–458, 1991.

3. ORAL MEDICINE

Dale Potter, D.D.S.

Now keep this straight:
You take the white penicillin tablet every 6 hours and

1 red pill every 2 hours

and ½ a yellow pill before every meal and

2 speckled orange pills between lunch and dinner

followed by 3 green pills before bedtime, unless you have
taken the oblong white tablet for pain, then. . . .

Any questions? Good luck.

Modified from unknown source.

DISORDERS OF HEMOSTASIS

1. How do you screen a patient for potential bleeding problems?
The best screening procedure for a bleeding disorder is a good medical history. If the review
of the medical history indicates a bleeding problem, a more detailed history is needed. The
following questions are basic:
1. Is there a family history of bleeding problems?
2. Has bleeding been noted since early childhood, or is the onset relatively recent?
3. How many previous episodes have there been?
4. What are the circumstances of the bleeding?
5. When did the bleeding occur? after minor surgery, such as tonsillectomy or tooth
extraction? after falls or participation in contact sports?
6. What medications was the patient taking when the bleeding occurred?
7. What was the duration of the bleeding episode(s)? Did the episode involve prolonged
oozing or a massive hemorrhage?
8. Was the bleeding immediate or delayed?
From Kupp MA, Chatton MJ: Current Medical Diagnosis and Treatment. East Norwalk, CT,
Appleton & Lange, 1983, p 324.

2. What laboratory tests should be ordered if a bleeding problem is suspected?
Platelet count: Normal values = 150,000–450,000
Bleeding time: Normal value = < 9 minutes
Prothrombin time: Normal value = 10–13.5 seconds
Partial thromboplastin time: Normal value = 25–36 seconds
Normal values may vary from one laboratory to another. It is important to check the
normal values for the laboratory that you use. If any of the tests are abnormal, the patient
should be referred to a hematologist for evaluation before any treatment is performed.

**3. What are the clinical indications for the use of 1-deamino-8-D-arginine vasopressin
(DDAVP, Desmopressin) in dental patients?**
DDAVP is a synthetic antidiuretic hormone that controls bleeding in patients with type I von
Willebrand's disease, platelet defects secondary to uremia related to renal dialysis, and
immunogenic thrombocytopenic purpura (ITP). The dosage is 0.3 μg/kg. DDAVP should not
be used in patients under the age of 2 years; caution is necessary in the elderly and in patients
receiving intravenous fluids.

4. When do you use epsilon aminocaproic acid or tranexamic acid?

Epsilon aminocaproic acid (Amicar) and tranexamic acid are antifibrinolytic agents that inhibit activation of plasminogen. They are used to prevent clot lysis in patients with hereditary clotting disorders. For epsilon aminocaproic acid, the dose is 75–100 mg/kg every 6 hours; for tranexamic acid, it is 25 mg/kg every 8 hours.

5. What is the minimal acceptable platelet count for an oral surgical procedure?

Normal platelet count is between 150,000 and 450,000. In general, the minimal platelet count for an oral surgical procedure is 50,000 platelets. However, emergency procedures may be done with as few as 30,000 platelets if the dentist is working closely with the patient's hematologist and uses excellent techniques of tissue management.

6. For a patient on warfarin (Coumadin), a dental surgical procedure can be done without undue risk of bleeding if the prothrombin time is below what value?

Warfarin affects clotting factors II, VII, IX, and X by impairing the conversion of vitamin K to its active form. The normal prothrombin time (PT) for a healthy patient is 10.0–13.5 seconds with a control of 12 seconds. Oral procedures with a risk of bleeding should not be attempted if the PT is greater than 1½ times the control or above 18 seconds with a control of 12 seconds.

7. Is the bleeding time a good indicator of peri- and postsurgical bleeding?

The bleeding time is used to test for platelet function. However, studies have shown no correlation between blood loss during cardiac or general surgery and prolonged bleeding time. The best indicator of a bleeding problem in the dental patient is a thorough medical history. The bleeding time should be used in patients with no known platelet disorder to help predict the potential for bleeding.

Source: Lind SE: The bleeding time does not predict surgical bleeding. Blood 77:2547–2552, 1991.

8. Should oral surgical procedures be postponed in patients taking aspirin?

Nonelective oral surgical procedures in the absence of a positive medical history for bleeding should not be postponed because of aspirin therapy, but the surgeon should be aware that bleeding may be exacerbated in a patient with mild platelet defect. However, elective procedures, if at all possible, should be postponed in the patient taking aspirin. Aspirin irreversibly acetylates cyclooxygenase, an enzyme that assists platelet aggregation. The effect is not dose-dependent and lasts for the 7–10-day life span of the platelet.

Source: Tierney LM, McPhee SJ, Papadakis MA, Schroeder SA: Current Medical Diagnosis and Treatment. Norwalk, CT, Appleton & Lange, 1993, p 440.

9. Are patients on nonsteriodal medications likely to bleed from oral surgical procedures?

Nonsteroidal antiinflammatory medications produce a transient inhibition of platelet aggregation that is reversed when the drug is cleared from the body. Again, patients with a preexisting platelet defect may have increased bleeding.

10. If a patient presents with spontaneous gingival bleeding, what diagnostic tests should be ordered?

A patient who presents with spontaneous gingival bleeding without a history of trauma, tooth brushing, flossing or eating, should be assessed for a systemic cause of the bleeding. Etiologies for gingival bleeding include inflammation secondary to localized periodontitis, platelet defect, factor deficiency, hematologic malignancy, and metabolic disorder. A thorough medical history should be obtained, and the following laboratory tests should be ordered:

1. Prothrombin time (PT)
2. Partial thromboplastin time (PTT)
3. Complete blood count (CBC)

INDICATIONS FOR PROPHYLACTIC ANTIBIOTICS

11. For what cardiac conditions is prophylaxis for endocarditis recommended in patients receiving dental care?

All patients with prosthetic cardiac valves, including both bioprosthetic and homograft valves

Any patient with a previous diagnosis of endocarditis, even in the absence of heart disease

Congenital cardiac malformations, except isolated secundum atrial septal defect

Rheumatic or other acquired valvular dysfunction

After surgical repair of valvular dysfunction

Hypertrophic cardiomyopathy

Mitral valve prolapse with valvular regurgitation

Source: Dajani AS, et al: Prevention of bacterial endocarditis recommendations by the American Heart Association. JAMA 264:2919–2922, 1990.

12. What cardiac conditions do *not* require endocarditis prophylaxis?

Isolated secundum atrial septal defect

Surgical repair (after 6 months) of secundum atrial septal defect, ventricular septal defect, or patent ductus arteriosus without residual murmur.

Coronary artery bypass graft surgery

Mitral valuve prolapse without valvular regurgitation

Physiologic, functional, or innocent heart murmur

History of rheumatic heart disease without valvular dysfunction

History of Kawasaki disease without valvular dysfunction

Cardiac pacemakers or implanted defibrillators

Source: Dajani AS, et al: Prevention of bacterial endocarditis recommendations by the American Heart Association. JAMA 264:2919–2922, 1990.

13. What are antibiotics and dosages recommended by the American Heart Association for the prevention of endocarditis from dental procedures?

The American Heart Association updates its recommendations every few years to reflect new findings. The dentist has an obligation to be aware of the latest recommendations. The patient's well-being is the dentist's responsibility. Even if a physician recommends an alternative prophylactic regimen, the dentist is liable if the patient develops endocarditis and the latest AHA recommendations were not followed.

Standard regimen

Amoxicillin   3.0 g orally 1 hour before procedure, then 1.5 g 6 hours after initial dose

For patients allergic to amoxicillin and penicillin

Erythromycin   Erythromycin ethylsuccinate 800 mg or erythromycin stearate 1.0 gm orally 2 hours before procedure; then one-half the dose 6 hours after initial dose

Clindamycin   300 mg orally 1 hour before procedure and 150 mg 6 hours after initial dose

Patients unable to take oral medications

Ampicillin   Intravenous (IV) or intramuscular (IM) administration of 2 g 30 minutes before procedure; then IV or IM administration of ampicillin 1 g or 1.5 g of amoxicillin orally 6 hours after initial dose

For patients allergic to ampicillin, amoxicillin, and penicillin

Clindamycin   Intravenous administration of 300 mg 30 minutes before procedure and an intravenous or oral administration of 150 mg 6 hours after initial dose

Patients considered at high risk and noncandidates for standard regimen

Ampicillin, gentamicin, amoxicillin

IV or IM administration of ampicillin 2 g plus gentamicin 1.5 mg/kg (not to exceed 80 mg) 30 minutes before procedure; then amoxicillin 1.5 g orally 6 hours after initial dose

For patients allergic to ampicillin, amoxicillin, and penicillin

Vancomycin   IV administration of 1.0 g over 1 hour before procedure; no repeat dose is necessary

Source: Dajani AS, et al: Prevention of bacterial endocarditis recommendations by the American Heart Association. JAMA 264:2919–2922, 1990.

14. What precautions should you take when treating a patient with a central line such as a Hickman or Portacath?

Patients with central venous access are usually receiving either intensive antibiotic therapy, chemotherapy, or nutritional support. It is imperative to consult with the patient's physician before performing any dental procedures. If it is determined that the dental procedure is necessary, the patient should receive antibiotic prophylaxis to protect the central venous access line from infection secondary to transient bacteremias. The same antibiotic regimen recommended for the prevention of endocarditis should be prescribed.

15. Should a patient with a prosthetic joint be placed on prophylactic antibiotics before dental treatment?

Case studies support the hematogenous seeding of prosthetic joints. However, it is questionable whether organisms from the oral cavity are a source for late deep infections of prosthetic joints. Most orthopedists recommend the premedication of dental patients with prosthetic joints. Patients should be premedicated with the same antibiotic regimen used for the prevention of endocarditis.

16. Should a patient who has had a coronary bypass operation be placed on prophylactic antibiotics before dental treatment?

Elective dental care for the patient who has had coronary bypass surgery should be postponed for at least 1 month post surgery. After 1 month, prophylactic antibiotics are not necessary. If emergency dental care is necessary before 1 month, the patient should be premedicated with the same regimen used for the prevention of endocarditis.

17. Is it necessary to prescribe prophylactic antibiotics for a patient on renal dialysis?

Patients on dialysis with arteriovenous (AV) shunts should be premedicated before any dental treatment that has the potential of producing a transient bacteremia. The regimen for the prevention of endocarditis is modified to reflect the patient's lack of kidney function. The dosage changes for the antibiotic coverage are as follows:

Standard regimen

Amoxicillin   3.0 g orally 1 hour before procedure; a second dose is not needed in the patient on renal dialysis

For patients allergic to amoxicillin and penicillin

Erythromycin   Erythromycin ethylsuccinate 800 mg or erythromycin stearate 1.0 g orally 2 hours before procedure; then one-half the dose 6 hours after initial dose

Clindamycin   300 mg orally 1 hour before procedure and 150 mg 6 hours after initial dose

Patients unable to take oral medications

Ampicillin   Intravenous (IV) administration 2 g 30 minutes before procedure; a second dose is not needed in the patient on renal dialysis

For patients allergic to ampicillin, amoxicillin, and penicillin

Clindamycin	Intravenous administration of 300 mg 30 minutes before procedure and an intravenous or oral administration of 150 mg 6 hours after initial dose; there is no change for patients on renal dialysis

Patients considered at high risk and noncandidates for standard regimen

Ampicillin, gentamicin

IV ampicillin 2 g plus gentamicin 1.5 mg/kg (not to exceed 80 mg) 30 minutes before procedure; a second dose is not needed in the patient on renal dialysis (The dialysis unit should be notified so that the patient is placed on the correct dialysis machine to remove the gentamicin.)

For patients allergic to ampicillin, amoxicillin, and penicillin

Vancomycin	IV administration of 500 mg over 1 hour before procedure; no repeat dose is necessary

Source: Bennett WM, et al: Drug Prescribing in Renal Failure, 2nd ed. Philadelphia, American College of Physicians, 1991.

TREATMENT OF HIV-POSITIVE PATIENTS

18. What are the considerations in treating a patient infected with the HIV virus and treated with azidothymidine?
Azidothymidine (AZT) is an antiviral widely used in patients infected with the human immunodeficiency virus (HIV). The drug is toxic to the hematopoietic system and may result in anemia, granulocytopenia, or thrombocytopenia. Patients on AZT should have a complete blood count (CBC) every 2 weeks. Before oral surgical procedures, a CBC should be done to determine whether the patient is neutropenic or thrombocytopenic.

Source: Deglin JH, et al: Davis's Drug Guide for Nurses, 2nd ed. Philadelphia, F.A. Davis, 1991.

19. A patient with HIV infection requires an oral surgical procedure to remove teeth after severe bone loss due to HIV-related localized perodontitis. What precautions should be taken?
It is estimated that 10–15% of patients with HIV develop immunogenic thrombocytopenic purpura (ITP). The antiplatelet antibodies appear to be found more frequently in advanced stages of the disease. Affected patients should have a CBC before any oral surgical procedure. If the platelets are low (below 150,000), the procedure should be done only after consultation with the patient's physician and with the knowledge that bleeding may be increased. The patient may require platelet transfusions to control post-operative bleeding.

Source: Magnac C, et al: Platelet antibodies in serum of patients with human immunodeficiency virus (HIV) infection: AIDS Res Hum Retroviruses 6:1443–1449, 1990.

20. Are there any contraindications to restorative dentistry procedures in patients with HIV infection?
If the patient is not neutropenic or thrombocytopenic, there are no contraindications to preventive and restorative dental care. In fact, patients should receive aggressive dental care to reduce the oral cavity as a source of infection. They should be placed on a 3–6-month recall to maintain optimal oral health and followed closely for opportunistic infections and HIV-related oral conditions.

CARDIOVASCULAR DISEASE

21. What is the appropriate response if a patient with a history of cardiac disease develops chest pain during a dental procedure?
The response should be as follows:
1. Discontinue treatment immediately.

2. Take and record vital signs (blood pressure, pulse, respiration), and question the patient about the pain. Chest pain from ischemia may be either substernal or more diffused. Patients often describe the pain as crushing, pressure, or heavy; it may radiate to the shoulders, arms, neck, or back.

3. If the patient has a history of angina and takes nitroglycerin, give the patient either his or her own nitroglycerin or a tablet from your emergency cart. Continue to monitor the patient's vial signs. If the pain does not stop after 3 minutes, give the patient a second dose. If after 3 doses in a 10-minute period the pain does not subside, contact the medical emergency service and have the patient transported to an emergency department to rule out a myocardial infarction.

4. If the patient does not have a history of heart disease and persistent chest pain for greater than 2 minutes, the medical emergency service should be contacted and the patient transported to a hospital emergency department for evaluation.

22. At what blood pressure should elective dental care be postponed?
Elective dental care should be postponed if the systolic blood pressure is > 160 mmHg or the diastolic pressure is > 100 mmHg.

23. At what blood pressure should emergency dental care be postponed and the patient treated palliatively until the blood pressure is controlled?
Emergency dental treatment should be postponed if the systolic pressure is > 180 or the diastolic pressure is > 110. Patients must be referred for care immediately to prevent morbidity if they have either (1) asymptomatic severe hypertension with a systolic pressure > 240 mmHg or diastolic pressure > 130 mmHg or (2) symptomatic hypertension, headache, heart failure, angina, or elevated perioperative blood pressure, with a systolic pressure of > 200 mmHg or diastolic pressure of > 120.

Source: Tierney LM, McPhee SJ, Papadakis MA, Schroeder SA: Current Medical Diagnosis and Treatment. Norwalk, CT, Appleton & Lange, 1993, p 366.

24. How long should dental care be postponed after a heart attack?
Dental treatment in a patient who has had a myocardial infarction should be done only after consultation with the patient's physician. Cintrin et al. showed that patients treated within 2 weeks of an uncomplicated myocardial infarction experienced no significant hemodynamic changes or complications related to local anesthesia, vigorous dental prophylaxis, or dental extraction. The general guidelines for a patient without angina or heart failure is to wait 6 months for elective dental care.

Source: Cintron G, et al: Cardiovascular effects and safety of dental anesthesia and dental interventions in patients with recent uncomplicated myocardial infarction. Arch Intern Med 146:2203–2204, 1986.

25. How do you differentiate between stable and unstable angina?
Unstable angina is characterized by a change in the pattern of pain. The pain occurs with less exertion or at rest, lasts longer, and is less responsive to medication. Dental care for such patients must be postponed and the patient referred to his or her physician immediately for care. Patients are at increased risk for myocardial infarction. If emergency dental care is necessary before the patient is stable, it should be attempted only with cardiac monitoring and sedation.

Source: Tierney LM, McPhee SJ, Papadakis MA, Schroeder SA: Current Medical Diagnosis and Treatment. Norwalk, CT, Appleton & Lange, 1993, p 298.

26. What precautions should be taken when treating a patient with recent onset of angina?
Patients with recent onset of angina less than 30 days' duration are at increased risk for myocardial infarction and sudden death. The angina may not be severe and may occur only with exercise. However, even though symptoms are mild, dental treatment should be postponed until the patient has had a medical evaluation.

Source: Kilmartin C, Munroe CO: Cardiovascular diiseases and the dental patient. J Can Dent Assoc 6:513–518, 1986.

27. Is the use of a vasoconstrictor in local anesthetics contraindicated in the patient with cardiac disease?

The use of vasoconstrictors is not contraindicated in the patient with cardiovascular disease. According to conservative recommendations, epinephrine should not exceed 0.04 mg, which equates to 4 carpules of 1/200,000 or 2 carpules of 1/100,000.

Source: Holroyd SV, Wynn RL, Requa-Clark B (eds): Clinical Pharmacology in Dental Practice, 4th ed. St. Louis, Mosby, 1988.

28. Should retraction cord that contains epinephrine be used in a patient with cardiovascular disease?

The concentration of epinephrine in impregnated cord is high, and systemic absorption occurs. Impregnated cord should not be used in patients with cardiac disease, hypertension, or hyperthyroidism. Malamed argues that epinephrine-containing retraction cord should not be used in dental practice.

Source: Kilmartin C, Munroe CO: Cardiovascular diseases and the dental patient. J Can Dent Assoc 6:513–518, 1986.

29. When should vasoconstrictors not be used in either local anesthetic or retraction cord?

Vasoconstrictors should not be used in patients with uncontrolled hypertension or hyperthyroidism. Epinephrine should not be used in dental patients under general anesthesia when either halogenated hydrocarbons or cyclopropane are used for anesthesia.

Source: Holroyd SV, Wynn RL, Requa-Clark B (eds): Clinical Pharmacology in Dental Practice, 4th ed. St. Louis, Mosby, 1988, p 58.

30. Is it safe to treat a patient who has had a heart transplant in an outpatient dental office?

Dental treatment should be done only after consultation with the patient's cardiologist. If the patient is stable without rejection, there are no contraindications to dental treatment. Such patients do not require prophylactic antibiotics for dental procedures unless the transplanted heart has valvular pathology. The patient most likely will be taking prednisone and cyclosporine. For restorative and preventive dental procedures and simple extractions, it is not necessary to increase the corticosteroids. Erythromycin and ketoconazole should not be prescribed for a patient on cyclosporine. Erythromycin and ketoconazole inhibit the metabolism of cyclosporine.

METABOLIC DISORDERS

31. What precautions do you need to take in treating a patient with insulin-dependent diabetes mellitus (IDDM)?

The major concern for the dental practitioner treating the patient with IDDM is hypoglycemia. It is important to question the patient for changes in insulin dosage, diet, and exercise routine before undertaking any outpatient dental treatment. A decrease in dietary intake or an increase in either the normal insulin dosage or exercise may place the patient at risk for hypoglycemia.

Source: Tierney LM, McPhee SJ, Papadakis MA, Schroeder SA: Current Medical Diagnosis and Treatment. Norwalk, CT, Appleton & Lange, 1993, p 928.

32. What are the symptoms of hypoglycemia?

1. Tachycardia   4. Tremulousness
2. Palpitations   5. Nausea
3. Sweating   6. Hunger

The symptoms may progress to coma and convulsions without intervention.

33. What should the dentist be prepared to do for the patient who has a hypoglycemic reaction?

The dental practitioner should have some form of sugar readily available—packets of table sugar, candy, or orange juice. Also available are 3-mg tablets of glucose (Dextrosol). If a patient develops symptoms of hypoglycemia, the dental procedure should be discontinued immediately; if conscious, the patient should be given some form of oral glucose.

If the patient is unconscious, the emergency medical service should be contacted. Then 1 mg of glucagon can be injected intramuscularly, or 50 ml of 50% glucose solution can be given by rapid intravenous infusion. The glucagon injection should restore the patient to a conscious state within 15 minutes; then some form of oral sugar can be given.

Source: Tierney LM, McPhee SJ, Papadakis MA, Schroeder SA: Current Medical Diagnosis and Treatment. Norwalk, CT, Appleton & Lange, 1993, p 932.

34. Is the diabetic patient at greater risk for infection after an oral surgical procedure?

It is important to minimize the risk of infection in diabetic patients. They should have aggressive treatment of dental caries and periodontal disease and then be placed on frequent recall examinations and oral prophylaxis.

After oral surgical procedures, endodontic procedures, and treatment of suppurative periodontitis, diabetic patients should be placed on antibiotics to prevent infection secondary to delayed healing. Antibiotics of choice are potassium phenoxymethyl penicillin, 500 mg, or erythromycin, 250 mg, 4 times/day for 7–10 days.

Source: Sonis ST, et al: Principles and Practice of Oral Medicine. Philadelphia, W.B. Saunders, 1984, p 157.

35. When is it necessary to increase the dose of prednisone in patients taking corticosteroids?

Patients with heart transplants who are on long-term prednisone therapy undergo cardiac biopsy without either intravenous sedation or stress doses of corticosteroids. For restorative dentistry, dental hygiene, mucogingival surgery, and simple extractions, it is not necessary to increase the patient's corticosteroids. However, it is important that the patient has taken the usual dose.

For multiple extractions or extensive mucogingival surgery, the dose of corticosteroids should be doubled on the day of surgery. If the patient is treated in the operating room under general anesthesia, stress level doses of cortisone, 100 mg intravenously or intramuscularly, should be given preoperatively.

36. Should antibiotics be prescribed for oral surgical procedures in patients receiving corticosteroids?

As with the diabetic patient, it is important to minimize the risk of infection in the patient on corticosteroids. Patients on long-term therapy, such as organ transplant recipients, should receive aggressive treatment to eliminate the oral cavity as a source of infection and then be placed on frequent recall examinations and oral prophylaxis.

Patients on corticosteroid therapy should be placed on antibiotic therapy after oral surgical procedures. Antibiotics should be started on the day of the procedure and continued for 5–7 days postoperatively. The antibiotic of choice is potassium phenoxymethyl penicillin, 500 mg 4 times/day. If the patient is allergic to penicillin and not taking cyclosporine, then erythromycin, 250 mg 4 times/day for 5–7 days, should be prescribed. If the patient is allergic to penicillin and taking cyclosporine, clindamycin, 300 mg 3 times/day for 5–7 days, is the antibiotic of choice.

37. What are the clinical symptoms of hypothyroidism? What dental care can safely be provided?

The clinical symptoms of hypothyroidism are weakness, fatigue, intolerance to cold, changes in weight, constipation, headache, menorrhagia, and dryness of the skin. Dental care should be deferred until after a medical consultation in a patient with or without a history of thyroid disease who experiences a combination of the above signs and symptoms. If the patient is myxedematous, he or she should be treated as a medical emergency and referred immediately for medical care. It is important *not* to prescribe opiates for palliative treatment of the myxedematous patient. The myxedematous patient may be unusually sensitive and die from normal doses of opiates.

Source: Tierney LM, McPhee SJ, Papadakis MA, Schroeder SA: Current Medical Diagnosis and Treatment. Norwalk, CT, Appleton & Lange, 1993, pp 863, 865.

ALLERGIC REACTIONS

38. What would you prescribe for the patient who develops a mild soft-tissue swelling of the lips under the rubber dam?

The patient probably has a contact allergic reaction from the latex. If the reaction is mild (slight swelling with no extension into the oral cavity) and self-limiting, the patient should be given 50 mg of oral diphenhydramine and observed for at least 2 hours for possible delayed reaction. If the reaction is moderate to severe, the patient should be given 50 mg of diphen-hydramine, either intramuscularly or intravenously, and closely monitored. Emergency services should be contacted to transport the patient to the emergency department for treatment and observation.

With the advent of the epidemic of HIV infection, latex gloves and condoms are now widely used. Allergic patients should be instructed to inform health care providers of their latex allergy and referred to an allergist.

39. What should you do if a patient for whom you have prescribed the prophylactic antibiotic amoxicillin approximately 1 hour ago now reports urticaria, erythema, and pruritus (itching)?

If the reaction is delayed (longer than 1 hour) and limited to the skin, the patient should be given 50 mg of diphenhydramine, intramuscularly or intravenously, then observed for 1–2 hours before being released. If no further reaction occurs, the patient should be given a prescription for 25–50 mg of diphenhydramine to be taken every 6 hours until symptoms are gone.

If the reaction is immediate (less than 1 hour) and limited to the skin, 50 mg of diphenhydramine should be given immediately either intravenously or intramuscularly. The patient should be monitored and emergency services contacted to transport the patient to the emergency department. If other symptoms of allergic reaction occur, such as conjunctivitis, rhinitis, bronchial constriction, or angioedema, 0.3 cc of aqueous 1/1000 epinephrine should be given by subcutaneous or intramuscular injection. The patient should be monitored until emergency services arrive. If the patient becomes hypotensive, an intravenous line should be started with either Ringer's lactate or 5% dextrose/water.

Source: Malamed SF, Sheppard GA: Medical Emergencies in the Dental Office, 4th ed. St. Louis, Mosby, 1992.

40. What are the signs and symptoms of anaphylaxis? How should it be managed in the dental office?

Anaphylaxis is characterized by bronchospasm, hypotension or shock, and urticaria or angioedema. It is a medical emergency in which death may result from respiratory obstruction, circulatory failure, or both. With the first indication of anaphylaxis, 0.2–0.5 cc of 1/1000 aqueous epinephrine should be injected subcutaneously or intramuscularly, and emergency services should be contacted. The injection of epinephrine may be repeated every 20–30 minutes, if necessary, for as many as 3 doses. Oxygen at a rate of 4 L/minute must be delivered with a face mask. The patient must be continuously monitored and an intravenous line containing either Ringer's lactate or normal saline should be infused at 100 cc/hour. If the patient becomes hypotensive, the intravenous infusion should be increased. If airway obstruction occurs from edema of the larynx or hypopharynx, a cricothyrotomy must be done. If the airway obstruction is due to bronchospasm, then an albuterol or terbutaline nebulizer should be administered or intravenous aminophylline, 6 mg/kg, infused over 20–30 minutes.

Source: Tierney LM, McPhee SJ, Papadakis MA, Schroeder SA: Current Medical Diagnosis and Treatment. Norwalk, CT, Appleton & Lange, 1993, p 634.

HEMATOLOGY/ONCOLOGY

41. What are the normal values for a complete blood count (CBC)?

General Values for a Normal CBC

White cell count		Hematocrit (HCT) *(Cont.)*	
18 years and older	4,000–10,000/μl	12–17 years	
12–17 years	4,500–13,000/μl	Male and female	36–39%
6 months to 11 years	4,500–13,500/μl	6 months to 11 years	
Red blood cell count		Male and female	34–45%
18 years and older		**Hemoglobin (HGB)**	
Male	4.5–6.4 M/μl	18 years and older	
Female	3.9–6.0 M/μl	Male	13.5–18.0 g/dl
12–17 years		Female	11.5–16.4 g/dl
Male and female	4.1–5.3 M/μl	12–17 years	
6 months to 11 years		Male and female	12.0–16.0 g/dl
Male and female	3.7–5.3 M/μl	6 months to 11 years	
Hematocrit (HCT)		Male and female	10.5–14.0 g/dl
18 years and older		**Platelet count (PLT)**	
Male	40–54%	8 days and older	150,000–450,000/μl
Female	36–48%	Up to 7 days	150,000–350,000/μl

42. What precautions should be taken when providing dental care to a patient with sickle-cell anemia?

1. Patients with sickle-cell disease should not receive dental treatment during a crisis, except for the relief of dental pain and the treatment of acute dental infections. Dental infections should be treated aggressively; if facial cellulitis develops, the patient should be admitted to the hospital for treatment.

2. The patient's physician should be consulted about the patient's cardiovascular status. These patient's often have myocardial damage secondary to infarctions and iron deposits.

3. Patients with sickle-cell anemia are at increased risk for bacterial infections and should receive prophylactic antibiotics before any dental procedure that may cause a transient bacteremia. The prophylactic antibiotic regimen used for the prevention of endocarditis should be followed. After a surgical procedure, antibiotics (500 mg penicillin VK qid or erythromycin, 250 mg qid, for penicillin-allergic patients) should be continued for 7–10 days postoperatively.

Sources: Sams DR, et al: Managing the dental patient with sickle cell anemia: A review of the literature. Pediatr Dent 12(5):317–320, 1990; Smith HB, et al: Dental management of patients with sickle cell disorders. J Am Dent Assoc 114:85, 1987.

43. Can local anesthetic with a vasoconstrictor be used in a patient with sickle-cell disease?

Because of the possibility of impairing local circulation, the use of vasoconstrictors in patients with sickle-cell disease is controversial. It is recommended that the planned dental procedure dictate the choice of local anesthetic. If the planned procedure is a routine, short procedure that can be performed without discomfort by using an anesthetic without a vasoconstrictor, then the vasoconstrictor should not be used. However, if the procedure requires long, profound anesthesia, 2% lidocaine with 1/100,000, epinephrine is the anesthetic of choice.

Source: Smith HB, et al: Dental management of patients with sickle cell disorders. J Am Dent Assoc 114:85, 1987.

44. Can nitrous oxide be used to help manage anxiety in the patient with sickle-cell anemia?

Nitrous oxide can be safely used in the patient with sickle-cell anemia as long as the concentration of oxygen is greater than 50%, the flow rate is high, and the patient is able to ventilate adequately.

Source: Smith HB, et al: Dental management of patients with sickle cell disorders. J Am Dent Assoc 114:85, 1987.

45. Can a dental infection cause a crisis in a patient with sickle-cell anemia?

Preventive dental care—routine scaling and root planing, topical fluorides, sealants and treatment of dental caries—is important in the patient with sickle-cell anemia. The literature reports two cases of a sickle-cell crisis precipitated by periodontal infections.

Source: Sams DR, et al: Managing the dental patient with sickle cell anemia: A review of the literature. Pediatr Dent 12(5):317–320, 1990.

46. What are the oral symptoms of acute leukemia?

Over 65% of patients with acute leukemia have oral symptoms. The symptoms result from myelosuppression due to the overwhelming numbers of malignant cells in the bone marrow and/or large numbers of circulating immature cells (blasts).

1. Symptoms from thrombocytopenia: gingival oozing, petechiae, hematoma, and ecchymosis

2. Symptoms from neutropenia: recurrent or unrelenting bacterial infections, lymphadenopathy, oral ulcerations, pharyngitis, and gingival infection

3. Symptoms from circulating immature cells (blasts): gingival hyperplasia from blast infiltration

Patients with the above signs or symptoms should be evaluated to rule out a hematologic malignancy. The dentist should consider carefully whether the symptoms can be explained by local factors or are disproportionate to the local factors. If a hematologic malignancy is suspected, a complete blood count with a differential white cell count should be ordered.

Source: Sonis ST, et al: Principles and Practice of Oral Medicine. Philadelphia, W.B. Saunders, 1984, p 327.

47. Is it safe to extract a tooth in a patient who is receiving chemotherapy?

The major organ system affected by cytotoxic chemotherapy is the hematopoietic system. When a patient receives chemotherapy, the white cell count and platelets may be expected to decrease in about 7–10 days. If the patient's absolute neutrophil count (calculated by multiplying the white cell count by the number of neutrophils in the differential count and divided by 100) drops below 500 neutrophils, the patient is considered neutropenic and at risk for infection. If the platelet count drops below 50,000, the patient is at risk for bleeding.

Dental procedures should be scheduled, if possible, 2 weeks before planned chemotherapy or after the counts begin to recover, usually 14 days for white cells and 21 days for platelets. Dental treatment should be attempted only after consultation and in coordination with the patient's physician and after the patient has had a complete blood count.

48. What precautions should be taken when treating a patient who has received bone marrow transplantation for a hematologic malignancy?

It is important to determine whether the patient has had either an autologous (native marrow) or allogenic (donor marrow) transplant. Dental care should be done only in consultation with the patient's physician. For the patient with autologous bone marrow transplant, elective dental treatment should be postponed for 6 months after transplant. For the patient with allogenic bone marrow transplant, elective dental care should be postponed for 1 year. If dental care must be done before the recommended postponement, a CBC should be checked and if the results are acceptable (platelets > 50,000 and neutrophils > 500), the patient should be premedicated with the same regimen used for the prevention of endocarditis.

49. What should be done if a patient has enlarged lymph nodes?

Lymphadenopathy may be secondary to a sore throat or upper respiratory infection or the initial presentation of a malignancy. A thorough history and clinical examination help to determine the etiology of the lymphadenopathy.

Patients with lymphadenopathy and an identifiable inflammatory process should be re-examined in 2 weeks to determine whether the lymphadenopathy has responded to treatment. If no inflammatory process can be identified or if the lymphadenopathy does not resolve after treatment, the patient should be referred to a physician for further evaluation and possible biopsy.

	INFLAMMATORY PROCESS	GRANULOMATOUS DISEASE/NEOPLASIA
Onset	Acute, then regression	Progressive enlargement
Pain on palpation	Tender	Neoplasia: asymptomatic Granulomatous: Painful
Symmetry	Bilateral for systemic, unilateral for localized infections	Usually unilateral
Consistency	Firm, movable	Firm, nonmovable

Source: Sonis ST, et al: Principles and Practice of Oral Medicine. Philadelphia, W.B. Saunders, 1984, p 332.

KIDNEY DISEASE

50. What precautions should be taken before beginning treatment of a patient on dialysis?
Patients typically receive dialysis three times/week, usually on a Monday, Wednesday, Friday schedule or a Tuesday, Thursday, Saturday schedule. Dental treatment for a patient on dialysis should be done on the day between dialysis appointments. Patients with an arteriovenous shunt should be premedicated to prevent infection of the shunt whenever the risk of transient bacteremia is present.

51. What adjustments in the dosage of oral antibiotics would you make for a patient on renal dialysis who has a dental infection?

Penicillin:	500 mg every 6 hours, dose after hemodialysis
Amoxicillin:	500 mg orally every 24 hours, dose after hemodialysis
Ampicillin:	250 mg to 1 g orally every 12–24 hours, dose after hemodialysis
Erythromycin:	250 mg orally every 6 hours; it is not necessary to dose after hemodialysis
Clindamycin:	300 mg every 6 hours; it is not necessary to dose after hemodialysis

Source: Bennett WM, et al: Drug Prescribing in Renal Failure, 2nd ed. Philadelphia, American College of Physicians, 1991.

52. What pain medications can be safely prescribed for patients on dialysis?
Codeine is safe to use in dialysis but may produce more profound sedation. The dose should be titrated beginning with one-half the normal dose for patients on dialysis and one-half to three-fourths the normal dose for patients with severely decreased renal function.

Acetaminophen is nephrotoxic in overdoses. However, it may be prescribed in patients on dialysis at a dose of 650 mg every 8 hours. For patients with decreased renal function, the regimen should be 650 mg every 6 hours.

Aspirin should be avoided in patients with severe renal failure and in patients on renal dialysis because of the possibility of potentiating hemorrhagic diathesis.

Propoxyphene (Darvon) should not be prescribed for a patient on renal dialysis. The active metabolite norpropoxyphene accumulates in patients with end-stage renal disease.

Meperidine (Demerol) should not be prescribed in patients on renal dialysis. The active metabolite, normeperidine, accumulates and may cause seizures.

Source: Bennett WM, et al: Drug Prescribing in Renal Failure, 2nd ed. Philadelphia, American College of Physicians, 1991.

53. What changes do you expect to see in the dental radiographs of a patient on renal dialysis?
The most common changes are decreased bone density with a ground-glass appearance, increased bone density in the mandibular molar area compatible with osteosclerosis, loss of lamina dura, subperiosteal cortical bone resorption in the maxillary sinus and the mandibular canal, and brown tumor.

Source: Spolnik KJ: Dental radiographic manifestations of end-stage renal disease. Dent Radiogr Photogr 54(2):21–31, 1981.

54. What precautions should be taken in treating a patient after renal transplantation?
After renal transplant patients are on immunosuppressive drugs and have an increased susceptibility to infection. Dental infections should be treated aggressively. Prophylactic antibiotics should be considered whenever the risk of bacteremia is present. Erythromycin should not be prescribed for any patient on cyclosporine.

55. What antibiotic, used often in dentistry, would you avoid in a patient on cyclosporine?
Cyclosporine is used to prevent organ rejection in renal, cardiac, and hepatic transplantation and to prevent graft versus host disease in patients with bone marrow transplants. Erythromycin should not be prescribed for patients taking cyclosporine. Erythromycin increases the levels of cyclosporine by decreasing its metabolism.

PULMONARY DISEASE

56. What precautions should be taken in treating a patient with chronic obstructive pulmonary disease?
Patients with chronic obstructive pulmonary disease (COPD) and a history of hemoptysis should be prescribed drugs with antiplatelet activity (aspirin and nonsteroidals) with caution. Hemoptysis has been reported after the use of aspirin in patients with COPD.
    Source: Tierney LM, McPhee SJ, Papadakis MA, Schroeder SA: Current Medical Diagnosis and Treatment. Norwalk, CT, Appleton & Lange, 1993, p 197.

57. What antibiotic should not be prescribed for patients with chronic pulmonary disease who take theophylline?
Erythromycin should not be prescribed for the patient taking theophylline. Erythromycin decreases the metabolism of theophylline and may cause toxicity.
    Source: Deglin JH, et al: Davis's Drug Guide for Nurses, 2nd ed. Philadelphia, F.A. Davis, 1991.

58. What intervention is appropriate for a dental patient who has an asthma attack in the office?
The medical history should provide an indication of the severity of the asthma and the medications that the patient takes for an asthma attack. The symptoms of an acute asthma attack are shortness of breath, wheezing, dyspnea, anxiety, and, with severe attacks, cyanosis. As with all medical emergencies, the first two steps are (1) to discontinue treatment and (2) to remain calm and not increase the patient's anxiety. Patients should be allowed to position themselves for optimal comfort and then placed on oxygen, 2–4 L/minute. If patients have their own nebulizer, they should be allowed to use it. If the patient does not have a nebulizer, he or she should be given either a metaproterenol or albuterol nebulizer from the emergency cart or case and take 2 inhalations.

    If the symptoms do not subside or increase in severity, emergency services should be contacted; the patient must be closely monitored and given either 0.3–0.5 ml of a 1:1000 solution of epinephrine subcutaneously or intravenous aminophylline, 5.6 mg/kg in 150 ml of either D-5 ½ normal saline or normal saline infused over 30 minutes. (To calculate kg weight, divide the patient's weight in pounds by 2.2.) The dose of epinephrine may be repeated every 30 minutes for as many as 3 doses. Epinephrine should not be used in patients with severe hypertension, severe tachycardia, or cardiac arrhythmias. Aminophylline should not be used in patients who have had theophylline in the past 24 hours.

59. Can nitrous oxide be used safely to sedate a patient with chronic obstructive pulmonary disease?
Sedation with nitrous oxide should be avoided in patients with COPD. The high flow of oxygen may depress the respiratory drive. Low-flow oxygen via a nasal cannula may be safely used without risk of respiratory depression.
    Source: Little JW, Falace DA: Dental Management of the Medically Compromised Patient, 4th ed. St. Louis, Mosby, 1993, p 237.

LIVER DISEASE

60. What laboratory blood tests should be ordered for a patient with alcoholic hepatitis?
Alcoholic hepatitis is the most common cause of cirrhosis, which is one of the most common causes of death in the United States. There are a number of concerns in treating the patient with alcoholic hepatitis:

1. Increased risk of peri- and postoperative bleeding, secondary to a decrease in vitamin K–dependent coagulation factors
2. Qualitative and quantitative effects of alcohol on platelets
3. Anemia secondary to dietary deficiencies and/or hemorrhage

Before attempting a surgical procedure, the minimal laboratory tests are prothrombin time, partial thromboplastin time, complete blood count, and bleeding time.

61. What precautions should be taken with patients on anticonvulsant medications?
It is important to obtain a detailed history of the seizure disorder to determine whether the patient is at risk for seizures during dental treatment. Important information includes the type and frequency of seizures, the date of the last seizure, prescribed medications, the last blood test to determine therapeutic ranges, and activities that tend to provoke seizures. For patients on valproic acid or carbamazepine, periodic tests for liver function should be performed. Blood counts on patients taking carbamazepine and ethosuximide should be done by the patient's physician. Both liver function and blood counts should be checked before any oral surgical procedure is planned.

Sources: Deglin JH, et al: Davis's Drug Guide for Nurses, 2nd ed. Philadelphia, F.A. Davis, 1991.

Little JW, Falace DA: Dental Management of the Medically Compromised Patient, 4th ed. St. Louis, Mosby, 1993, p 331.

Tierney LM, McPhee SJ, Papadakis MA, Schroeder SA: Current Medical Diagnosis and Treatment. Norwalk, CT, Appleton & Lange, 1993.

Seizure Medications and Precautions for the Dental Practitioner

MEDICATION	ADVERSE REACTIONS	INTERACTIONS
Valproic acid Heparin	Prolonged bleeding time, leukopenia, thrombocytopenia	Increased risk of bleeding with aspirin and NSAIDs or warfarin. Additive depression of CNS with other depressants, including narcotic analgesics and sedative/hypnotics
Carbamazepine (Tegretol)	Aplastic anemia, agranulocytosis, thrombocytopenia, leukopenia, leukocytosis	Erythromycin increases levels of carbamazepine and may cause toxicity
Phenytoin (Dilantin)	Aplastic anemia, agranulocytosis, leukopenia, thrombocytopenia	Additive depression of CNS with other depressants, including narcotics and sedative/hypnotics
Phenobarbital		Additive depression of CNS with other depressants, including narcotics and sedative/hypnotics. May increase the risk of hepatic toxicity of acetaminophen
Primidone	Blood dyscrasias, orthostatic hypotension	Additive depression of CNS with other depressants, including narcotics and sedative/hypnotics
Ethosuximide	Aplastic anemia, granulocytosis, leukopenia	Additive depression of CNS with other depressants
Clonazepam	Anemia, thrombocytosis, leukopenia	Additive depression of CNS with other CNS depressants

62. What emergency procedures should be taken for a patient having a seizure?

It is important to determine whether the patient has a history of seizure disorder. Any patient who has a seizure in the dental office without a history of seizures must be treated as a medical emergency. The emergency medical service should be contacted as the dentist proceeds with management. There are two stages of a seizure: the ictal phase and the postictal phase. The management of each is described below.

Ictal phase

1. Place the patient in a supine position away from hard or sharp objects to prevent injury; a carpeted floor is ideal. If the patient is in the dental chair, it is important to protect the patient by moving equipment as far as possible out of the way.

2. Airway must be maintained and vital signs monitored during the tonic stage. If suctioning equipment is available, it should be ready with a plastic tip for suctioning secretions to maintain the airway. The patient may experience periods of apnea and develop cyanosis. The head should be extended to establish a patent airway, and oxygen should be administered. Vital signs, pulse, respiration and blood pressure must be monitored throughout the seizure.

3. If the ictal phase of the seizure lasts more than 5 minutes, emergency services should be called. Tonic-clonic status epilepticus is a medical emergency. If the dentist is trained to do so, an intravenous line should be initiated, and a dose of 25–50 ml of 50% dextrose should be given immediately in case the etiology of the seizure is hypoglycemia. If there is no response, the patient should be given 10 mg of diazepam intravenously over a 2-minute period. The patient's vital signs must be monitored, because the diazepam may cause respiratory depression. The dose of diazepam may be repeated after 10 minutes, if necessary.

Postictal phase

1. Once the seizure activity has stopped and the patient enters the postictal phase, it is important to continue to monitor the vital signs and, if necessary, to provide basic life support. If respiratory depression is significant, emergency services should be called, the airway maintained, and respiration supported. Blood pressure may be initially depressed but should recover gradually.

2. If, from the postictal phase, the patient recovers without basic life support or other complications, the patient's physician should be contacted, and the patient, if stable, should be discharged from the dental office, accompanied by a responsible adult.

Source: Malamed SF, Sheppard GA: Medical Emergencies in the Dental Office, 4th ed. St. Louis, Mosby, 1992, pp 233–236.

63. What dental considerations must be considered in treating a patient with seizure disorders?

If the patient is taking phenytoin, he or she is at risk for gingival hyperplasia. Tissue irritation from orthodontic bands, defective restorations, fractured teeth, plaque, and calculus accelerate the hyperplasia.

The dental practitioner should consider the patient's seizure status. A rubber dam with dental floss tied to the clamp should be used for all restorative dental procedures to enable the rapid removal of materials and instruments from the patient's oral cavity. Fixed prosthetics, when indicated, should be fabricated rather than removable prosthetics. If removable prosthetics are indicated, they should be fabricated with metal for all major connectors. Acrylic partial dentures should be avoided because of the risk of breaking and aspiration during seizure activities. Unilateral partial dentures are contraindicated. Temporary crowns and bridges should be laboratory-cured for strength.

64. What are the common causes of unconsciousness in dental patients?

The most common cause of loss of consciousness in the dental office is syncope. The signs and symptoms are diaphoresis, pallor, and loss of consciousness. The management of syncope is to place the patient in the supine position with the feet elevated, to monitor vital signs, and to give oxygen, 3–4 L/minute, via nasal cannula.

RADIATION THERAPY

65. What are the risk factors for the development of osteoradionecrosis?
Bone exposed to high radiation therapy is hypovascular, hypocellular, and hypoxic tissue. Osteoradionecrosis develops because the radiated tissue is unable to repair itself. The risk for osteoradionecrosis increases as the dose of radiation increases from 5,000 rads to over 8,000 rads. Tissues receiving less than 5,000 rads are at low risk for necrosis. In addition, the risk increases with poor oral health. Oral surgical procedures after radiation therapy place the patient at high risk for developing osteoradionecrosis. Soft-tissue trauma from dentures and oral infections from periodontal disease and dental caries also put the patient at risk.

66. How should the dentist prepare the patient for radiation therapy of the head and neck?
The dentist should consult with the radiotherapist to determine what oral structures will be in the field as well as the maximal radiation dose. If teeth are in the field and the dose is greater than 5,000 rads, periodontally involved teeth and teeth with periapical lucencies should be extracted at least 2 weeks before radiation therapy begins.

The dentist should prepare the patient for postradiation xerostomia, provide custom fluoride trays, and prescribe 0.4% stannous flouride gel to be used for 3–5 minutes twice daily. The patient must be placed on a 2–3-month recall schedule. On recall, the teeth must be carefully examined for root caries, and instruction in oral hygiene should be reviewed.

BIBLIOGRAPHY

1. Bennett WM, et al: Drug Prescribing in Renal Failure, 2nd ed. Philadelphia, American College of Physicians, 1991.
2. Cintron G, et al: Cardiovascular effects and safety of dental anesthesia and dental interventions in patients with recent uncomplicated myocardial infarction. Arch Intern Med 146:2203–2204, 1986.
3. Dajani AS, et al: Prevention of bacterial endocarditis recommendations by the American Heart Association. JAMA 264:2919–2922, 1990.
4. Deglin JH, et al: Davis's Drug Guide for Nurses, 2nd ed. Philadelphia, F.A. Davis, 1991.
5. Holroyd SV, Wynn RL, Requa-Clark B (eds): Clinical Pharmacology in Dental Practice, 4th ed. St. Louis, Mosby, 1988.
6. Kilmartin C, Munroe CO: Cardiovascular diseases and the dental patient. J Can Dent Assoc 6:513–518, 1986.
7. Kupp MA, Chatton MJ: Current Medical Diagnosis and Treatment. Norwalk, CT, Appleton & Lange, 1983.
8. Lind SE: The bleeding time does not predict surgical bleeding. Blood 77:2547–2552, 1991.
9. Little JW, Falace DA: Dental Management of the Medically Compromised Patient, 4th ed. St. Louis, Mosby, 1993.
10. Magnac C, et al: Platelet antibodies in serum of patients with human immunodeficiency virus (HIV) infection: AIDS Res Hum Retroviruses 6:1443–1449, 1990.
11. Malamed SF, Sheppard GA: Medical Emergencies in the Dental Office, 4th ed. St. Louis, Mosby, 1992.
12. Sams DR, et al: Managing the dental patient with sickle cell anemia: A review of the literature. Pediatr Dent 12(5):317–320, 1990.
13. Smith HB, et al: Dental management of patients with sickle cell disorders. J Am Dent Assoc 114:85, 1987.
14. Sonis ST, et al: Principles and Practice of Oral Medicine. Philadelphia, W.B. Saunders, 1984.
15. Spolnik KJ: Dental Radiographic manifestations of end-stage renal disease. Dent Radiogr Photogr 54(2):21–31, 1981.
16. Tierney LM, McPhee SJ, Papadakis MA, Schroeder SA: Current Medical Diagnosis and Treatment. Norwalk, CT, Appleton & Lange, 1993.

4. ORAL PATHOLOGY

Sook-Bin Woo, D.M.D., M.M.Sc.

DEVELOPMENTAL CONDITIONS

Tooth-related Problems

1. Describe the different types of dentinogenesis imperfecta.

Dentinogenesis imperfecta (DI) causes the teeth to be opalescent and affects both the primary and permanent dentition.

Type I: DI with osteogenesis imperfecta

Type II: DI without osteogenesis imperfecta

Type III: Brandywine type, which also occurs in the absence of osteogenesis imperfecta but is clustered within a racial isolate in Maryland. In addition to classic findings of DI, radiographs may exhibit multiple periapical radiolucencies, and large pulp chambers may lead to multiple pulp exposures.

2. What is the difference between fusion and concrescence? Between twinning and gemination?

Fusion is a more complete process than concrescence and may involve either (1) merging of the entire length of two teeth (enamel, dentin, and cementum) to form one large tooth, with one less tooth in the arch, or (2) fusion of the root only (dentin and cementum) with the maintenance of two clinical crowns. **Concrescence** involves fusion of cementum only.

Twinning is more complete than gemination and results in the formation of two separate teeth from one tooth bud (one extra tooth in the arch). In **gemination**, separation is attempted, but the two teeth share the same root canal.

3. What is a Turner's tooth?

A Turner's tooth is a solitary, usually permanent tooth with signs of enamel hypoplasia or hypocalcification. This phenomenon is caused by trauma or infection to the overlying deciduous tooth that damages the ameloblasts of the underlying tooth bud and thus leads to localized enamel hypoplasia or hypocalcification.

4. What are "bull teeth"?

Bull teeth, also known as taurodonts, have long anatomic crowns, large pulp chambers, and short roots, resembling teeth found in bulls. They are most dramatic in permanent molars but may affect teeth in either dentition. They occur more frequently in certain syndromes, such as Klinefelter's syndrome.

5. What is the difference between dens evaginatus and dens invaginatus?

Dens evaginatus occurs primarily in persons of mongoloid descent and affects the premolars. Evagination of the layers of the tooth germ results in the formation of a tubercle that arises from the occlusal surface and consists of enamel, dentin, and pulp tissue. This tubercle tends to break when it occludes with the opposing dentition and may result in pulp exposure and subsequent pulp necrosis. Dens invaginatus occurs mainly in maxillary lateral incisors and ranges in severity from an accentuated lingual pit to a "dens in dente." This phenomenon is caused by invagination of the layers of the tooth germ. Food traps in the pit, and caries begin early.

6. What are the causes of generalized intrinsic discoloration of teeth?

Amelogenesis imperfecta	Fluorosis	Porphyria
Dentinogenesis imperfecta	Rh incapatibility	Biliary atresia
Tetracycline staining		

7. Why do teeth discolor from ingestion of tetracycline during odontogenesis?
Tetracycline binds with the calcium component of bones and teeth and is deposited at sites of active mineralization, causing a yellow-brown endogenous pigmentation of the hard tissues. Because teeth do not turn over like some bone tissues, this stain becomes a permanent "label" that fluoresces under ultraviolet light.

8. Which teeth are most commonly missing congenitally?
Third molars, maxillary lateral incisors, and second premolars.

9. What conditions are associated with multiple supernumerary teeth?
Gardner's syndrome and cleidocranial dysplasia.

10. What are the most common sites for supernumerary teeth?
Midline of the maxilla (mesiodens), posterior maxilla (fourth molar or paramolar), and mandibular bicuspid areas are the most common sites.

Intrabony Lesions

11. A 40-year-old African American woman presents with multiple radiolucencies and radiopacities. What is the diagnosis?
The African-American population is prone to developing benign fibro-osseous lesions of various kinds. They may range from localized lesions, such as periapical cemental dysplasia involving one tooth (usually mandibular anterior) to florid cemento-osseous dysplasia, involving all four quadrants. The second condition also has been referred to as familial gigantiform cementoma, multiple enostoses, and sclerotic cemental masses.

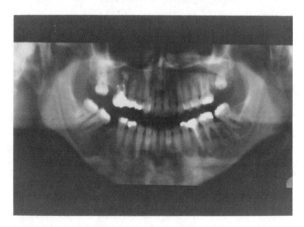

Florid cemento-osseous dysplasia affecting at least three quadrants.

12. Are fibrous dysplasias of bone premalignant lesions?
Fibrous dysplasia, a developmental malformation of bone, is of unknown etiology and is not premalignant. The monostotic form often affects the maxilla unilaterally. The polyostotic form is associated with various other abnormalities, such as skin pigmentations and endocrine dysfunction (Albright and Jaffe-Lichtenstein syndromes). Cherubism, which used to be termed familial fibrous dysplasia, is probably not a form of fibrous dysplasia. In the past, fibrous dysplasia was treated with radiation, which caused the development of osteosarcoma.

13. The globulomaxillary cyst is a fissural cyst. True or false?
False. Historically, the globulomaxillary cyst was classified as a nonodontogenic or fissural cyst thought to form as a result of enclavement of epithelial rests along the line of fusion

between the lateral maxillary and the nasomedial processes. Current thinking puts it in the category of odontogenic cysts, probably of developmental origin and possibly related to the development of the lateral incisor or the canine. The two embryonic processes mentioned above do not fuse. The fold between them fills in and becomes erased by mesodermal invasion so that there is no opportunity for trapping of epithelial rests. This cyst occurs between the roots of the maxillary lateral incisor and cuspid, both of which are vital.

14. The median palatal cyst is a true fissural cyst. True or false?
True. The epithelium of this intrabony cyst arises from proliferation of entrapped epithelium when the right and left palatal shelves fuse in the midline. The soft-tissue counterpart, which also occurs in the midline of the palate and is known as the palatal cyst of the newborn (Epstein's pearl), is congenital and exteriorizes on its own. The histology is similar to that of dental lamina cysts of the newborn (see below).

15. A neonate presents with a few white nodules on the mandibular alveolar ridge. What are they?
They are most likely dental lamina cysts of the newborn (Bohn's nodules). The epithelium of these cysts arises from remnants of dental lamina on the alveolar ridge after odontogenesis. Dental lamina cysts of the newborn tend to involute and do not require treatment.

16. A boy presents to the dental clinic with multiple jaw cysts and a history of jaw cysts in other family members. What syndrome does he most likely have?
The boy most likely has the bifid rib–basal cell nevus–jaw cyst syndrome, which is inherited as an autosomal dominant trait. The cysts are odontogenic keratocysts, which have a higher incidence of recurrence than other odontogenic cysts. Other findings include palmar pitting, palmar and plantar keratosis, calcification of the falx cerebri, hypertelorism, ovarian tumors, and neurologic manifestations such as mental retardation and medulloblastomas.

17. Are all jaw cysts that produce keratin considered odontogenic keratocysts?
Yes and no. The odontogenic keratocyst is a specific histologic entity. The epithelial lining exhibits corrugated parakeratosis, uniform thinness (unless altered by inflammation) and palisading of the basal cell nuclei. The recurrence rate is high, and the condition is associated with the basal cell–bifid rib nevus syndrome. Odontogenic cysts that produce orthokeratin do not show the basal cell nuclei changes, do not have the same tendency to recur, and are not associated with the syndrome. However, some pathologists use the term "orthokeratinized variant" after odontogenic keratocyst to denote the difference, whereas others use the term orthokeratinizing odontogenic cyst. The clinical differences are important.

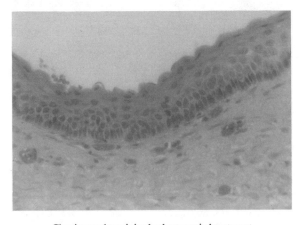

Classic parakeratinized odontogenic keratocyst.

18. What neoplasms may arise in a dentigerous cyst?
Ameloblastoma, mucoepidermoid carcinoma, and squamous cell carcinoma may arise in a dentigerous cyst. Odontogenic tumors that may arise in a dentigerous relationship, although not within a dentigerous cyst, include adenomatoid odontogenic tumor and calcifying epithelial odontogenic tumor (Pindborg tumor).

19. What is the difference between a lateral radicular cyst and a lateral periodontal cyst?
A lateral radicular cyst is an **inflammatory cyst** in which the epithelium is derived from rests of Malassez (as in a periapical or apical radicular cyst). It is in a lateral rather than an apical location because the inflammatory stimulus emanates from a lateral canal. The associated tooth is always nonvital. The lateral periodontal cyst is a **developmental cyst** in which the epithelium probably is derived from rests of dental lamina. It is usually located between the mandibular premolars, which are vital.

20. What is the incidence of cleft lip and/or cleft palate?
Cleft lip and cleft palate should be considered as two entities: (1) cleft palate alone and (2) cleft lip with or without cleft palate. The former is more common in women and the latter in men. The incidence of cleft palate is 1 in 2,000–3,000 births, whereas the incidence of cleft lip and/ or cleft palate is 1 in 700–1,000 births. Of all cases, 25% are cleft palate alone and 75% are cleft lip with or without cleft palate.

Soft-Tissue Conditions

21. Name the organism that colonizes lesions of median rhomboid glossitis.
Candida colonizes the lesions but probably is not the cause because in many instances, even with elimination of candida, the area of papillary atrophy persists. Some investigators have reverted to the original hypothesis that median rhomboid glossitis is a developmental malformation, possibly caused by failure of the tuberculum impar to retract completely.

22. Is benign migratory glossitis ("geographic tongue") associated with any systemic conditions?
Most cases of benign migratory glossitis occur in the absence of a systemic condition, although some cases have been associated with fissured tongue. However, patients with psoriasis, especially generalized pustular psoriasis, have a higher incidence of benign migratory glossitis.

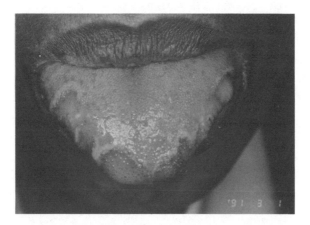

Benign migratory glossitis.

23. What predisposes to the formation of a hairy tongue?
Xerostomia, broad-spectrum antibiotics, systemic steroids, and oxygenating mouth rinses predispose to the formation of a hairy tongue. The "hairs" represent filiform papillae with

multiple layers of keratin that fail to shed adequately. The papillae are putatively colonized by chromogenic bacteria, so that the tongue may appear black, brown, or even green.

INFECTIONS

Fungal

24. How many clinical forms of candidiasis are there?
Acute forms: pseudomembranous candidiasis (the typical type with curdy white patches) and atrophic candidiasis (often seen in patients infected with human immunodeficiency virus [HIV], angular cheilitis)
Chronic forms: hyperplastic candidiasis (leukoplakialike patches that do not wipe off easily), atrophic candidiasis (denture sore mouth), mucocutaneous candidiasis (associated with skin candidiasis and an underlying systemic condition such as an endocrinopathy)

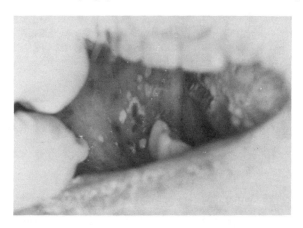

Acute pseudomembranous candidiasis.

25. What factors predispose to candidal infection?
Predisposing factors include (1) poor immune function, which may be due to age (very young and very old), malignancies, immunomodulating drugs, endocrine dysfunction, or HIV infection; (2) malnutrition; (3) antibiotics that upset the normal balance of flora; and (4) dental prostheses, especially dentures.

26. A culture performed on an oral ulcer grows candida. Does this mean the patient has candidiasis?
No. Approximately one-half the adult population harbors candida in the mouth. These persons grow candida on culture in the complete absence of a candidal infection.

27. How do you make a diagnosis of candidiasis?
Good clinical judgment. Pseudomembranous plaques of candidiasis wipe off, leaving a raw, bleeding surface.
Potassium hydroxide (KOH) preparation. The plaque is scraped, and the scrapings are put onto a glass microscopic slide. A few drops of KOH are added, the slide is warmed over an alcohol flame for a few seconds, and a coverslip is placed over the slide. The hyphae, if present, can be seen under a microscope.
Biopsy to show hyphae penetrating the tissues (too invasive for routine use).
Cultures. Although this is not the ideal way to diagnose candidiasis, the quantity of candida that grows on culture correlates somewhat with clinical candidiasis.

28. What are common antifungal agents for treating oral candidiasis?
Polyenes: nystatin (topical), amphotericin (topical, systemic)
Imidazoles: chlortrimazole, ketoconazole
Triazoles: fluconazole

29. Actinomycosis represents a fungal infection. True or false?
False. Actinomycetes is a gram-positive bacillus. Do not be fooled by the suffix -mycosis.

30. What are sulfur granules?
These yellowish granules (hence the name) are seen within the pus of lesions of actinomycosis.
They represent aggregates of *Actinomyces israelii*, which are invariably surrounded by neutrophils.

31. Name two opportunistic fungal disease that often present in the orofacial region.
Aspergillosis and mucormycosis often present in the orofacial region. Both tend to infect
immunocompromised hosts, with the latter causing rhinocerebral infections in patients with
diabetes mellitus.

32. Name two deep fungal infections that are endemic in North America.
Histoplasmosis (caused by *Histoplasma capsulatum*) is endemic in the Ohio-Mississippi basin,
and coccidioidomycosis (caused by *Coccidioides immitis*) is endemic in the San Joaquin Valley
in California.

Viruses

**33. Name the four most common viruses of the Herpesviridae family that are pathogenic in
humans.**
Herpes simplex virus (HSV 1 and 2, ?6)   Varicella zoster virus (VZV)
Cytomegalovirus (CMV)   Epstein-Barr virus (EBV)

34. Antibodies against HSV protect against further outbreaks of the disease. True or false?
False. The herpes viruses are unique in that they exhibit latency. Once one has been infected
by HSV, the virus remains latent within nerve ganglia for life. When conditions are favorable
(for the virus, not the patient), HSV travels along nerve fibers and causes a mucocutaneous
lesion at a peripheral site, such as a cold sore on the lip. A positive antibody titer (IgG)
indicates that the patient has been previously exposed, and at the time of reactivation the titer
may rise.

35. How do you differentiate between recurrent aphthous ulcers and recurrent herpetic ulcers?
Clinically, recurrent aphthous ulcers (minor) occur only on the *nonkeratinized* mucosae of the
labial mucosa, buccal mucosa, sulci, ventral tongue, soft palate, and faucial pillars. Recurrent
herpetic ulcers occur on the vermilion border of the lips (cold sores or fever blisters) (see figure,
opposite page) and on the *keratinized* mucosae of the palate and attached gingiva. A culture
confirms the presence of virus. In immunocompromised hosts, however, recurrent herpetic
lesions can occur on both the keratinized and nonkeratinized mucosae.

**36. An elderly patient with long-standing rheumatoid arthritis presents with a history of upper
respiratory tract infection, ulcers of the right hard palate, and right facial weakness and
vertigo. What does he have?**
The patient has herpes zoster infection, which typically is unilateral. The patient also has
Ramsay Hunt syndrome, which is caused by infection of cranial nerves VII and VIII with
herpes zoster, leading to facial paralysis, tinnitus, deafness, and vertigo.

37. List lesions associated with the Epstein-Barr virus that can present in the orofacial region.
Infectious mononucleosis   Nasopharyngeal carcinoma
Burkitt's lymphoma (African type)   Hairy leukoplakia

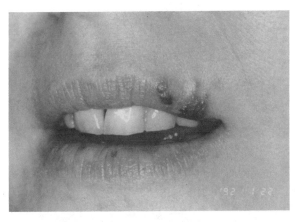

Recurrent herpes labialis (cold sores or fever blisters).

38. Describe the oral presentation of infectious mononucleosis.
Infectious mononucleosis usually presents as multiple, painful, punctate ulcers of the posterior hard palate and soft palate in young adults or teenagers. It is often associated with regional lymphadenopathy and constitutional signs of a viral illness.

39. What oral lesions have been associated with infection by human papillomavirus (HPV)?

Focal epithelial hyperplasia   Verruca vulgaris
  (Heck's disease)   Squamous papilloma
Oral condylomas   Some squamous cell and verrucous carcinomas

The benign conditions are usually associated with HPV 6 and 11; the malignant ones with HPV 16 and 18.

40. What oral conditions does coxsackievirus cause?
Herpangina and hand-foot-mouth disease are caused by the type A coxsackievirus and generally affect children, who then develop oral ulcers associated with an upper respiratory tract viral prodrome.

41. What are Koplik spots?
Koplik spots are early manifestations of measles or rubeola (therefore also called herald spots). They are 1–2 mm, yellow-white, necrotic ulcers with surrounding erythema that occur on the buccal mucosa, usually a few days before the body rash of measles is seen. Koplik spots are not seen in German measles.

Others

42. What are the organisms responsible for noma?
Noma, which is a gangrenous stomatitis resulting in severe destruction of the orofacial tissues, is usually encountered in areas where malnutrition is rampant. The bacteria are similar to those associated with acute necrotizing ulcerative gingivitis, i.e., spirochetes and fusiform bacteria.

43. What are the oral findings in syphilis?
Primary: oral chancre
Secondary: mucous patches, condyloma latum
Tertiary: gumma, glossitis
Congenital: enamel hypoplasia, mulberry molars, notched incisors

44. What is a granuloma?

A granuloma is a collection of epithelioid histiocytes, often associated with multinucleated giant cells. In granulomas of tuberculosis, giant cells are called Langhans cells. Many infectious agents, including fungi (such as histoplasmosis) and those causing tertiary syphilis and cat-scratch disease, can produce granulomatous reactions. Foreign body reactions are often granulomatous. Some granulomatous disease, such as cheilitis granulomatosa, Crohn's disease, and sarcoidosis, have no known etiology at present.

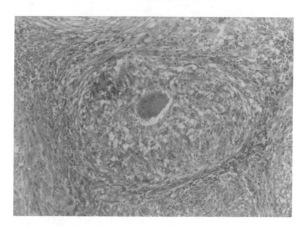

Tuberculous granuloma with Langhans giant cell.

45. What are Langhans cells?

Langhans cells are multinucleated giant cells seen in granulomas, usually those caused by *Mycobacterium tuberculosis*. Their nuclei have a characteristic horseshoe distribution. Do not confuse them with Langerhans cells, which are antigen-processing cells.

REACTIVE, HYPERSENSITIVITY, AND AUTOIMMUNE CONDITIONS

Intrabony Lesions

46. The periapical granuloma is composed of a collection of histiocytes, that is, a true granuloma. True or false?

False. The periapical granuloma is a tumorlike (-oma) proliferation of granulation tissue found around the apex of a nonvital tooth. It is associated with chronic inflammation from pulp devitalization. The inflammation can stimulate proliferation of the epithelial rests of Malassez to form a cyst, either apical radicular or periapical (see figure, opposite page).

47. What is condensing osteitis?

Condensing osteitis, a relatively common condition, manifests as an area of radiopacity in the bone, usually adjacent to a tooth that has a large restoration or a root canal, although occasionally it may lie adjacent to what appears to be a sound tooth. Condensing osteitis is asymptomatic. Histologically, it consists of dense bone with little or no inflammation. It probably arises as a bony reaction to a low-grade inflammatory stimulus from the adjacent tooth. Condensing osteitis also has been referred to as idiopathic osteosclerosis, bone scar, and focal sclerosing osteomyelitis.

48. What are the etiologic difference among the wearing down of teeth caused by attrition, abrasion, and erosion?

    Attrition: tooth-to-tooth contact
    Abrasion: a foreign object-to-tooth contact, e.g., toothbrush bristles, bobby pins, nails
    Erosion: a chemical agent-to-tooth contact, e.g., lemon juice, gastric juices

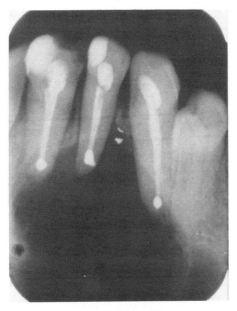

Apical radicular cyst.

Soft-Tissue Conditions

49. Aphthous ulcers may be associated with certain systemic conditions. Name them.

Iron, folate or vitamin B12 deficiency   Reiter's disease
Inflammatory bowel disease   HIV infection
Behçet's disease   Conditions predisposing to neutropenia

50. An aphthous ulcer is the same as a traumatic ulcer. True or false?

False but with reservations. A traumatic ulcer is the most common form of oral ulcer and, as its name suggests, occurs at the site of trauma, such as the buccal mucosa, lateral tongue, lower labial mucosa, or sulci. It follows a history of trauma such as mastication or toothbrush injury. An aphthous ulcer may occur at the same sites, but often with no history of trauma. However, patients prone to developing aphthae tend to do so after episodes of minor trauma.

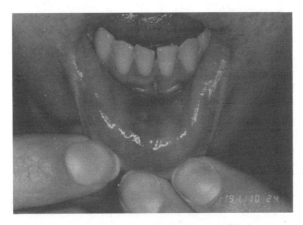

Recurrent aphthous ulcer (minor) of lower labial mucosa.

51. A child returns one day after a visit to the dentist at which several amalgam restorations were placed. He now has ipsilateral ulcers of the lateral tongue and buccal mucosa. What is your diagnosis?
The diagnosis is factitial injury. Children may inadvertently chew their tongues and buccal mucosae while tissues are numb from local anesthesia, because the tissues feel strange to the child. Children and parents should be advised to be on the look-out for such behavior.

52. Is the mucocele a true cyst?
It depends. The term mucocele refers loosely to a cystlike lesion that contains mucus and usually occurs on the lower lip or floor of the mouth. However, it may occur wherever mucus glands are present. In most cases, it is not a true cyst because it is not lined by epithelium. It is caused by escape of mucus into the connective tissue when an excretory salivary duct is traumatized. Therefore, the mucocele is lined by fibrous and granulation tissue. In a small number of cases, it is caused by distention of the excretory duct due to a distal obstruction. In such a case, the mucocele is a true cyst, because the lining is the epithelium of the duct.

53. What is the etiology of necrotizing sialometaplasia?
This painless ulcer usually develops on the hard palate but may occur wherever salivary glands are present. It represents vascular compromise and subsequent infarction of the salivary gland tissue, with reactive squamous metaplasia of the salivary duct epithelium that may mimic squamous cell carcinoma. The lesion resolves on its own.

54. Name the major denture-related findings in the oral cavity.
    Chronic atrophic candidiasis, especially of the palate (denture sore mouth)
    Papillary hyperplasia of the palatal mucosa
    Fibrous hyperplasia of the sulcus impinged upon by a denture flange
      (epulis fissuratum)
    Traumatic ulcers from overextension of flanges
    Angular cheilitis from overclosure
    Denture-base hypersensitivity reactions

55. A patient is suspected of having an allergy to denture materials. What can you recommend?
The patient should be patch-tested by an allergist or dermatologist to a panel of denture base materials, which includes both metals and products of acrylic polymerization. Usually, the lesions resolve with topical steroids

56. What is a gum boil (parulis)?
A gum boil is an erythematous nodule usually located on the attached gingiva. It may have a yellowish center that drains pus and may be asymptomatic. The nodule consists of granulation tissue and a sinus tract that usually can be traced to the root of the tooth beneath with a thin gutta percha point. It indicates an infection of either pulpal or periodontal origin (see figure, opposite page).

57. What is plasma cell gingivitis?
Plasma cell gingivitis, reported in the 1970s, presented as an intensely erythematous gingivitis and was likely due to an allergic reaction to a component of chewing gum or other topical allergen.

58. Some patients have a reaction to tartar-control toothpaste. What is the offending ingredient?
The offending ingredient is cinnamaldehyde. Susceptible patients develop burning of the mucosa and sometimes bright red gingivitis, akin to plasma cell gingivitis, after using the product. They often also have a reaction to chewing gum that contains cinnamon.

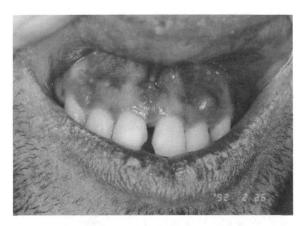

Two parulides. The one on the left is about to drain.

59. What is the differential diagnosis for desquamative gingivitis? What special handling procedures are necessary if you obtain a biopsy?

Desquamative gingivitis, which usually affects middle-aged women, is characterized by red, eroded, and denuded areas of the gingiva. Definitive diagnosis requires immunoreactive studies of the gingiva with various commerically available antibodies directed against autoantibodies, usually with direct immunofluorescence techniques. To preserve the integrity of immune-reactants, the biopsy specimen should be split: one-half should be submitted in formalin for routine histopathology, and the other half in Michel's solution or fresh on ice. The immunofluorescence patterns show that 50% are cicatricial pemphigoid, 25% are lichenoid reactions or lichen planus, 20% have nonspecific immunoreactivity, and 5% are bullous pemphigoid and pemphigus vulgaris. Occasionally, other conditions such as lupus erythematosus, linear IgA disease, and epidermolysis bullosa acquisita may present as desquamative gingivitis.

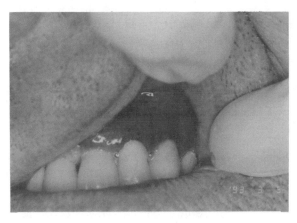

Desquamative gingivitis.

60. What is the Grinspan syndrome?

As reported by Grinspan, this syndrome consists of hypertension, diabetes mellitus, and lichen planus. Current thinking suggests that the lichen planus is caused by medications that the patients take for hypertension (especially hydrochlorothiazides) and diabetes mellitus.

61. What drugs can give a lichen planuslike (lichenoid) mucosal reaction?

A lichenoid mucosal reaction may result from (1) drugs for treating hypertension, such as hydrochlorothiazide, captopril, and methyldopa; (2) hypoglycemic agents such as chlorpropamide, and tolazamide; (3) antiarthritic agents, such as penicillamine; (4) antigout agents, such as allopurinol; and (5) nonsteroidal antiinflammatory drugs.

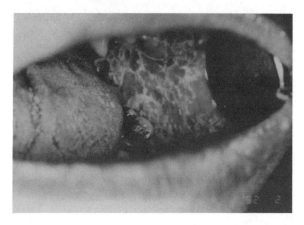

Lichenoid stomatitis associated with hydrochlorothiazide.

62. Name the drugs that can be used to treat symptomatic lichen planus.

Most of the drugs involved are immunomodulating agents. The most commonly used are corticosteroids, applied topically, injected intralesionally, or taken systemically. Dapsone, azathioprine, and cyclosporine A have been used with some success. More recently, retinoids also have been prescribed with limited success.

63. What is galvanism?

Galvanism is the process by which different metals in contact with each other (as in amalgam) set up cells and currents. In susceptible individuals, it may lead to electro-galvanically-induced keratoses and lichenoid lesions of the mucosa in contact with amalgam restorations.

64. What are the typical skin lesions of erythema multiforme called?

The typical skin lesions are called target, iris, or bull's-eye lesions. Erythema multiforme is an acute mucocutaneous inflammatory process that may recur periodically. It may be idiopathic but also may occur after ingestion of drugs or after a herpes simplex virus infection.

65. Name the common factors responsible for recurrent erythema multiforme.

The most common factors are herpes simplex virus reactivation and hypersensitivity to certain foods, such as benzoates. Do not expect to be able to culture herpes simplex virus from the lesions of recurrent erythema multiforme, which is a hypersensitivity reaction to some component of the virus. Usually the viral infection precedes the lesions of erythema multiforme.

66. What is Stevens-Johnson syndrome?

Stevens-Johnson syndrome is a severe form of erythema multiforme with extensive involvement of the mucous membranes of the oral cavity, eyes, genitalia, and occasionally the upper gastrointestinal and respiratory tracts. Desquamation and ulceration of the lips, with crusting, is usually dramatic. Typical target lesions may be seen on the skin.

67. What is the difference between pemphigus and pemphigoid?

Both are autoimmune, vesiculobullous diseases. In pemphigus (usually vulgaris), autoantibodies attack desmosomal plaques of the epithelial cells, leading to acantholysis and formation of an intraepithelial bulla. In pemphigoid (usually cicatricial), autoantibodies attack the junction between the epithelium and connective tissue, leading to the formation of a subepithelial bulla.

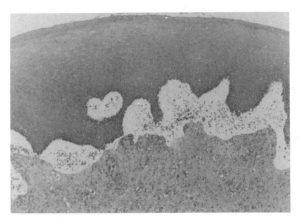

Subepithelial bulla formation in cicatricial pemphigoid.

68. What two forms of pemphigoid involve the oral cavity?

Cicatricial pemphigoid (formerly known as mucous membrane pemphigoid) and bullous pemphigoid involve the oral cavity. These autoimmune, vesiculobullous diseases have antigens located in the lamina lucida of the basement membrane. Cicatricial pemphigoid presents primarily with oral mucosal and ocular lesions and occasionally with skin lesions, whereas bullous pemphigoid presents primarily with skin lesions and occasionally with mucosal lesions.

69. Differentiate between a Tzanck test and a Tzanck cell.

The **Tzanck test** entails direct examination of cells to diagnose a herpes simplex virus infection. The test is done by scraping the lesion (which may be a vesicle, ulcer, or crust) and smearing the debris on a slide. The slide is then stained and examined under a microscope for virally infected cells, which show multinucleation and "ground-glass" nuclei. **Tzanck cells** are acantholytic cells seen within the bulla of lesions of pemphigus vulgaris.

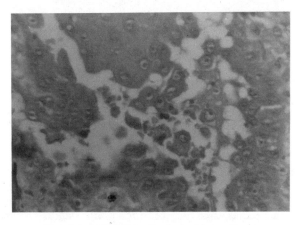

Tzanck (acantholytic) cells of pemphigus vulgaris.

70. What is the difference between systemic lupus erythematosus (SLE) and discoid lupus erythematosus (DLE)?
SLE is the prototypical multisystem, autoimmune disease characterized by circulating antinuclear antibodies; the principal sites of injury are skin, joints, and kidneys. The oral mucosa also is often involved, and the lesions may appear lichenoid, with white striae, and atrophic or erythematous. DLE is the limited form of the disease; most manifestations are localized to the skin and mucous membranes with no systemic involvement. DLE does not usually progress to SLE, although certain phases of SLE are clinically indistinguishable from DLE. The oral findings are similar in both.

71. What is the midline lethal granuloma?
This term is used to describe a destructive, ulcerative process, usually located in the midline of the hard palate, which may lead to palatal perforation. Although the clinical picture is dramatic and ominous, the histologic picture may be somewhat nonspecific, showing only inflammation and occasionally vasculitis. Some authorities believe that midline lethal granuloma may be a localized form of an inflammatory condition known as Wegener's granulomatosis. Other conditions that may present in a similar fashion include fungal infections, syphilitic gummas, and malignant neoplasms such as lymphomas.

CHEMOTHERAPY AND HIV DISEASE

72. What are the common oral manifestations of patients who have undergone chemotherapy?
Chemotherapy can produce direct stomatotoxicity by acting on mitotically active cells in the basal cell layer of the epithelium. The mucosa becomes atrophic and, when traumatized, ulcerates. The chemotherapeutic agents also act on other rapidly dividing cells in the body, such as hematopoietic tissues. The results are neutropenia, anemia, and thrombocytopenia. Neutropenia may have an indirect stomatotoxic effect by allowing oral bacteria to colonize the ulcers. Usually, these ulcers develop in the period of profound neutropenia and resolve when neutrophils reappear in the blood circulation. In addition, patients are at increased risk for developing oral candidiasis, oral herpetic lesions, and deep fungal infections. Thrombocytopenia may cause oral petechiae, ecchymoses, and hematomas, especially at sites of trauma.

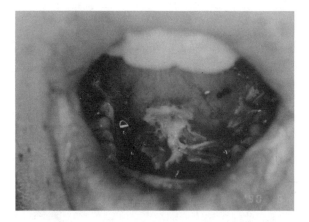

Chemotherapy-associated oral ulcerative mucositis.

73. A patient who underwent cancer chemotherapy now has recurrent intraoral herpetic lesions but no history of cold sores or fever blisters. Is this likely?
Yes. Many people have been exposed to herpes simplex virus without their knowledge and are completely asymptomatic. The virus becomes latent within sensory ganglia and reactivates to

give rise to recurrent or recrudescent herpetic lesions. The prevalence of individuals who have been exposed to HSV increases with age.

74. What are the complications of leukemia in the oral cavity, aside from those associated with chemotherapy?
Leukemic infiltration of the bone marrow leads to reduced production of functional components of the marrow. Granulocytopenia results in more frequent and more aggressive odontogenic infections; thrombocytopenia results in petechiae, ecchymoses, and hematomas in the oral cavity, which is subject to trauma from functional activities. The patient may have a more than adequate white cell count, but many of these white cells are malignant and do not necessarily function like normal white cells. In addition, some leukemias, especially acute monocytic leukemia, have a propensity to infiltrate the gingiva, causing localized or diffuse gingival enlargement.

75. A patient underwent a matched allogenic bone marrow transplantation for the treatment of leukemia. Three months later he has erosive and lichenoid lesions in his mouth. What is your diagnosis?
The likely diagnosis is chronic oral graft-versus-host disease. The allogenic bone marrow transplant or graft contains immunocompetent cells that recognize the host cells as foreign and attacks them. The oral lesions of chronic graft-versus-host disease resemble the lesions of lichen planus.

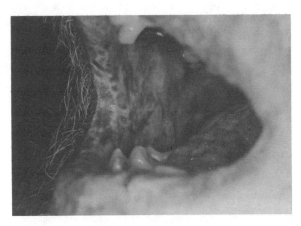

Chronic oral graft-versus-host disease of buccal mucosa.

76. What are the effects of radiation on the oral cavity?
Short-term: oral erythema and ulcers, candidiasis, dysgeusia, parotitis, acute sialadenitis
Long-term: xerostomia, dental caries, osteoradionecrosis, epithelial atrophy and fibrosis

77. What factors predispose to osteoradionecrosis?
This necrotic process affects bone that has been in the radiation field. Predisposing factors include high total dose of radiation (especially if >6,500 cGys), presence of odontogenic infection (such as periapical pathosis and periodontal disease), trauma (such as extractions), and site (the mandible is less vascular and more susceptible than the maxilla).

78. What is the basic cause of osteoradionecrosis?
The breakdown of hypocellular, hypovascular, and hypoxic tissue readily results in a chronic, nonhealing ulcer that can be secondarily infected. Some reports show that the infection is for the most part superficial.

79. What are the common oral manifestations of HIV infection?

Soft tissue: candidiasis, recurrent herpetic infections, deep fungal infections, aphthous ulcers, hairy leukoplakia

Periodontium: nonspecific gingivitis, acute necrotizing ulcerative gingivitis, severe and rapidly destructive periodontal disease, often with unusual pathogens

Tumors: Kaposi's sarcoma, B-cell lymphoma, squamous cell carcinoma

80. A patient who has tested positive for HIV antibodies presents with a CD4 count of 150 but has never had an opportunistic infection or been symptomatic. Does he have AIDS?

Yes. By the new CDC definition (February 1993), patients with CD4 counts below 200 are considered to have AIDS.

81. Like other leukoplakias, hairy leukoplakia has a tendency to progress to malignancy. True or false?

False. Hairy leukoplakia is associated with EBV infection and usually a superimposed hyperplastic candidiasis. HPV has also been associated with hairy leukoplakia, which is not a premalignant condition. However, patients infected with HIV are more susceptible to oral cancer in general.

82. Are HIV-associated aphthous ulcers similar to recurrent major aphthae?

Yes. They tend to be greater than 1 cm, persist for long periods of time (weeks to months), and are difficult to treat.

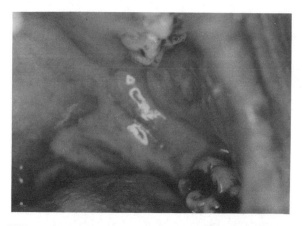

HIV-associated aphthous ulcers of the soft palate and oropharynx.

83. Should HIV-associated aphthous ulcers be routinely cultured?

Yes. Very often the culture is positive for HSV or even CMV, and the patient needs to be treated appropriately.

84. Kaposi's sarcoma (KS) is seen equally in the different population risk groups. True or false?

False. Over 90% of the epidemic cases of KS are diagnosed in homosexual or bisexual men. KS is an AIDS-defining lesion that is seen much less frequently in the other risk groups (see figure, opposite page).

85. Other than infection control and diagnosis of oral lesions, what other management issues should you keep in mind when treating patients with AIDS?

Hematologic dysfunction is common. HIV infection is associated with autoimmune thrombocytopenic purpura, granulocytopenia, and anemia. In addition, antiretroviral agents such as zidovudine are myelosuppressive, as are drugs used as prophylaxis against *Pneumocystis carinii* pneumonia, such as trimethoprim-sulfamethoxazole. The patient's blood picture should be known before treatment, especially surgical procedures, begins.

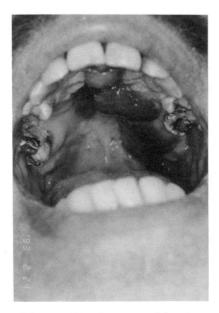

HIV-related Kaposi's sarcoma of the palate.

86. How do you treat intraoral Kaposi's sarcoma?
Treatment consists of surgical excision, intralesional injections of vinca alkaloids, radiation, and possibly interferon.

BENIGN NEOPLAMS AND TUMORS

Odontogenic Tumors

87. Name the benign odontogenic tumors that are purely epithelial.
Ameloblastoma
Calcifying epithelial odontogenic tumor (Pindborg tumor)
Adenomatoid odontogenic tumor
Solid variant of the calcifying odontogenic cyst
Squamous odontogenic tumor
Clear-cell odontogenic tumor (rare)

88. Which odontogenic tumor is associated with amyloid production? with ghost cells?
Calcifying epithelial odontogenic tumor (Pindborg tumor) is associated with amyloid production; calcifying epithelial odontogenic cyst (Gorlin cyst) is associated with ghost cells.

89. Which two lesions, one in the long bones and one in the cranium, resemble the ameloblastoma?
In the long bones, adamantinoma resembles ameloblastoma; in the cranium, craniopharyngioma does.

90. Do all forms of ameloblastoma behave aggressively and tend to recur?
No. A form of ameloblastoma that occurs in teenagers and young adults behaves less aggressively and has a lower tendency to recur. It is called the unicystic ameloblastoma.

91. Because the ameloblastoma is so aggressive, it can be considered a malignancy. True or false?
False. The ameloblastoma is a locally destructive lesion that has no tendency to metastasize. However, it has two malignant counterparts: ameloblastic carcinoma and malignant ameloblastoma.

92. To which teeth are cementoblastomas usually attached?
Cementoblastomas usually are attached to the mandibular permanent molars.

93. Name two odontogenic tumors that produce primarily mesenchymal tissues.
Odontogenic fibroma and odontogenic myxoma produce primarily mesenchymal tissues.

94. A teenager presents with a mandibular radiolucency with areas that histologically resemble ameloblastoma as well as dental papilla. What is your diagnosis?
The diagnosis is ameloblastic fibroma, one of the rare odontogenic tumors that has both a neoplastic epithelial and mesenchymal component.

Fibro-osseous Tumors

95. Ossifying fibromas arise from bone cells, and cementifying fibromas are odontogenic in origin. True or false?
In real life and real pathology, the line of demarcation between the two is not so clear. They are clinically indistinguishable. Histologically, although pure ossifying and pure cementifying fibromas exist, it is much more common to see a mixture of bone/osteoid and cementum in any given lesion, with either predominating or in equal proportions. Many pathologists use the term cemento-ossifying fibroma as a unifying concept. The cell of origin is likely to be a mesenchymal cell in the periodontal ligament that is capable of producing either bone or cementum, therefore duplicating the two anchoring sites for Sharpey's fibers.
From that point of view, both are odontogenic in origin.

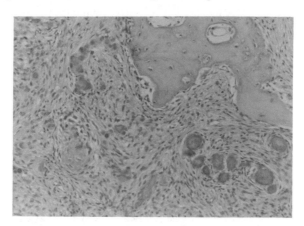

Central cemento-ossifying fibroma with round globules of cementum and trabeculae of osteoid.

96. Is it possible to distinguish histologically fibrous dysplasia and central ossifying fibroma?
No. The clinical and radiographic findings are the most important for differentiating between the two. Fibrous dysplasia tends to occur in the maxilla of young people and presents as a poorly defined radiolucent or radiopaque area that is nonencapsulated. The radiographic appearance has been described as "ground glass." The central ossifying fibroma is a well-demarcated radiolucency, often with a distinct border, and may contain areas of radiopacity within the lesion. It is more common in the mandible.

Soft-Tissue Tumors

97. Is fibroma of the oral cavity a true neoplasm?
It depends on your definition of neoplasm. As the name (-oma) suggests, fibroma of the oral cavity is a tumor composed of fibrous tissue. It tends to occur as a result of trauma and therefore usually presents on the buccal mucosa, lower labial mucosa, and lateral tongue. It is nonencapsulated and grows as long as the inciting factor, such as trauma, is present. By Willis's definition of neoplasm ("new growth"), the growth, once established, continues in an excessive manner even after cessation of the stimuli that first evoked the change. Some pathologists therefore prefer the term fibrous hyperplasia to fibroma because it more accurately reflects the nature of the lesion. The pathogenesis is similar to that of fibrous hyperplasias caused by poorly fitting dentures.

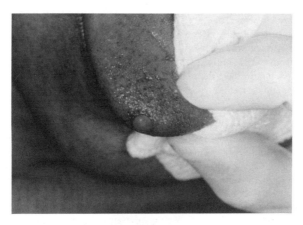

Fibroma of tongue.

98. What are Verocay bodies?
Verocay bodies are amorphous-looking, eosinophilic material that forms between parallel groups of nuclei in the schwannoma. They actually represent duplicated basement membrane produced by Schwann cells and are an important component of Antoni A tissue.

99. What is the cell of origin of the granular cell tumor? How is it different from the cell of origin of the congenital epulis of the newborn?
The cell of origin of the granular cell tumor is probably a neural cell, such as the Schwann cell. This tumor used to be called the granular cell myoblastoma because it was believed that the cell of origin was a myocyte. The cell appears granular because it contains many lysosomes. By light microscopy, the cells resemble cells of the congenital epulis of the newborn. Whereas the granular cell tumor stains for S-100 protein—a marker for neural tissues, among others—the congenital epulis does not.

100. A patient presents with multiple neuromas of the lips and tongue. What do you suspect?
The patient probably has multiple endocrine neoplasia type III, which is inherited as an autosomal dominant defect. Such patients also have pheochromocytomas, cafe-au-lait macules, neurofibromas of the skin, and medullary carcinoma of the thyroid. Recognition of the oral findings may lead to early diagnosis of the thyroid carcinoma.

101. What are venous lakes?
Venous lakes are purplish-blue nodules or papules, often present on the lips of older individuals, that represent dilated venules or varices.

102. What is the most common benign salivary gland tumor?
The most common benign salivary gland tumor is pleomorphic adenoma.

103. Why is pleomorphic adenoma sometimes called the benign "mixed tumor"?
Pleomorphic adenoma is called a "mixed tumor" because histologically it may have a mixture of both epithelial- and connective-tissue components. In fact pleomorphic adenoma is an epithelially derived tumor. The connective-tissue components may be prominent because one of the cells responsible for the tumor is the myoepithelial cell, which, as its name suggests, has properties of both epithelial and connective tissue. This cell is responsible for the areas of cartilage and bone formation as well as for the myxoid nature of many "mixed tumors." In addition, there are areas of epithelial-cell proliferation in the form of ducts, islands, and sheets of cells.

104. What is the brown tumor?
The brown tumor is histologically a central giant-cell granuloma associated with hyperparathyroidism. It appears brown when excised because it is a highly vascular lesion. Because it is indistinguishable from banal central giant-cell granuloma, all patients diagnosed with central giant-cell granuloma should have their calcium levels checked.

MALIGNANT NEOPLASMS

105. What percentage of the population has leukoplakia? What percentage of leukoplakias have dysplasia or carcinoma when first biopsied, compared with erythroplakias?
Leukoplakia occurs in 3–4% of the population. About 15–20% of leukoplakias have dysplasia or carcinoma at the time of biopsy, whereas 90% of erythroplakias show such changes at the time of biopsy.

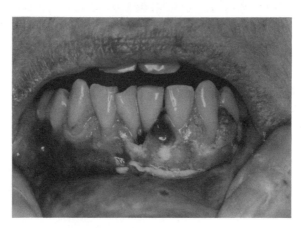

Squamous cell carcinoma presenting as leukoplakia with erythematous and verrucous areas.

106. What is proliferative verrucous leukoplakia?
Proliferative verrucous leukoplakia is a clinically aggressive and progressive form of leukoplakia with a higher rate of malignant transformation than banal leukoplakia.

107. What is the prevalence of oral cancer in the United States? Which country in the world has the highest prevalence of oral cancer?
Oral cancer comprises 3–5% of all cancers in the United States if one includes oropharyngeal lesions. India has the highest prevalence of oral cancer, which is the most common cancer in that country and is related to the use of betel nut and tobacco products.

108. What are the risk factors for oral cancer?
Tobacco products
Alcohol (especially in conjunction with smoking)
Betel nut products (especially in East Indians and some South East Asian cultures)
Sunlight (especially for cancer of the lip in men)
History of syphilitic glossitis
History of submucous fibrosis
Immunosuppression
History of oral cancer or other cancer
Preexisting oral mucosal dysplasia
Low levels of vitamin A (controversial)

109. What do snuff-associated lesions look like?
At the site where the snuff is placed (usually the sulcus), the mucosa is whitened with a translucent hue, and linear white ridges run parallel to the sulcus.

110. What is the difference in prognosis between a squamous cell carcinoma and a verrucous carcinoma?
Approximately one-half of squamous cell carcinomas have metastasized at the time of diagnosis. The larger they are, the more likely that metastases will develop. Verrucous carcinomas do not tend to metastasize despite the rather large size of some lesions. They are locally aggressive lesions. Whereas many squamous cell carcinomas are radiosensitive, verrucous carcinomas have been reported to become extremely aggressive and histologically anaplastic when treated with radiation.

111. What is a "rodent ulcer"?
A rodent ulcer refers to a basal cell carcinoma that, despite its insignificant rate of metastasis, erodes adjacent tissues like the gnawing of a rodent and through persistence may cause destruction of the facial complex.

112. What are the three most common intraoral malignant salivary gland tumors?
Mucoepidermoid carcinoma, polymorphous low-grade adenocarcinoma, and adenoid cystic carcinoma are the three most common types. The polymorphous low-grade adenocarcinoma also has been reported under the names of terminal duct carcinoma and lobular carcinoma.

113. Which two salivary gland tumors often show perinuclear invasion (neurotropism)?
Adenoid cystic carcinoma and polymorphous low-grade adenocarcinoma often show perinuclear invasion. However, any malignancy (particularly carcinomas) can show perinuclear invasion that may represent invasion of the lymphatics around a nerve.

114. The benign lymphoepithelial lesion of Sjögren's syndrome is an innocuous autoimmune sialadenitis. True or false?
False. The "benign" lymphoepithelial lesion is not so benign. Many experts feel that these lesions are premalignant. Affected patients have a higher incidence of lymphoma than the general population.

115. A patient with Sjögren's syndrome is referred for a labial salivary gland biopsy to identify a benign lymphoepithelial lesion. Does this sound right?
No. The benign lymphoepithelial lesion of Sjögren's syndrome is found in the major glands, mainly the parotid, especially if parotid enlargement is present. A labial salivary gland biopsy will show an autoimmune sialadenitis characterized by lymphocytic infiltrates that form foci. The more foci, the more likely the diagnosis of an autoimmune sialadenitis, which is much less specific than the lymphoepithelial lesion.

116. Do lymphomas of the oral cavity occur outside Waldeyer's ring?

Yes. Oral lymphomas are most common in Waldeyer's ring, but they can occur in the palate (a condition formerly described as lymphoproliferative disease of the palate), buccal mucosa, tongue, floor of the mouth, and retromolar areas. They are not infrequently primary in the jaw bones.

117. What does a monoclonal plasma cell proliferation mean?

Plasma cells produce immunoglobulin that contains heavy and light chains. Each plasma cell and its progeny produces either kappa or lambda light chains. A group of plasma cells that produces only kappa or lambda light chains but not both is most likely due to a proliferation of a single malignant clone of plasma cells, such as a plasmacytoma or multiple myeloma. The presence of both light chains in a plasma cell proliferation is more in keeping with a polyclonal proliferation, which characterizes inflammatory lesions.

118. Name the different epidemiologic forms of Kaposi's sarcoma.

1. Classic or European form: usually Eastern European men (often Jewish); multiple red papules on the lower extremities, with rare visceral involvement and a more indolent course.

2. Endemic or African form: young men or children in equatorial Africa; frequent visceral involvement that can be fulminant.

3. Epidemic form: HIV-associated; may be widely disseminated to mucocutaneous and visceral sites; variable course.

4. Renal transplant-associated: patients who have undergone renal transplantation with immunosuppressive therapy; lesions usually regress when immunosuppressive therapy is discontinued.

119. A patient has a suspected metastatic tumor to the mandible. What are the likely primary tumors?

Lung	Kidney
Breast	Thyroid
Prostate	Skin
Gastointestinal tract	

120. Osteosarcoma of the jaws occurs in younger patients than osteosarcoma of the long bones. True or false?

False. Patients with osteosarcoma of the jaws are 1–2 decades older than patients with osteosarcoma of the long bones.

121. What conditions predispose to osteosarcoma?

Many cases of osteosarcoma in young adults occur de novo. However, there are well-documented cases of osteosarcoma arising in association with Paget's disease, chronic osteomyelitis, a history of retinoblastoma, and prior radiation to the bone for fibrous dysplasia.

NONVASCULAR PIGMENTED LESIONS

122. What drugs can cause mucosal pigmentation?

Oral contraceptives	Minocycline
Antimalarials agents (e.g., plaquenil)	Zidovudine (possible)

123. Why does heavy metal poisoning cause primary staining of the gingiva?

Heavy metals such as lead, bismuth, and silver can cause a grayish black line to appear on the gingival margins, especially in patients with poor oral hygiene. Plaque bacteria can produce hydrogen sulfide, which combines with the heavy metals to form heavy metal sulfides that are usually black.

124. What can cause mucosal melanosis?
Benign: physiologic pigmentation, postinflammatory hyperpigmentation (especially in dark-skinned individuals), oral melanotic macule, smoking, mucosal nevus
Malignant: melanoma
Systemic conditions: Peutz-Jegher's syndrome, Albright's syndrome, Addison's disease, neurofibromatosis

125. What are the different forms of oral melanocytic nevi?
Intramucosal nevus: tends to be elevated, papular or nodular
Junctional nevus: tends to be macular
Compound nevus: tends to be papular
Blue nevus: tends to be macular

126. What is the most common site for oral melanoma?
The most common site for oral melanoma is the hard palate.

127. What is the difference between a melanocyte and a melanophage?
A melanocyte is a neuroectodermally-derived dendritic cell that contains the intracellular apparatus to manufacture melanin. A melanophage is a macrophage that has phagocytosed melanin pigment and therefore can look like a melanocyte because it contains melanin. In fact, however, it lacks the enzymes to produce melanin.

METABOLIC LESIONS ASSOCIATED WITH SYSTEMIC DISEASE

128. What are the three presentations of Langerhans cell disease or histiocytosis (histiocytosis X)?
Chronic localized: eosinophilic granuloma; usually in adults.
Chronic disseminated: limited to a few organ systems in adults; Hand-Schuller-Christian disease is a well-recognized form, characterized by exophthalmos; diabetes insipidus and bony lesions; as well as skin and visceral involvement.
Acute disseminated: Letterer-Siwe disease in children; widespread involvement of multiple organ systems, especially skin; usually runs a rapidly progressive, often fatal course; considered a malignancy for the most part.

129. What are Birbeck granules?
Birbeck granules are racket-shaped cytoplasmic inclusions seen in Langerhans cells of histiocytosis X.

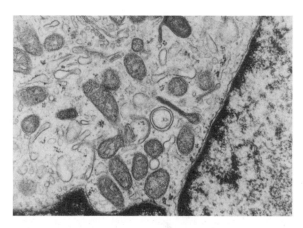

Racket-shaped Birbeck granule of Langerhans cell histiocytosis.

130. What are the oral changes associated with pregnancy?
Oral changes associated with pregnancy include gingivitis and pyogenic granuloma (epulis gravidarum).

131. An elderly man complains that his jaw seems to be getting too big for his dentures and that his hat does not fit him anymore. What do you suspect?
The likely diagnosis is Paget's disease (osteitis deformans), a metabolic bone disease in which initial bone resorption is followed by haphazard bone repair, with resulting marked sclerosis. This condition may lead to narrowing of skull base foramina and neurologic deficits. The maxilla is often affected; a cotton-wool appearance has been described on radiographs.

132. What oral lesions are associated with gastrointestinal disease?
The most common gastrointestinal disease associated with oral signs is inflammatory bowel disease, especially Crohn's disease. Patients may manifest with cobblestoning of the mucosa and papulous growths, which represent granulomatous inflammation similar to what is seen in the gastrointestinal tract. Occasionally, patients also develop a pyostomatitis vegetans. In addition, they may also have aphthouslike ulcers as well as symptoms of glossitis associated with B12 deficiency if part of the ileum has been resected for the disease. Patients with gluten-sensitive enteropathies may also present with aphthouslike ulcers.

133. What is primary and secondary Sjögren's syndrome?
Primary Sjögren's syndrome, which used to be called the sicca syndrome, consists of dry eyes (keratoconjunctivitis sicca) and dry mouth (xerostomia) in the absence of other systemic conditions. Secondary Sjögren's syndrome consists of primary Sjögren's syndrome plus a connective-tissue disorder such as rheumatoid arthritis, systemic lupus erythematosus, progressive systemic sclerosis, or polymyositis. Most patients with Sjögren's syndrome have circulating autoantibodies.

134. What is the dental significance of the Sturge-Weber syndrome?
The Sturge-Weber syndrome is characterized by vascular malformations of the leptomeninges, facial skin innervated by the fifth nerve (nevus flammeus), and the corresponding ipsilateral areas in the oral mucosa and bone. Bleeding is therefore an important consideration in dental treatment. Patients also may exhibit mental retardation and seizure disorders. Treatment may include dilantin.

DIFFERENTIAL DIAGNOSES AND GENERAL CONSIDERATIONS

Intrabony Lesions

135. What are pseudocysts of the jaw bones? Give examples.
These conditions appear cystlike on radiograph but are not true cysts at all. Examples include:

Traumatic (simple) bone cyst:	empty at surgery
Aneurysmal bone cyst:	giant cells and blood-filled spaces
Static bone cyst (Stafne bone cavity):	salivary gland depression
Hematopoietic marrow defect:	hematopoietic marrow

136. What is the differential diagnosis for a multiloculated radiolucency?
Dentigerous cyst
Odontogenic keratocyst
Ameloblastoma
Vascular malformations, such as hemangiomas
Odontogenic myxoma
Intraosseous salivary gland tumors
Lesions that contain giant cells, such as aneurysmal bone cyst, central giant cell granuloma, and cherubism

Soft-Tissue

137. What is the differential diagnosis for an upper lip nodule?
Salivary gland lesion: sialolith, benign salivary gland tumor (especially pleomorphic adenoma and canalicular adenoma), malignant salivary gland tumor
Vascular lesion: hemangioma, lymphangioma, other vascular anomaly
Neural lesion: neurofibroma, schwannoma, neuroma
Skin appendage tumors

138. What can cause diffuse swelling of the lips?
Vascular malformations, such as lymphangiomas and hemangiomas
Angioneurotic edema
Hypersensitivity reactions
Cheilitis glandularis
Cheilitis granulomatosa (e.g., Melkersson-Rosenthal syndrome)
Crohn's disease

139. What is the differential diagnosis for a solitary gingival nodule?
The most common diagnoses are fibroma or fibrous hyperplasia, pyogenic granuloma (especially in pregnant patient), peripheral giant-cell granuloma, and peripheral ossifying fibroma (essentially a fibrous hyperplasia with metaplastic bone formation). Other less common conditions include benign and malignant tumors, especially of odontogenic origin, and (in elderly patients) metastatic tumors.

140. What can cause generalized overgrowth of gingival tissues?
Common causes include plaque accumulation; drugs such as phenytoin, cyclosporine A, sodium valproate, diltiazem, and nifedipine (the last two are calcium channel blockers); fibromatosis gingivae; and leukemic infiltrate.

141. A labial salivary gland biopsy is useful for diagnosis of certain systemic conditions. What are they?
Sjögren's syndrome
Autoimmune sialadenitis associated with connective-tissue disease
Graft-versus-host disease
Amyloidosis
Sarcoidosis

142. What can cause chronic xerostomia?
Common causes include many anticholinergic drugs, autoimmune sialadenitis (such as Sjögren's syndrome and graft-versus-host disease), aging (although many experts believe this to be drug-related), depression, chronic illness, radiation to the gland, primary neurologic dysfunction, and nutritional deficiencies (e.g., vitamin A, vitamin B, and iron).

143. Name possible causes of bilateral parotid swelling.
Mumps	Malnutrition
Sjögren's syndrome	Alcoholism
Radiation-induced acute parotitis	Bulimia
Diabetes mellitus	Warthin's tumor

144. What may cause depapillation of the tongue?
Vitamin B deficiency	Median rhomboid glossitis (focally)
Iron deficiency	Syphilis
Folate deficiency	Plummer-Vinson syndrome
Benign migratory glossitis (focally)	

145. What may cause diffuse enlargement of the tongue?

Congenital macroglossia	Cretinism
Lymphangioma	Acromegaly
Hemangioma	Trisomy 21
Neurofibromatosis	Amyloidosis
Hyperpituitarism	Hypothyroidism

146. What is the differential diagnosis of midline swellings of the floor of the mouth?

Ranula (mucocele)	Dermoid cyst
Epidermoid cyst	Benign lymphoepithelial cyst

147. What may cause diffuse white plaques in the oral cavity?

Lichen planus (especially plaquetype)	Pachyonychia congenita
Cannon's white sponge nevus	Dyskeratosis congenita
Leukedema	Extensive leukoplakia (especially proliferative
Hereditary benign intraepithelial	verrucous leukoplakia)
dyskeratosis	Candidiasis

148. Name the conditions that may give rise to papillary lesions of the oral cavity.

Possible underlying conditions include papilloma, verruca vulgaris, condyloma, papillary hyperplasia of the palatal mucosa (denture injury), Heck's disease, oral florid papillomatosis, verrucous carcinoma, papillary squamous cell carcinoma, pyostomatitis vegetans (associated with inflammatory bowel disease), and verruciform xanthoma.

149. What lesions may occur in the oral cavity of neonates?

Lesions in the oral cavity of neonates include neuroectodermal tumor of infancy, congenital epulis of the newborn, gingival cyst of the newborn (if located on the alveolar ridge, they are known as Bohn's nodules; if located on the midline of the palate, they are known as Epstein's pearls), lymphangiomas of the alveolar ridge, and natal teeth.

150. What may cause "burning mouth" syndrome?

This sensation usually results from mucosa that is atrophic or inflamed, which, in turn, may be caused by candidiasis (especially atrophic candidiasis of the tongue or of the palate caused by dentures), xerostomia, allergies (especially to denture materials), and specific inflammatory mucosal lesions, such as lichen planus and migratory glossitis. Sometimes a psychological component may be involved.

151. What may cause oral paresthesia?

Oral paresthesia may be caused by manipulation or inflammation of a nerve or tissues around a nerve, direct damage to a nerve or tissues around a nerve, tumor impinging on or invading a nerve, primary neural tumor, and central nervous system tumor.

152. Why do lesions appear white in the oral cavity?

Lesions appear white because the epithelium has been changed, usually thickened, causing the underlying blood vessels to be deeper, as in hyperkeratosis, epithelial hyperplasia (acanthosis), and swelling of the epithelial cells (Cannon's nevus, leukedema). Lesions may appear white if exudate or necrosis is present in the epithelium (candidiasis, ulcers) or if there are fewer vessels in the connective tissue (scar). Finally, a change in the intrinsic nature of the epithelial cell, such as epithelial dysplasia, may cause the mucosa to appear white (leukoplakia).

153. Why do lesions appear red in the oral cavity?

Lesions appear red because the epithelium is thinned and the underlying vessels are now closer to the surface, as in epithelial atrophy, desquamative conditions, healing ulcers, and loss of the keratin layer. Redness also may be caused by an increase in the number or dilatation of blood vessels in the connective tissue, as in inflammation. Finally, a change in the intrinsic nature of the epithelial cell, such as epithelial dysplasia, may cause the mucosa to look red (erythroplakia).

154. Distinguish macules, papules, and plaque.
A macule is a localized lesion that is not raised and is better seen than felt. It is often used to describe localized pigmented lesions, such as amalgam tattoos and melanotic macules. Both papules and plaque are raised lesions; the papule is <5 mm, and the plaque is larger.

155. What is the difference between a bulla and vesicle?
The bulla is usually >5 mm in size; the vesicle is <5 mm.

156. Differentiate between a hamartoma and a choristoma.
A hamartoma is a tumorlike growth consisting of an overgrowth of tissues that histologically appear mature and are native to the area (e.g., hemangioma, odontoma). A choristoma is a tumorlike growth consisting of an overgrowth of tissues that histologically appear mature but are not native to the area (e.g., cartilaginous choristoma or bony choristoma of the tongue). A hamartoma of the skin and mucosa is sometimes called a nevus (e.g., vascular, epidermal, or melanocytic nevus).

157. What are oncocytes?
Oncocytes are eosinophilic, swollen cells found in many salivary gland tumors, such as oncocytomas and Warthin's tumor, and in oncocytic metaplasia of salivary ducts. They are swollen because they contain many mitochondria.

158. What are Russell bodies?
Russell bodies are round, eosinophilic bodies found in reactive lesions and represent globules of immunoglobulin within plasma cells.

BIBLIOGRAPHY

Developmental Conditions
 1. Christ TF: The globulomaxillary cyst: An embryologic misconception. Oral Surg 30:515, 1970.
 2. Cohen DA, et al: The lateral periodontal cyst. J Periodontol 55:230, 1984.
 3. Waldron CA: Fibro-osseous lesions of the jaws. J Oral Maxillofac Surg 43:249, 1985.
 4. Wright JM: The odontogenic keratocyst: Orthokeratinized variant. Oral Surg 51:609, 1981.

Infections
 5. Dismukes WE: Azole antifungal drugs: Old and new. Ann Intern Med 109:177, 1988.
 6. Lehner T: Oral candidosis. Dent Pract Dent Res 17:209, 1967.
 7. Scully C, et al: Papillomaviruses: The current status in relation to oral disease. Oral Surg Oral Med Oral Pathol 65:526, 1988.
 8. Weathers DR, Griffin JW: Intraoral ulcerations of recurrent herpes simplex and recurrent aphthae: Two distinct clinical entities. J Am Dent Assoc 81:81, 1970.

Reactive, Hypersensitivity, and Autoimmune Conditions
 9. Bean SF, Quezada RK: Recurrent oral erythema multiforme. Clinical experience with 11 patients. JAMA 249:2810, 1983.
10. Kerr DA, McClatchey KD, Regezi JA: Idiopathic gingivostomatitis. Oral Surg Oral Med Oral Pathol 32:402, 1971.
11. Nisengard RJ, Rogers RS III: The treatment of desquamative gingival lesions. J Periodontol 58:167, 1987.
12. Rennie JS: Recurrent aphthous stomatitis. Br Dent J 159:361, 1985.
13. Schiodt M, Halberg P, Hentzer B. A clinical study of 32 patients with oral discoid lupus erythematosus. Int J Oral Surg 7:85, 1978.
14. Silverman S, Lozada-nur F: A prospective follow-up study of 570 patients with oral lichen planus: Persistence, remission, and malignant association. Oral Surg Oral Med Oral Pathol 60:30, 1985.

Chemotherapy and HIV Disease

15. Greenberg MS, et al: Oral herpes simplex infections in patients with leukemia. J Am Dent Assoc 1145:483, 1987.
16. Libman H, Witzburg RA (eds): HIV Infection: A Clinical Manual. Boston, Little, Brown, 1993.
17. Marks RE, Johnson RP: Studies in the radiobiology of osteoradionecrosis and their clinical significance. Oral Surg Oral Med Oral Pathol 64:379, 1987.
18. Peterson DE, Elias EG, Sonis ST (eds): Head and Neck Management of the Cancer Patient. Boston, Martinus Nijhoff, 1986, p 351.
19. Schubert MM, et al: Oral manifestations of chronic graft-v.-host disease. Ann Intern Med 144:1591, 1984.

Benign Neoplasms and Tumors

20. Ellis GL, Auclair PL, Gnepp DR: Surgical Pathology of the Salivary Glands. Philadelphia, W.B. Saunders, 1991.
21. Eversole LR, Leider AS, Nelson K: Ossifying fibroma: A clinicopathologic study of 64 cases. Oral Surg Oral Med Oral Pathol 60:505–511, 1985.
22. Hansen LS, Eversole LR, Green TL, Powell NB: Clear cell odontogenic tumor—A new histologic variant with aggressive potential. Head Neck Surg 8:115, 1985.
23. Robinson L, Martinez MG: Unicystic ameloblastoma: A prognostically distinct entity. Cancer 40:2278, 1977.

Malignant Neoplasms

24. Batsakis JG: The pathology of head and neck tumors: The lymphoepithelial lesion and Sjögren's syndrome. Head Neck Surg 5:150, 1982.
25. Batsakis JG, et al: The pathology of head and neck tumors: Verrucous carcinoma. Head Neck Surg 5:29, 1982.
26. Freedman PD, Lumerman H: Lobular carcinoma of intraoral minor salivary glands. Oral Surg Oral Med Oral Pathol 56:157, 1983.
27. Hansen L, Olson J, Silverman S: Proliferative verrucous leukoplakia. Oral Surg Oral Med Oral Pathol 60:285, 1985.
28. Waldron CA, Shafer WG: Leukoplakia revisited. Cancer 36:1386, 1975.

Nonvascular Pigmented Lesions

29. Argenyi ZB, et al: Minocycline-related cutaneous hyperpigmentation as demonstrated by light microscopy, electron microscopy, and x-ray energy spectroscopy. J Cutan Pathol 14:176, 1987.
30. Buchner A, Hansen L: Pigmented nevi of the oral mucosa. Oral Surg Oral Med Oral Pathol 63:566, 1987.

Metabolic Lesions Associated with Systemic Disease

31. Beitman RG, Frost SS, Roth JLA: Oral manifestations of gastrointestinal disease. Digest Dis Sci 26:741, 1981.
32. Little JW, Falace DA: Dental Management of the Medically Compromised Patient, 3rd ed. St. Louis, C.V. Mosby, 1988, p 325.
33. Writing Group of the Histiocytosis Society: Histiocytosis syndromes in children. Lancet i:208, 1987.

Differential Diagnoses and General Considerations

34. Regezi JA, Sciubba JJ: Oral Pathology: Clinical-Pathologic Correlations, 2nd ed. Philadelphia, W.B. Saunders, 1993.
35. Shafer WG, Hine MK, Levy BM: A Textbook of Oral Pathology, 4th ed. Philadelphia, W.B. Saunders, 1983.

5. ORAL RADIOLOGY

Richard Valachovic, D.M.D., M.Sc.

RADIATION PHYSICS AND BIOLOGY

1. How are x-rays produced?

X-rays are produced by "boiling off" electrons from a filament, the cathode, and accelerating the electrons to the target at the anode. The accelerated x-rays are decelerated by the target material, resulting in bremsstrahlung. Characteristic x-rays are produced when the incoming electrons knock out an inner K- or L-shell electron in the target and an electron from the L or M shell falls in to fill the void.

2. At the energies typically used in dental radiography, what interactions do the x-rays undergo with tissues?

X-rays undergo three interactions with tissue: elastic scatter, Compton scatter (also known as inelastic or incoherent scatter), and photoelectric absorption. Pair production occurs at much higher energy values (1.02 megaelectron volts [MeV]) than are used in dentistry.

3. Which of the interactions is primarily responsible for patient dose?

In the photoelectric process the incoming x-ray transfers all its energy to the tissue. Photoelectric absorption, therefore, contributes the most to patient dose.

4. Why are filters used?

Filters are used to remove the low-energy x-rays, which are primarily responsible for photoelectric interactions and patient dose. Removing these x-rays increases the average energy of the beam and reduces the likelihood of photoelectric interactions, thereby reducing patient dose.

5. Why are intensifying screens used in extraoral radiography? How do they work?

Intensifying screens are used to reduce patient dose. They do so by converting x-rays to light. The light then interacts with the x-ray film, which is much more sensitive to light than to x-rays.

6. What radiosensitive organs are in the field of typical dental x-ray examinations?

The thyroid is an extremely radiosensitive organ, as well as lymphoid tissue and bone marrow in the exposed areas.

7. What evidence suggests a risk of carcinogenesis from exposures to low levels of ionizing radiation such as those in dentistry?

No single study proves the association between carcinogenesis and exposure to x-rays at the low levels used in dentistry. Many studies that follow patients exposed to higher levels, however, provide evidence of a link. Populations that have been studied include atomic bomb survivors in Nagasaki and Hisoshima, radium watch-dial painters, patients exposed to multiple fluoroscopies for tuberculosis, and others.

8. What units are used to describe radiation exposure and dose? What do they measure?

1. The roentgen (R) is the basic unit of radiation exposure for x- and gamma radiation. It is defined in terms of the number of ionizations produced in air.

2. The RAD (roentgen absorbed dose) is a measure of the amount of energy absorbed by an organ or tissue. Different organs or tissues absorb a different amount of energy when exposed to the same amount of radiation or roentgens.

3. The Rem (roentgen equivalent man or mammal) is a measure of the degree of damage caused to different organs or tissues. Different organs or tissues show differing amounts of damage even when they have absorbed the same amounts of rads. The International System of Units (SIs) are the coulomb/kilogram, the Gray, and the Sievert for the roentgen, rad, and rem, respectively.

9. What are the effects of ionizing radiation on the cell?

Radiation damage to the cell is divided into direct and indirect effects. A direct effect takes place when the radiation interacts directly with a biologic molecule to produce damage:

1. $RH \longrightarrow RH^+ + e$

2. $RH^+ \longrightarrow R^+ + H^+$

An indirect effect occurs when the radiation interacts with a nonbiologic molecule, which then interacts with a biologic molecule and results in cell damage:

1. $H_2O \longrightarrow H_2O^+ + e^-$

2. $H_2O^+ \longrightarrow OH^0$

3. $RH + OH^0 \longrightarrow R + H_2O$

10. What is the difference between density and contrast?

Density refers to the overall degree of blackening of a film. Contrast refers to the differences in densities between adjacent areas of the film.

11. Which technique factors control film density?

The longer a film is exposed, the darker it will be; hence, time of exposure controls density. The milliampere (mA) determines how hot the filament gets and how many electrons are boiled off. The greater the filament current, the hotter the filament and the more electrons are boiled off to reach the anode and to produce x-rays. As a result of the kilovolt peak (kVp), which is the potential voltage difference between the cathode (filament) and anode, electrons that are boiled off are accelerated to the anode. The greater the potential difference between the cathode and anode, the greater the acceleration of the electrons toward the anode. Electrons that hit the anode at greater speed result in x-rays with higher energies. X-rays with higher energies are more likely to reach the film and blacken it. Thus, kVp also controls film density. The distance from the source to the film also has a great effect on film density (see question 17).

12. Which technique factors control film contrast? How do they affect contrast?

Contrast is controlled by the kVp only. The higher the kVp, the lower the contrast, and vice versa. Time, mA, and distance affect only density and not contrast.

13. Assume that you manually develop your x-ray films and that you do not know the developing time. What is the best way to ensure an acceptable film?

If you do not know the developing time, the best option is to develop by sight. Remove the film from the developer from time to time and visually determine whether you have sufficient density (assuming that the exposure was made correctly). Be careful not to expose the film to daylight.

14. Assuming that you have manually developed the film, how long should you fix it?

A general rule of thumb is to fix the film for at least twice the developing time. Thus, you should know how long you took to develop the film and then fix it for at least double that time.

15. How is the latent image on an x-ray film converted into a visible image?

When a film is developed, the exposed silver halide crystals are converted to metallic silver, which blackens film and thus makes the image visible.

16. How would you trouble-shoot a dental radiograph that is too dark or too light?

Changes in radiographic quality most commonly result from errors in processing and less commonly, but not rarely, from errors in the technique factors. Check the exposure factors (kVp, mAs) to ensure that they were appropriate for the patient. Check the chemicals to ensure that they are the correct temperature, that they have been stirred, and that they are fresh. If all of these factors are satisfactory, evaluation of the x-ray unit or film may be necessary. A problem with either, especially the films, is rare.

17. What is the inverse square law?

The intensity or exposure rate of radiation at a given distance from the source is inversely proportional to the square of the distance. If we double the distance from the source, for example, the intensity of the radiation is reduced fourfold.

18. How do we control scatter radiation?

In intraoral radiography, we do not control scattered x-rays that result from the interaction of x-rays with the patient. We do try, however, to minimize the scatter by use of a lead-lined long cone. In extraoral radiography, such as cephalometric radiography, scattered radiation is controlled by the use of a grid that is situated between the patient and the x-ray film.

19. What is meant by film speed? How is film speed expressed?

Film speed refers to the amount of radiation required to produce a particular density. Thus, the faster a film, the less radiation is needed to produce the same density than for a slower film. The speed of a film is expressed as the reciprocal value of the number of roentgens required to produce a density of one. Thus, if 5 roentgens are required to produce a density of one, the film speed is 0.20. If 8 roentgens are required to produce a density of one, the film speed is 0.125.

20. What is meant by the terms sensitivity, specificity, and predictive value when applied to the efficacy of radiographic examinations?

Sensitivity refers to the ability of a test, in this case a radiograph, to detect disease in patients who have disease. Thus, sensitivity is a measure of the frequency of positive (true-positive rate) and negative (false-negative rate) test results in those patients with disease. **Specificity** refers to the ability of a test to screen out patients who do not in fact have the disease. Thus, specificity is a measure of the frequency of negative (true-negative rate) and positive (false-positive) test results in patients without disease. The **predictive value** of a radiograph is the probability that a patient with a positive test result actually has the disease (positive predictive value) or the probability that a patient with a negative test result actually does not have the disease (negative predictive value).

21. What is the basic technology behind magnetic resonance imaging (MRI)?

Atoms in the body act like bar magnets. In the MRI procedure, the area to be examined is subjected to an external magnetic field. The atoms line up with the magnetic field so that their long axes point in the same direction, just as one finds when bar magnets are subjected to a magnetic field. Once the atoms are so aligned, they are also subjected to a radio wave. The atoms absorb some of the radio wave's energy and lean over. When the radio wave is turned off, the atoms "relax" and emit the energy that they absorbed. This energy can be picked up by appropriate receivers and converted into a picture.

RADIOGRAPHIC TECHNIQUES

22. What are the advantages of using the paralleling technique?

In the paralleling technique the film is placed parallel to the object or tooth, and the central ray is directed perpendicular to both the object and the film. The result is an image with relatively minimal distortion. In the bisecting angle technique by contrast, the film is not parallel to the tooth, and the central beam is directed at 90° to an imaginary line bisecting the angle formed by the long axes of the tooth and film. The result is a more distorted image.

23. What are the advantages of the long-cone technique?
The long-cone technique has two primary benefits. The long cone reduces patient dose by reducing the field size. It also increases the target-film distance, thereby reducing magnification.

24. Why is it important to obtain right-angle views of any radiographic abnormality?
Radiographs are two-dimensional representations of three-dimensional objects. To obtain a three-dimensional view with film, one needs to obtain views at right angles to each other. For example, a periapical film suggesting a cyst of the mandible should be supplemented with an occlusal view and a posteroanterior (PA) view of the mandible.

25. If you intend to remove a tooth surgically—for example, an impacted second bicuspid—how can you determine whether the impacted tooth lies buccal or lingual to the erupted teeth?
A periapical view shows only the mesiodistal location of a tooth relative to other teeth. To determine its buccolingual relation, you need a view at right angles to the periapical view. An occlusal view is generally the easiest view to take and is the only intraoral view that you can take at 90° to the periapical view. In areas where it may not be possible to get an occlusal view, such as the third molar region, a PA mandibular film may be the best solution. This, of course, is an extraoral view. You could also determine the impacted tooth's buccolingual relation by exposing a second periapical view with the tube positioned either more mesially or distally than in the first periapical exposure. By applying the buccal object rule, you can then determine the impacted tooth's buccolingual relation to the erupted teeth.

26. What are the indications for an occlusal film?
Indications for an occlusal film include the following: to determine the buccolingual position of an impacted tooth; to demonstrate the buccal and lingual cortices, particularly in the mandible; to visualize the intermaxillary suture; to demonstrate arch form; and to replace periapical films in young children. An occlusal film may also be used when one wishes to visualize on one film a lesion that is too large to fit on a single periapical film.

27. What operator error results in a foreshortened image?
Foreshortening results when the vertical angulation of the tube is too great—that is, the tube is angled too steeply. Elongation, by contrast, results from a vertical angle that is too shallow. A good way to remember cause and effect is to think of the sun and your shadow. Your shadow is shortest at noon when the sun is highest in the sky (a very steep vertical angle) and longest in the late afternoon when the sun is low in the sky (a very shallow vertical angle).

28. Is it preferable to err on the side of foreshortening or elongation? Why?
If one is going to err, it is best to foreshorten. Think again of the sun and shadows. The short shadows produced by the high-noon sun have crisp, well-delineated margins, whereas the long shadows produced by the low late-afternoon sun disappear into the distance with ill-defined margins. It is better to have a foreshortened image that is crisp rather than an elongated image that is difficult to read. This is particularly true when one is examining the apical area.

29. Which radiographic view is considered the primary view for evaluating the alveolar bone for periodontal disease? What are the radiographic manifestations of periodontal disease?
The bitewing view is the primary view for evaluating radiographic changes consistent with periodontal disease, which include loss of crestal cortication, changes in the contour of the interdental bone, horizontal and angular bone loss, and furcation involvement. The bitewing film is superior to a periapical film because distortion, including elongation or foreshortening, is slight. The reasons are simple: the vertical angle is zero, and the central ray is directed at right angles to the film.

30. Is there a generally accepted protocol for the frequency of radiographic evaluation to the adult dental patient?

Yes. The United States Food and Drug Administration, in cooperation with the American Dental Association and other major organizations, has developed and disseminated protocols for exposing dental patients to x-ray examinations. These protocols require a history and clinical examination before prescribing an individualized radiographic examination.

31. How should radiographic protocols be altered for the pregnant dental patient?

With the use of standard radiation protection, there should be no additional risk to the fetus from x-ray exposures commonly used in dentistry. However, because of the concerns many women have during pregnancy, it is advisable to limit x-ray exposures to the necessary minimum.

32. In a patient who has trismus and whose teeth you wish to examine, what alternatives to the standard bitewing and periapical views may be used?

Intraorally, buccal bitewings can be used. For buccal bitewings, insert a standard no. 2 film into the buccal vestibule with the tube side facing the teeth. Direct the cone from the opposite side and increase the time exposure by two steps. If the patient can open even slightly, an occlusal view also can be done. The lateral occlusal film can give an excellent view of the teeth, including the periapical regions. Extraorally, a lateral oblique film can be obtained. Although not giving as detailed information as an occlusal film, the lateral oblique also depicts the teeth and surrounding periapical regions. A panoramic film has less resolution than the occlusal film and possibly even less than the lateral oblique (depending on the screen-film combination). Thus it provides less detail than either of the two.

33. What are the differences between standard intraoral radiography (bitewings and periapicals) and panoramic radiography?

1. Bitewing and periapical techniques use direct-exposure film while the panoramic technique uses intensifying screens.

2. The panoramic view uses a tomographic technique that results in loss of detail and resolution.

34. What imaging techniques are available to evaluate the soft-tissue components of the temporomandibular joints (TMJs)?

Three imaging procedures are available for evaluation of the soft-tissue components of the TMJs: arthrography, computed tomography (CT), and MRI. MRI studies are becoming more widely used because they image soft tissue well, do not employ ionizing radiation, and are noninvasive. Arthrography is the most invasive and involves the introduction of contrast into one or both joint spaces.

35. Name the paranasal sinuses and the radiographic views commonly used to evaluate the sinuses.

The paranasal sinuses are the frontal sinuses, the maxillary sinuses, the sphenoid sinuses, and the ethmoid sinuses. The views used to evaluate them are the Waters view (maxillary sinus), the Caldwell view (maxillary and frontal sinus), the lateral view (maxillary and frontal sinus), and the submentovertex view (sphenoid and ethmoid sinus). A panoramic film, which is in fact a form of tomography rather than a plain film, can be used as an adjunct to these views. The panoramic film shows the maxillary sinus.

The view of choice depends on precisely what is under examination. For example, the submentovertex view permits excellent visualization of the lateral wall of the maxillary sinus, whereas Waters view depicts the medical, lateral, and inferior borders of the maxillary sinus.

36. What plain film views may be used to visualize the TMJ?

The transpharyngeal or Parma view provides an image mainly of the lateral aspect of the condyle. The lateral transcranial view also provides an image mainly of the lateral aspect of the condyle. Its main purpose is to depict the condyle–glenoid fossa relationship. The Zimmer or trans- or perorbital view provides a mediolateral image of the condyle as well as the condylar neck. A reverse Towne view is useful for visualizing the condylar neck. Keep in mind that tomography provides better visualization of the TMJ than plain film views. The above views, however, are relatively easy to take.

37. What are the indications for a panoramic film?
There is no specific indication for the panoramic film. Virtually any structure that is portrayed on a panoramic film can be displayed by another view, which often provides greater detail. For example, the panoramic film is often used to visualize impacted third molars. A lateral oblique view of the jaws provides the same information with greater detail. A Waters view provides greater information about the maxillary and other sinuses than a panoramic film.

38. Which intraoral view is best for visualizing the greater palatine foramina?
The greater palatine foramina cannot be visualized on any intraoral film. On some maxillary occlusal films, a foramen can be seen in the area of the second or third molars. This foramen is the nasolacrimal canal and not the greater palatine foramen.

39. What are the names of the major salivary glands? How are they studied radiographically?
The three major salivary glands are the parotid, submandibular, and sublingual glands. Because the salivary glands consist of soft tissue, they cannot be seen on radiographs unless special steps are taken to make them visible. In a technique called sialography, a radiopaque dye or contrast is injected through the duct openings into the gland. Iodine is the agent normally used to provide contrast. Calcifications of the duct may be seen on intraoral films, especially calcifications of Wharton's duct, the submandibular gland duct. The stones or sialoliths may be seen on either periapical or more commonly on occlusal films.

40. What are the contraindications to sialography?
As stated above, iodine compounds are normally used as the contrast medium. It cannot be used, however, in allergic patients. In such patients, another contrast agent must be used.

41. What are the typical magnifications of radiographs commonly used in dentistry?
The magnification of periapical and bitewing films is about 4%; of cephalometric filsm, about 10%; and of panoramic films, 20–25%.

BASIC RADIOLOGIC INTERPRETIVE CONCEPTS

42. What are the radiographic features of any lesion or area of interest on the film that always should be defined and recorded?
1. Location of the lesion as exactly as possible
2. Size
3. Shape
4. Appearance of borders
5. Density, with particular attention to whether it is radiolucent, radiopaque or mixed
6. Effects of the lesion on adjacent structures

43. Once the radiographic features of the area of interest are described, what is the first decision to be made about that area?
The first and most important determination is to decide whether the area is normal or abnormal. Simple as this may sound, this determination is the biggest challenge that you will face on a daily basis in clinical practice.

44. What is by far the most likely interpretation of a bilaterally symmetric radiographic appearance in the jaws?
A bilateral symmetric appearance, with extremely few exceptions, is indicative of normality. Among the few exceptions to this rule are cherubism and infantile cortical hyperostosis (Caffey's disease).

45. The location of a lesion may be a clue to its origin. What single anatomic structure in the mandible is most useful in differentiating between a lesion of possible odontogenic vs. non-odontogenic origin?

The mandibular or inferior alveolar canal is extremely useful in distinguishing between a lesion of odontogenic versus non-odontogenic origin. Because one does not expect to find odontogenic tissues below the canal, it is most unlikely that lesions situated below the canal are odontogenic in origin. Indeed, the lesion of odontogenic origin rarely, if ever, begins below the canal. Of course, any lesion, including one of odontogenic origin, may begin above the canal and extend below it.

46. What is the most likely tissue of origin for a tumor in the mandibular canal?

Because a nerve and a blood vessel run in the canal, the tissue of origin is most likely to be either neural or vascular, resulting in tumors such as neurolemmoma, neurofibroma, traumatic neuroma, or hemangioma.

47. What broad categories of possible disease entities need to be considered in developing a differential diagnosis of any abnormality noted during a radiographic examination?

   Trauma
   Metabolic, nutritional and endocrinologic diseases
   Congenital anomalies and abnormalities of growth and development
   Iatrogenic lesions
   Neoplastic diseases (benign and malignant)
   Inflammation and infection

48. What general radiographic features or principles permit the diagnosis of an underlying systemic cause for a particular condition or appearance?

When a systemic cause underlies a problem, both the mandible and maxilla are affected. Furthermore, the jaws are typically affected bilaterally, often symmetrically. One would expect the teeth, if the condition affects them too, also to be affected in a bilaterally symmetrical fashion.

49. What technique can be used to determine the track of a fistula that exits on the soft tissue adjacent to the teeth?

Insert a gutta percha point into the fistula, and allow it to track as far as it can. Obtain a periapical view with the gutta percha point in place.

50. What are the usual radiographic signs of inflammatory disease involving the paranasal sinuses?

Mucous membrane thickening	Presence of a soft-tissue mass
Air-fluid levels	Changes in the cortical margins of a sinus
Opacification of a sinus cavity	

51. What common radiographic signs help to distinguish among a cyst, benign neoplasm, or malignant neoplasm?

Cysts tend to be radiolucent and round or oval in shape and to have intact cortical margins. Benign neoplasms are more variable than cysts in density, shape, and definition of margins. Malignant neoplasms of the jaws tend to be aggressive, with ragged margins and poor definition of shape and borders. Malignant lesions often grow quickly, leaving roots of teeth in position and giving the appearance of roots floating in space. Both cysts and benign neoplasms are more likely than malignant neoplasms to resorb tooth roots.

52. When should bitewing views first be obtained for the typical child?

The first bitewing views should be obtained after the establishment of contacts on the posterior teeth.

53. How do primary teeth differ from permanent teeth radiographically? How does the difference affect the radiographic evidence of caries in primary teeth?
Primary teeth are smaller and have relatively larger pulp chambers with pulp horns in closer proximity to the external surface of the crown. The enamel layer is thinner in dimension. Primary teeth are slightly less opaque on film because of a higher inorganic content. As a result, caries in primary teeth tends to progress more rapidly from initial surface demineralization to involvement of the dentin. Thus careful interpretation is especially important in evaluating the primary dentition.

54. What is the correlation between the histologic and radiographic progress of dental caries?
There must be 30–60% loss in mineralization before caries is radiographically evident with standard D- and E-speed intraoral films. Therefore, the histologic or clinical progress of a carious lesion is advanced, sometimes significantly, compared with its radiographic progress.

55. What is the Rule of 3's for radiographic assessment of the development of permanent teeth?
It takes approximately 3 years for a permanent tooth bud to calcify after matrix formation is complete, approximately 3 more years for the tooth to erupt after calcification is complete, and about 3 more years after initial eruption for root formation to be complete.

56. What is the difference in the progress of pit and fissure caries and proximal or smooth-surface caries on a radiograph?
Pit and fissure caries start at the pit or fissure and develop a triangular appearance, with the base of the triangle at the amelodentinal junction and the apex directed toward the surface. The lesion then continues into the dentin. Once the caries have extended into the dentin, a new triangle is formed, with the base of the apex now at the amelodentinal junction and the apex pointed toward the deeper aspect of the tooth. Smooth-surface caries penetrate the outermost part of the enamel on a narrow front and then expand in all directions, resulting in a hemispheric zone with the apex of the hemisphere directed toward the dentin.

57. In pathology of the maxilla, what feature is most useful in determining whether the pathology arose inside or outside the sinus?
The floor of the sinus is the most useful feature. If the pathology arose inside the sinus, the floor is intact and in its normal position or perhaps depressed inferiorly. If the pathology arose outside the sinus, the floor of the sinus is intact and in its normal position or moved or pushed superiorly. If the sinus floor has been destroyed, then it may not be possible to determine whether the pathology arose from without or within the sinus.

58. Foramina may be superimposed over the apices of teeth, mimicking the presence of periapical disease. What radiographic features are most useful in distinguishing between normal structures and apical pathology?
If the lucency is due to the superimposition of a foramen, then the periodontal ligament space and the lamina dura around the tooth are intact. The exposure of a second radiograph, with the tube in a different position from the first exposure, also is frequently useful. If the lucency moves relative to the apex of the tooth, then the lucency is not associated with the tooth and is not due to periapical pathology. This exercise, however, does not rule out the possibility that the lesion is abnormal; it means merely that the lesion is not related to the tooth.

59. A radiolucency normally surrounds the crown of an unerupted tooth. What is it called?
The radiolucent area is called the follicle space.

60. Is it possible for a patient to be in acute pain as a result of a periapical abscess, yet to have a completely normal periapical film?
This finding is not unusual because 30–60% of mineralization must be lost before bone destruction is radiographically evident. In an acute situation, there frequently has not been

sufficient time for this amount of bone destruction to occur. Thus, the radiograph lags behind the clinical picture. The same may be true in the healing phase. A patient may be improving clinically yet still show radiographic signs of pathology.

61. Is a widened periodontal ligament space at the apex of a tooth always indicative of pathology?

No. When a radiolucency such as the mental foramen or mandibular canal is superimposed over the periodontal ligament space, the ligament space appears to be widened. Such a widening is purely artifactual. The periodontal ligament space also may appear wider at the neck of a tooth. If the lamina dura is normal in this area, then the widened periodontal ligament space is probably a variant of normal.

62. Can a patient refuse an x-ray examination that is considered necessary, given signs and symptoms, and sign a release of responsibility in the chart?

A patient may legally refuse to undergo a radiographic examination. Such patients probably waive their right to seek damages later if an adverse event occurs that may have been detected by the radiograph. The patient's decision to refuse a radiographic examination is a matter of informed consent. The dentist may not be protected from suit if the record reflects merely that the patient was told of the need for an x-ray and declined to undergo the examination. The record should show clearly that the patient was told why the examination was necessary, what information the dentist needed, and how the lack of that information may lead to improper diagnosis and/or treatment.

63. What are the radiographic manifestations in the jaws of patients infected with the human immunodeficiency virus (HIV)?

There are no unique oral or maxillofacial radiographic manifestations of HIV infection, although infected patients are at a significantly higher risk for aggressive periodontal disease.

64. What is the efficacy of dental radiographs?

Studies of standard dental radiography (bitewing, periapical, and panoramic views) show considerable variance in the abilities to detect common dental diseases such as caries, periodontal disease, and apical periodontitis. Radiographs should not be considered to be perfect, but are most valuable when combined with a thorough history and clinical examination.

RADIOGRAPHIC INTERPRETATION

65. What is the earliest radiographic sign of periapical disease of pulpal origin?

The earliest radiographic sign is widening of the periodontal ligament space around the apex of the tooth.

66. What is the second most common radiographic sign of periapical disease of pulpal origin?

The second most common radiographic sign is loss of the lamina dura around the apex of the tooth.

67. Describe the radiographic differences that allow one to distinguish among periapical abscess, granuloma, radicular (periapical) cyst, and an apical surgical scar.

One cannot distinguish among periapical abscess, granuloma, or radicular (periapical) cyst on radiographic grounds alone. All these lesions are radiolucent with well-defined borders. Whereas an abscess may be expected to be less well corticated than a radicular cyst, this feature is not marked or constant enough to be of real utility. An apical surgical scar may be radiographically distinguishable from the other three lesions if there is radiographic evidence of surgery, such as a retrograde amalgam. Of course, a history should elicit the fact of surgery.

68. How does the radiographic appearance of pulpal pathology that has extended to involve the bone differ in primary posterior teeth from the picture commonly seen in permanent posterior teeth?

In permanent teeth, widening of the periodontal ligament space is seen around the apex of the tooth. In primary teeth, by contrast, the infection presents as widening of the periodontal ligament space or an area of lucency in the furcation area.

69. Does any radiographic sign permit the diagnosis of a nonvital tooth?

It is frequently stated that tooth vitality cannot be determined by radiographs alone, but this is not so. The presence of a root canal filling in a tooth provides virtually conclusive proof of its nonvitality, as does the presence of a retrograde filling, usually amalgam.

70. At times it may be difficult to distinguish between hypercementosis and condensing or sclerosing osteitis around the apex of a tooth. What radiographic feature permits a definitive diagnosis when one is confronted with this dilemma?

If hypercementosis is present, the periodontal ligament space is visible around the added cementum; that is, the cementum is contained within and is surrounded by the periodontal ligament space. Condensing osteitis, by contrast, is situated outside the periodontal ligament space.

71. What is the radiographic sign of an ankylosed tooth?

The radiographic sign of an ankylosed tooth is loss of the periodontal ligament space and lamina dura.

72. What is the earliest radiographic sign of periodontal disease?

The earliest radiographic sign of periodontal disease is loss of density of the crestal cortex, which is best seen in the posterior regions. In the anterior part of the mouth, the alveolar crests lose their pointed appearance and become blunted. In the posterior areas, the alveolar crests usually meet the lamina dura at right angles. In the presence of periodontal disease, these angles become rounded.

73. What is the earliest radiographic sign of furcation involvement due to periodontal disease?

In periodontal disease, one may see the loss of a cortical plate, either the buccal or lingual plate, on an intraoral film. The plate may be lost so that the crest now occupies a position apical to the furcation. This appearance, however, does not permit a diagnosis of furcation involvement. Widening of the periodontal ligament space in the furcation area is the earliest radiographic sign of furcation involvement.

74. What is the radiographic differential diagnosis of a radiolucency on the root of a periodontally healthy tooth?

Internal resorption, external resorption, and superimposition are the most common causes. Note that the question refers to a periodontally healthy tooth. If bone loss has resulted in exposure of the root, then caries and abrasion, among other potential possibilities, enter the picture.

75. How could you distinguish among the above radiolucencies on the root of a tooth?

In internal resorption, the canal is widened, whereas it is unaffected in external resorption. If the resorption began below the bone level, then it has to be internal resorption because without adjacent bone, there are no osteoclasts in the area to cause external resorption. Of course, if either internal or external resorption involves both the canal and other tooth structure, it is not possible to distinguish between the two conditions. A superimposed radiolucency moves relative to the root if another view is obtained with the tube in a different position. The most common such lucencies are normal anatomy, such as foramina, sinus, mandibular canal, and accessory or nutrient foramina or canals. Artifacts such as cervical burnout also may produce a lucency on the root at the junction of the enamel, cementum, and bone.

76. What is the radiographic differential diagnosis of a radiolucency on the crown of a tooth?
Caries, internal resorption, restorations, abrasions, erosions, and enamel hypoplasia are among
the more common possibilities. Caries typically have irregular margins; they may also have
typical shapes, such as the triangular appearance of interproximal caries. Internal resorption
has smooth, well-defined margins. The same is true of radiolucent restorations, which
frequently can be recognized by their shape and sometimes by the presence of an opaque base,
such as calcium hydroxide, lining the floor of the preparation. Abrasions, particularly at the
cervical margins, often have a V-shaped appearance. Other abrasions, such as those caused by
a clasp on a denture, typically have well-defined borders and straight lines, unlike most
naturally occurring phenomena. Erosions also have well-defined borders, and their shape is
typically round or oval. Hypoplasia usually is not a single lucency on a tooth but rather many
small lucencies.

77. What is the differential diagnosis of a root that appears short on the radiograph?
A root that appears short may indicate an incompletely formed tooth, which may be either
vital and still developing or nonvital; a short but otherwise normal root (the root may be
congenitally short or underdeveloped because of an acquired condition such as radiation); root
resorption; foreshortening; surgery, as in apicoectomy; or iatrogenic causes, as in orthodontic
treatment. In certain conditions, such as dentinogenesis imperfecta, the teeth also have short
roots.

**78. How can one distinguish between the various possibilities for a radiographically short-
appearing root?**
In a normal root, the canal is not radiographically visible to the apex and appears to end just
before the apex. In the case of a foreshortened normal root, the canal is not open at the apex.
Foreshortening can be distinguished from a normal short root by the fact that other structures
in the radiograph point to the steep angulation of the tube. Alternatively, a second film can be
exposed to ensure that the correct vertical angle is used. If the root still looks short, then it
cannot be due to foreshortening. In teeth with an open apex, the shape of the canal is
important. In a still-developing tooth, the ends of the canal diverge ("blunderbuss"), whereas
in resorption the walls of the canal converge. Surgical intervention is usually easily spotted by
the presence of a retrograde amalgam. The involvement of multiple teeth with short roots
points to a condition such as dentinogenesis imperfecta. A history of orthodontic treatment
confirms an iatrogenic cause.

**79. What other possibilities enter the picture if many or all of the teeth have pulps that are
reduced in size?**
Other possibilities include dentinogenesis imperfecta, amelogenesis imperfecta, and dentinal
dysplasia. On rare occasions, the cause of reduced pulp size in many teeth may be idiopathic.
In such cases, however, all of the teeth are unlikely to be affected, as with dentinogenesis
imperfecta, amelogenesis imperfecta, and dentinal dysplasia.

**80. What conditions should be considered in a differential diagnosis of generalized large pulp
chambers?**
Any condition that results in a disturbance in calcification of the tooth may result in enlarged
pulp chambers, including vitamin D-resistant rickets, hypophosphatasia, cystinosis, and hypo-
parathyroidism.

81. What are the radiographic signs of osteomyelitis?
A classic sign of osteomyelitis is a periosteal reaction or periostitis, which is typically seen in
the mandible but rarely, if ever, in the maxilla. The periosteum lays down bone on its deep
aspect, resulting in new bone formation, known as an involucrum formation. Cloacae, which
are drainage tracts for purulent material, may be visible on radiographs. Sequestra, which are
areas of bone separated from adjacent bone, are another typical feature.

82. What radiographic features help to differentiate a malignant lesion from osteomyelitis?
Malignant lesions destroy bone uniformly. In osteomyelitis, areas of radiographically normal-appearing bone are frequently seen between the areas of destruction. Sequestra are not present in malignant lesions. The nature of the periosteal response cannot be used to distinguish between malignancies and infection, with the possible exception of the sun-ray periosteal reaction described in osteogenic sarcoma.

83. What features of a periosteal reaction help to differentiate between infectious periostitis and a periosteal reaction due to malignant disease?
A periosteal reaction by itself does not permit a definitive diagnosis of either an infectious or malignant origin, notwithstanding comments to the contrary. Although some periosteal reactions are more suggestive than others of a particular origin (e.g., the sun-burst appearance in osteogenic sarcoma), none is definitive.

84. Both fluid and a soft-tissue mass present as opacification of the maxillary sinus on a Waters view. How can one distinguish radiographically between fluid or soft tissue in the sinus?
Take a second view with patient's head tilted upward, downward, or laterally relative to the position for the first Waters view. If the superior border of the opacity remains the same, one is dealing with soft tissue. If the superior surface changes, one is dealing with fluid because the fluid level changes when the head is tilted (as with water in a glass). This technique, of course, does not work when opacification of the sinus is complete. One cannot distinguish between fluid or soft tissue in the sinus on the basis of the degree of opacity on plain films.

85. Sometimes it is difficult to distinguish a tooth or part of a tooth embedded in bone from other opacities in the bone or from opacities in the sinus. What radiographic features are helpful in this predicament?
An opacity surrounded by a thin, relatively uniform radiolucent zone, which in turn is surrounded by a thin radiopaque line or cortex, is of inestimable value. The radiolucent zone and cortex provide conclusive proof that the opacity is not in the sinus. The uniform zone is suggestive of the periodontal ligament space, whereas the cortex is suggestive of the lamina dura. This general appearance is thus reminiscent of a tooth. The presence of a canal in the opacity is also useful. Whether the opacity is in fact tooth depends, among other things, on the density and uniformity of the opacity as well as on its shape and size. An odontoma, for example, has the general features of uniform radiolucent zone, surrounded by a cortex, yet it is a benign tumor. One may not be able to determine with certainty from a periapical view alone whether an opacity is inside or outside the sinus. A Waters view helps to clarify the situation.

86. List the radiographic signs of a fractures.
The radiographic signs of a fracture include a demonstrable radiolucent fracture line, displacement of a bony fragment, disruption in the continuity of the normal bony contour, and increased density (due to overlap of the adjacent fragments).

87. What radiographic sign helps to differentiate between a recent fracture and an older fracture?
The edges of an older fracture are typically rounded, whereas the edges of a recent fracture are sharp.

88. What plain film views are of greatest assistance in evaluating the jaws for fractures?
The Waters view provides the single best plain film view of the maxilla. The zygomatic arches are best examined with a basal or submentovertex view. A PA film of the mandible is helpful, as are lateral oblique films. Occlusal views are useful in both the mandible and maxilla. Periapical films provide the greatest detail about a fracture if the fracture line traverses an area that a periapical film is able to cover. A reverse Towne projection shows the condylar necks and condyles, as does the transorbital or periorbital view.

89. What radiographic features help to differentiate between the radicular cyst emanating from a maxillary central incisor and the nasopalatine or incisive canal cyst?

If the lesion crosses the midline, it is far more likely to be a nasopalatine cyst. An intact lamina dura around the teeth is indicative of vital teeth and effectively rules out a radicular cyst. The presence of large restorations on a central incisor supports the diagnosis of a radicular cyst, but this feature is overridden by an intact lamina dura.

90. To what extent do the amount and degree of calcification in a tumor point to its benign or malignant nature?

Calcification has no significance in predicting the benign or malignant nature of a tumor. Both benign tumors (e.g., odontomas, adenomotoid odontogenic tumors, ossifying fibromas) and malignant tumors (e.g., osteogenic sarcoma) produce bone or calcifications. To determine the benign or malignant nature of a tumor, one must look to other features.

91. Which lesions may present with a soap-bubble or honeycomb appearance?

Ameloblastoma
Aneurysmal bone cyst
Giant cell lesions
Hemangioma

92. What are the radiographic features of degenerative joint disease (DJD) or osteoarthritis involving the TMJs?

The changes of DJD include subchondral sclerosis, flattening of the articular surfaces of the condyle, and osteophyte formation. Osteophyte formation occurs in the later stages of the disease process. Small erosions, called Ely cysts, may be seen on the articulating surfaces. A narrowing of the joint space is another common finding. The eminence may be flattened or hollowed and may also show osteophyte formation.

93. Why is it important to visualize both TMJs on radiograph even when a patient has signs and symptoms only on one side?

The unique nature of the TMJs—both are part of a common mandible—often results in functional symptoms on one side while the osseous pathology may be on the other side. Once the decision to radiograph a joint has been made, both sides should be examined.

94. What common intracranial calcifications may be observed on a radiographic view of the skull, such as a cephalometric view? What intracranial calcifications represent pathology and should be further evaluated?

Physiologic calcifications include those of the pineal gland, the choroid plexus, dura (falx cerebri, tentorium, vault), ligaments (petroclinoid, interclinoid), habenular commissure, basal ganglia, and dentate nucleus. **Pathologic calcifications** include calcifications in tumors (meningioma, craniopharyngioma, glioma), cysts (dermoid cyst), and infections (parasitic, as in cysticercosis; tuberculosis)

BIBLIOGRAPHY

1. Christensen EE: Christensen's Introduction to the Physics of Diagnostic Radiology, 3rd ed. Philadelphia, Lea & Febiger, 1984.
2. Goaz PW, White SC: Oral Radiology Principles and Interpretation, 3rd ed. St. Louis, C.V. Mosby, 1994.
3. Langlais RP, Kasle MJ: Exercises in Oral Radiographic Interpretation, 3rd ed. Philadelphia, W.B. Saunders, 1992.
4. Som PM, Bergeron RT: Head and Neck Imaging, 2nd ed. St. Louis, C.V. Mosby, 1991.
5. Stafne EC, Gibilisco JA: Oral Roentgenographic Diagnosis, 4th ed. Philadelphia, W.B. Saunders, 1985.
6. Wood NK, Goaz PW: Differential Diagnosis of Oral Lesions. St. Louis, C.V. Mosby, 1985.
7. Worth HM: Principles and Practice of Oral Radiologic Interpretation. Chicago, Year Book Medical Publishers, 1963.

ILLUSTRATIONS

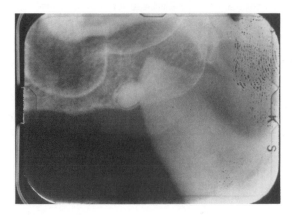

Root. A small, rounded, uniformly opaque structure is visible in the left posterior maxilla. The opacity is surrounded by a small, uniform radiolucent zone, which in turn is surrounded by a thin, uniform radiopaque line or cortex. The radiopacity is reminiscent of tooth structure, the radiolucent zone of the periodontal ligament space and the cortex of the lamina dura. This radiographic appearance is virtually diagnostic of a tooth—in this case, a root that remained following extraction of a tooth. The triangular opacity is a normal structure, the coronoid process of the mandible.

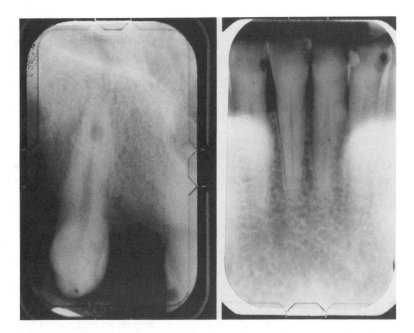

Left, **Tori.** Symmetrical opacities are visible in the premolar region of the mandible. The posterior borders of the opacities are not visible on the films; the anterior borders, however, are well defined. The teeth are unaffected by the opacities. The appearance is due to the presence of lingual tori. This radiograph illustrates the principle that bilateral, symmetrical opacities are, with rare exceptions, normal or variants of normal.

Right, **Radiolucency on root of a tooth.** This radiograph shows an example of external resorption. Note the intact canal, eliminating internal resorption as a possible cause. Other causes of a radiolucency on the root of a tooth include superimposition, caries, abrasion, and radiolucent restorations.

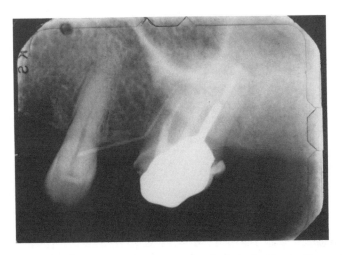

Fistulous tract. The patient presented with a complaint of pain in the left posterior maxilla. Clinical examination revealed drainage from the buccal sulcus around tooth no. 15. To determine the origin of the problem, a gutta percha point was inserted and a film exposed. Rather than being purely periodontal, the problem emanated from the apex of the mesiobuccal root.

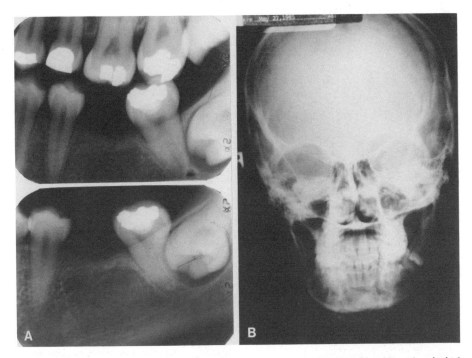

Buccal object rule. The radiographs above illustrate the buccal object rule. Bitewing and periapical films (*A*) show an impacted third molar on the left side. For the periapical exposure, the cone was moved distally in relation to the bitewing view. The impacted third molar moved mesially, that is, in the opposite direction in which the tube was moved. Applying the principles of the buccal object rule, we can determine that the impacted third molar lies buccal to the erupted second molar. The posteroanterior mandibular view (*B*) confirms this deduction. Note that in order to apply the rule, one must have a reference object—in this case, the erupted second molar.

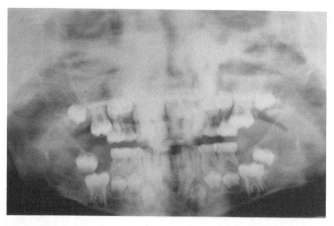

Cherubism. The panoramic radiograph above shows symmetrical, bilateral, multilocular radiolucent areas in the mandibular ramus. This is one of the rare exceptions to the general statement that symmetrical bilateral appearances are normal or variants of normal. The appearance indicates cherubism. Another exception to the general statement is infantile cortical hyperostosis or Caffey's disease.

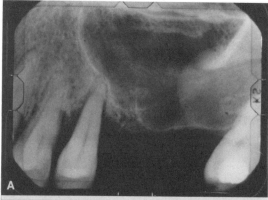

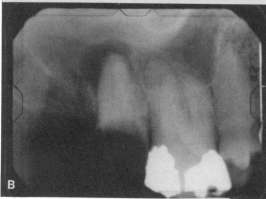

Pathology arising from within or without the sinus. The periapical radiograph (*A*) shows a dome-shaped opacity situated apical to the area of tooth no. 15. The well-defined and uncorticated opacity is situated above the sinus floor, which is intact. The intact sinus floor strongly suggests that the opacity arose inside the sinus rather than outside with subsequent invasion of the sinus. The radiographic appearance is consistent with a mucous retention phenomenon. The apical view (*B*) shows a radiolucent area apical to the root of tooth no. 2. The sinus floor is elevated but intact.

This appearance suggests that the problem originated outside the sinus and is consistent with rarefying osteitis and a concomitant periostitis, which occurs as the floor of the sinus attempts to confine the lesion by continually reforming. If the sinus floor is destroyed, it may be difficult and sometimes impossible to determine whether the lesion arose from within or without the sinus.

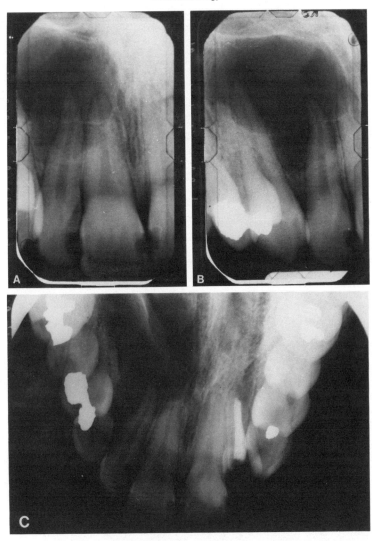

Radicular cyst. The large radiolucency in the right maxilla illustrates a radicular cyst arising from tooth no. 7. The lucency is well defined and partly corticated, features that are consistent with a benign lesion. The cortical borders of the sinus and nasal cavity are intact. Note that the lucency does not cross the midline. Another entity that should perhaps be considered is an incisive canal or nasopalatine cyst. With rare exceptions, however, the nasopalatine cyst crosses the midline.

Radiolucency on crown of a tooth. The radiographs (*right* and *following page*) illustrate different causes of a radiolucency on the crown of a tooth. The widened canal of the central incisor (*A*) is an example of internal resorption. *(Figure continues on next page.)*

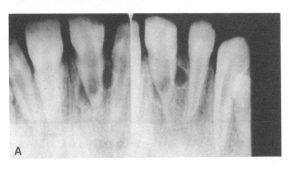

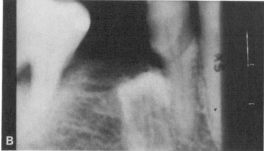

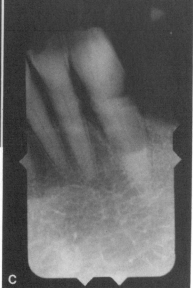

B, With external resorption in the impacted premolar, the canal is visible throughout the length of the tooth. The somewhat curved radiolucency across the first bicuspid results from abrasion caused by the clasp of a removable partial denture. Another example of abrasion due to a denture clasp is shown in C. Erosion, caries, radiolucent restorations, and enamel hypoplasia also may result in a radiolucency on the crown of an erupted tooth.

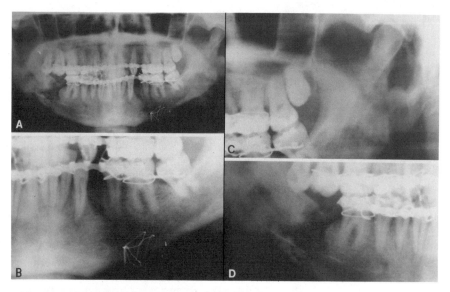

Fractures and osteomyelitis. The most obvious abnormality is the fracture in the premolar area of the left mandible (*A* and *B*). Also evident is a fracture of the right body of the mandible. Although single fractures of the mandible do occur, it is much more common for more than one to be present. Closer examination reveals that the left condyle also has sustained a fracture (*A* and *C*). More often than not, unilateral fracture of the condyle is associated with a fracture of the opposite side of the body of the mandible. Perhaps the greatest concern to the patient is the presence of osteomyelitis in the right body (*A* and *D*). This case illustrates eloquently a highly specific feature of osteomyelitis: the more or less rounded opacity surrounded by a radiolucent zone. The rounded opacity, situated at the inferior cortex, is a sequestrum. A larger, boat-shaped sequestrum is visible inferior to and partly surrounding the round sequestrum. This panoramic film illustrates a cardinal point: always examine the entire film. Once you have spotted an area of interest, be certain to examine the rest of the film. If necessary, cover the previously examined area so that your attention is not continually drawn to it.

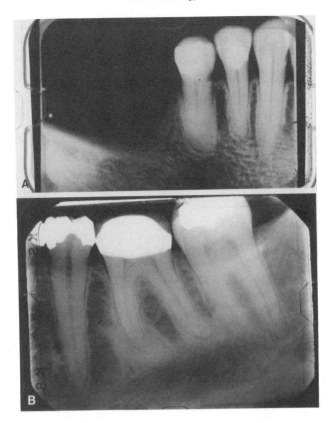

Hypercementosis and condensing osteitis. *A,* Enlarged root of tooth no. 29, particularly in the apical area. The root of tooth no. 28 also shows some widening. The periodontal ligament space surrounds the tissue that has been laid down, and the lamina dura is visible outside the periodontal ligament space. *B,* An opacity within which the periodontal ligament space is situated. *A* illustrates hypercementosis, whereas *B* is an illustration of condensing osteitis.

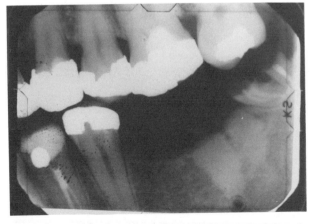

Extraction sockets. At times the appearance of a healing or healed extraction socket may present a problem. The sockets shown above have filled with dense bone. In some cases, such an appearance may be confused with a root. Features that may be of assistance in distinguishing between the two include the density of the socket, the presence or absence of a canal, and the presence or absence of a periodontal ligament space. At times, nonetheless, the diagnosis may be difficult indeed. For a good discussion and illustration of the problem, see Worth HM: Principles and Practice of Oral Radiologic Interpretation. Chicago, Year-Book, 1963, pp 310–316.

6. PERIODONTOLOGY

Mark Obernesser, D.D.S., M.M.Sc.

The Fundamentals of Gums and the Art of Gum Gardening—101
". . . 'tis better to have longer teeth than teeth no longer. . . "
— An anonymous periodontist

CLASSIFICATIONS AND ETIOLOGIES OF PERIODONTAL DISEASES

1. What are the etiologic agents in periodontal disease?
Contrary to old wives' tales, periodontal disease is not caused by occlusal trauma, vitamin deficiencies, or hypercholesterolemia. The cause is bacterial plaque—specifically, gram-negative bacteria.

2. What is the chief component of plaque?
Bacteria. Approximately 90–95% of the wet weight of plaque is bacteria. The other 5–10% consists of a few host cells, an organic matrix, and inorganic ions.

3. What are the basic types of plaque? How do they differ in composition?
The basic types of plaque are supragingival and subgingival. Supragingival plaque has a majority of aerobes and facultative bacteria (mostly gram-positive), whereas subgingival plaque consists mostly of anaerobic bacteria (frequently gram-negative).

4. What are the basic types of subgingival plaque?
The three basic types of subgingival plaque are hard-tissue, soft-tissue, and loose plaque. They all differ in composition. Hard-tissue plaque adheres to the cementum, dentin, and enamel; soft-tissue plaque adheres to the epithelial cells; and loose plaque floats inbetween. Loose plaque has come under a great deal of investigation because of its possible role in attachment loss.

5. What is a major factor in determining the different bacteria in supragingival and subgingival plaque?
The major factor is oxygen. The redox potential of the gingival sulcus greatly influences the bacterial composition.

6. What is calculus? How is it basically formed?
Calculus is mineralized plaque. It is formed by the bathing of the plaque in a supersaturated solution of Ca^{++} and PO_4^-—saliva.

7. Why is calculus frequently a dark color (e.g., black, brown, gray)?
After the plaque has been solidified to calculus and an inflammatory response has occurred, localized bleeding ensues. Red blood cells adhere to and permeate the calculus, hemolysis follows, and the hemoglobin/iron colors the calculus.

8. What terms are used to describe healthy gingiva?
Healthy gingiva have scalloped, knifelike margins and a firm, stippled texture. In white people they are salmon-pink in color. Afro-Americans, Indians, Asians, and Africans frequently have pigmented gingiva. Salmon-pink naturally does not apply, but the other terms do.

9. What terms are used to describe inflamed gingiva?
The key word is inflammation, and the cardinal signs of inflammation are calor rubor tumor and dolor. All may apply to inflamed gingiva. The margins are described as rolled, the gingiva

as erythematous and edematous. The stippling is absent, and the gingiva are frequently described as boggy.

10. What is gingivitis? What bacterial groups are generally associated with gingivitis?
Gingivitis is inflammation of the gingiva. The bacterial groups associated with gingivitis are spirochetes, *Actinomyces* (gram-positive filament), and *Eikenella* (gram-negative rod).

11. Is gingivitis a forerunner of periodontitis?
No. Gingivitis is not necessarily a forerunner of periodontitis. Chronic gingivitis may exist for long periods without advancing to periodontitis.

12. What causes the transition from gingivitis to periodontitis?
The exact cause of the progression is most likely multifactorial, including a pathogenic combination of bacteria and an abnormal host response.

13. What are the clinical signs of acute necrotizing ulcerative gingivitis (ANUG)?
ANUG is an acute, recurring infection of the gingiva characterized by necrosis of the papilla (leading to blunting), spontaneous bleeding, pain, and fetor oris. It has been theorized that the disease is stress-related (e.g., taking the National Dental Board examinations, practical examinations, being on death row at Alcatraz).

14. What bacteria are associated with gingivitis of pregnancy? Why?
Bacteria associated with gingivitis of pregnancy are the black-pigmenting *Bacteroides*, which crave steroid hormones for their own metabolism. Therefore, pregnancy essentially selects for these bacteria. Patients who use birth control pills or receive steroid therapy (chronic autoimmune diseases) are also at risk.

15. What bacteria are generally associated with active adult periodontitis?
The bacteria most frequently cultured from active adult periodontal lesions include *Prophyoromonas gingivalis, Actinobacillus actinomycetemcomitans, Wolinella recta, Fusobacterium nucleatum, Provetella intermedia, Bacteroides forsythus, Eikenella corrodens,* and *denticola.*

16. What are the clinical features of localized juvenile periodontitis?
The periodontal destruction is localized to the first permanent molars and/or the permanent central incisors. Clinical signs of inflammation are less acute than would be expected from the severity of destruction. Other features include familial pattern, paucity of plaque, onset during the circumpubertal period, and preponderance of *A. actinomycetemcomitans* when the sites are cultured.

17. What bacteria are associated with rapidly advancing periodontitis?
P. gingivalis
P. intermedia
Bacteroides capillus
E. corrodens

18. What bacteria are associated with refractory periodontitis?
The major infectious agents are *B. forsythus, F. nucleatum, Strep. intermedius, E. corrodens,* and *P. gingivalis.* Although the diseases listed above have clinically distinct manifestation, many of the same players show up in cultural studies again and again. When the diagnosis of refractory or rapidly progressive periodontitis is made, the patient's medical and family history should be thoroughly investigated. There may be underlying systemic medical problems. Do not hesitate to use the clinical medical laboratory and to refer the patient for a complete medical examination.

19. What is the first cellular line of defense of the body against the periopathogens?
Other than the epithelial cell barrier, the first line of defense is the polymorphonuclear neutrophil (PMN).

20. Which periodontal diseases may involve bacterial invasion of the connective tissue?
Localized juvenile periodontitis (LJP)
Gingivitis
Acute necrotizing ulcerative gingivitis (ANUG)

21. What bacteria may be associated with tissue invasion?
For LJP the answer is again *A. actinomycetemcomitans.* For gingivitis and ANUG the culprits are spirochetes.

22. What is meant by a burn-out lesion in a patient with LJP?
At one point the patient with LJP had an infection with periodontal lesions in which the chief etiologic agent was *A. actinomycetemcomitans.* A body responds with an immunologic response and controls the infection, but the bony defect remains. The deep pocketing now becomes inhabited with bacterial flora more characteristic of adult periodontal lesions.

23. What bacteria are associated with gingivitis and periodontitis related to infection with the human immunodeficiency virus (HIV)?
Studies indicate that the bacteria complex associated with HIV-related gingivitis and periodontitis are similar and include *A. actinomycetemcomitans, P. intermedia, P. gingivalis, W. recta,* and yeasts. A major difference may be the number of *W. recta* that are isolated. Concentrations of *W. recta* tend to be higher in HIV-related periodontitis. Enteric bacteria may also be isolated.

24. Patients with deep periodontal pockets and heavy deposits of plaque and calculus may develop an acute periodontal abscess after scaling. Why?
After scaling and root planing of deep sites the coronal tissue heals (contracts and reattaches), but there may be infective material below. The process is analogous to tightening a pursestring.

25. What is a perioendo abscess?
A perioendo abscess is a combined lesion in which periodontal and endodontic problems occur simultaneously. Symptoms may vary, but as a general rule the lesion demonstrates radiographic involvement of the periodontium and periapex with significant probing depths, percussion sensitivity, and pulpal sensitivity. Treatment may include scaling, root planing, periodontal surgery, and root-canal therapy.

26. What treatment is frequently used for a periodontal abscess?
Initial treatment may consist of the establishment of drainage and the removal of the etiologic agents (incision and drainage, scaling, root planing, irrigation), followed first by a course of antibiotic therapy and then by surgical treatment. Variations exist. Be careful of the endoperio abscess.

27. When is it safe to treat a pregnant woman's nonacute periodontal problem?
In general, the second trimester is the window of treatment for most dental procedures. If antibiotics or other medications are indicated, consult with the obstetrician and *Physician's Desk Reference.*

28. Which periodontal disease most nearly fulfills Koch's postulates?
Koch's postulates state that a pathogenic bacterium causes a disease, that the disease is transmissible through the bacteria, and that if you eliminate or control the bacteria, you eliminate the infection. LJP, caused by *A. actinomycetemcomitans,* most nearly fulfills Koch's postulates.

29. Why do most periodontal infections not fulfill Koch's postulates?
The answer lies in the preceding question. Most periodontal infections may be described as mixed anaerobic infections.

30. What is the paradox regarding an acute dental abscess?
The paradox basically pertains to bone loss associated with the lesion. An acute infection may involve rapid, extensive bone loss, but after the infection is eradicated, the lesion has great potential to heal completely.

31. What bacterial group is associated with root caries?
Root caries may be a problem for patients with gingival recession and xerostomia (whether induced by drugs, radiation, or some other agent). The bacteria associated with root caries are gram-positive rods and filaments, particularly *Actinomyces viscosus*.

CONCEPT OF DISEASE ACTIVITY

32. What is meant by active destructive disease?
Active destructive disease indicates a loss of periodontal attachment.

33. How is periodontal disease activity described?
In the past, periodontal disease was thought to be a slow, continuous process. Many of the older texts state that the disease progresses at a rate of 0.1 mm per year, but longitudinal studies have demonstrated otherwise. Current ideas revolve around the concept of random bursts of disease activity.

34. What is the nonspecific plaque hypothesis?
The hypothesis simply states that it is the quantity and not the quality of the plaque that causes periodontal disease.

35. What is meant by a shift in flora in comparing a healthy or diseased periodontal site?
The healthy periodontal site is characterized by a preponderance of gram-positive organisms and fewer gram-negative organisms. In the diseased state the opposite holds true.

36. What bacteria are associated with active destructive periodontal disease (adult periodontitis)?
The bacteria associated with destructive periodontal disease include *P. gingivalis*, *E. corrrodens*, *F. nucleatum*, *W. recta*, *B. forsythus*, and *A. actinomycetemcomitans*. The major player may be *P. gingivalis*.

37. What traditional clinical markers (other than a great change in attachment loss) may be significant in determining active periodontal disease?
One would think that the classic signs of inflammation (tumor, calor, rubor, and suppuration) would be predictors of pending attachment loss. Data demonstrate the sensitivity and specificity only of calor (temperature) for predicting attachment loss. However, it is difficult to leave inflamed gingiva untreated.

38. What two inflammatory mediators may be indicators of disease activity?
Interleukin 1-beta and tumor necrosis factor alpha may indicate disease activity.

PERIODONTAL DIAGNOSIS

39. What is periodontal pocketing?
Periodontal pocketing is the measurement from the crest of the gingiva to the depth of the pocket. Measurements range from <1–3 mm in the healthy state (without inflammation).

40. What sites are routinely probed during a thorough periodontal examination?
Six sites are commonly checked: the mesio-, mid-, and distobuccal sites as well as the corresponding lingual/palatal sites. Most periodontists sweep the probe continuously through the sulcus to get a better feel for the pocket depths as a whole.

41. What is periodontal pseudopocketing?
Pseudopocketing is a condition in which pocketing occurs without attachment loss. A classic example is phenytoin (Dilantin) hyperplasia.

42. How do you make the diagnosis of periodontal disease?
The classic definition for diagnosis of periodontal disease is radiographic evidence of bone loss.

43. Which is more important: attachment loss or periodontal pocketing?
Attachment loss is much more significant because supportive structures are being destroyed. Pocketing may increase or decrease, depending on the severity of gingival inflammation, without attachment loss. Frequently, extensive attachment loss and gingival recession, with poor prognosis of a tooth, may be accompanied by shallow periodontal pocketing.

44. How is attachment loss measured?
The most common way to measure attachment loss is with the periodontal probe, but there is one catch: you must establish a reference point, such as the cementoenamel junction or a restoration margin, from which you make your initial measurement. Probings are then repeated after appropriate intervals and the changes are noted. Other methods include radiographs (subtraction radiography) or automated probes.

45. What are the two most significant clinical parameters for the prognosis of a periodontal involved tooth?
The two most significant clinical parameters are mobility and attachment loss.

46. What is gingival hypertrophy?
Gingival hypertrophy indicates that the gingiva have increased in size and not number. Hypertrophy indicates inflammation, whereas hyperplasia may not.

47. What causes gingival recession?
The major causes are tooth brush or floss abrasion, parafunctional habits, periodontal disease, and orthodontics (if the bands are improperly placed).

48. Which area of the oral cavity has the least amount of attached gingiva?
The buccal, mandibular, premolar area commonly has the least amount of attached tissue.

49. What is a long junctional epithelium?
After a periodontal pocket has been scaled, root planed, and curetted, a soft tissue reattachment to the root surface may occur. This reattachment is called a long junctional epithelium. Pocket reduction is due to a gain in attachment, not to a decrease of inflammation. Fibrous reattachment is also possible.

50. What is the term for gingival cells that attach to the root cementum? How do they attach to the root?
The term is junctional epithelium; the cells attach by hemidesmisomes.

51. What is a mucogingival defect?
Mucogingival defects are defined by periodontal pocketing that goes beyond the mucogingival junction.

52. What are the major risk factors for periodontitis?
Major risk factors for periodontal disease include increased age, poor education, neglect of dental care, previous history of periodontal disease, tobacco use, and diabetes.

53. Which radiographs tend to be most useful for detecting and determining the severity of periodontal disease?
As with interproximal caries, bitewing x-rays tend to be most accurate in assessing bone loss. If the bone loss is extensive, vertical bitewings may be taken.

54. What is the crown-to-root ratio in a healthy dentition?
As a general rule, the crown-to-root ratio in a healthy dentition is 1:2 (for each tooth).

55. What root shapes generally have a more favorable prognosis?
As the preceding question suggests, the crown-to-root ratio is very important. Long, tapering roots are usually sturdier than short, conical roots.

56. What is the clinical significance of the crown-to-root ratios?
Teeth with poor crown-to-root ratios tend to have a worsened prognosis, especially if mobility is significant.

57. What is a fenestration?
If you studied the classical languages you would quickly surmise that fenestration refers to a window in the bone. Bony fenestrations are frequently treated surgically with grafts, with or without guided tissue regeneration.

58. What is positive bony architecture?
In the healthy state the bone contours follow the gingival contours, a pattern that is usually described as scalloping. Negative bony architecture is another story.

59. What is negative bony architecture?
As described above, the bony architecture usually follows the gingival tissue. Negative bony architecture denotes intrabony defect(s). Many periodontists believe that when osseous surgery is performed, it is necessary to recreate positive bony architecture, even at the expense of healthy supporting bone. Growing evidence suggests, however, that the recreation of positive bony architecture does not improve the periodontal prognosis.

60. What are the basic classifications of bony defects?
Bony defects are generally classified according to the number of bony walls that remain. For example, a one-wall defect has only one remaining wall of bone, two-wall defects have two remaining walls, and so on.

61. Which bony defect is most likely to repair or fill naturally after treatment?
Three-wall periodontal defects are most likely to repair naturally after therapy.

62. Why are three-wall defects most likely to repair after treatment?
Three-wall defects tend to be narrow, and three walls may contribute regenerative cells. Two- and one-wall defects lack that luxury.

63. Name the microbiologic methods of assessing bacterial plaque.
There are numerous ways to assess bacterial plaque. General categories include cultural, microscopic, enzymatic, and genetic methods.

64. How are furcations classified?
Furcations are classified according to probing. Class I furcations are found at the onset of probing: class II, approximately halfway into the furcation; and class III, throughout the furcation.

65. What periodontal pathology do diabetes, Papillon-LeFèvre, and Chediak-Higashi disease have in common?
With all of these diseases the normal cellular immunologic response is impaired. The white cells (PMNs) do not function properly. Therefore patients are susceptible to periodontal infections. Watch for abscesses.

66. What is gingival crevicular fluid (GCF)?
GCF is an ultrafiltrate of serum. Therefore, it contains many of the components of serum, particularly complement and antibody. The flow rates of GCF have been used in attempt to predict disease activity. Furthermore, investigators have been interested in GCF for other markers of periodontal breakdown (e.g., beta glucuronidase, interleukin, collagenase).

67. What enzymatic methods may be used to assess bacterial plaque? disease activity?
Some of the enzymatic methods used to assess bacterial plaque associated with active disease include BANA (benzoyl-arginine-naphthylamide) hydrolysis, collagenase, and beta-glucuronidase.

68. What genetically based techniques are used to assess bacterial plaque?
Most of these techniques are based on DNA/RNA homologies. DNA/RNA probes specific for a suspected periodontal pathogen are produced and used to analyze plaque. Commercial probes are on the market. A chairside probe already in use in Europe still awaits FDA approval for use in the United States.

69. Name the major immunologic techniques for assessing bacterial plaque.
The major techniques are fluorescent antibody staining, enzyme-linked immunosorbent assay (ELISA), and latex agglutination, all of which may have high-technology instrumentation applied to them. They are used most commonly as research tools.

ADJUNCTIVE PERIODONTAL THERAPY

70. What antibiotics are used frequently to treat a periodontal abscess?
After the establishment of drainage, whether it be via the sulcus or incision and drainage (I&D), penicillin or amoxicillin (500 mg q6h) provides adequate antibiotic coverage.

71. What antibiotics may be well advised for the treatment of adult periodontitis?
For adult periodontitis, with high concentrations of *P. gingivalis*, doxycycline (50–100 mg bid) provides adequate coverage. *P. gingivalis* tends to be more sensitive to doxycycline than to tetracycline.

72. What is the appropriate response to refractory periodontitis?
This is the time to call out the cavalry. Broad-spectrum antibiotic coverage may be indicated, such as clindamycin (300 mg tid) or amoxicillin/clavulanic acid (500 mg 6h) and metronidazole (250 mg tid). Other combinations exist.

73. How is localized juvenile periodontitis treated?
LJP has a preponderance of *A. actinomycetemcomitans* and is sufficiently treated with tetracycline (250 mg 6h).

74. In a patient who is allergic to penicillin and erythromycin, what is the next antibiotic to be used for prophylaxis for a heart murmur?
The next line of treatment is clindamycin, 300 mg 1 hour before treatment and 150 mg 6 hours later.

75. Why are third-generation cephalosporins frequently contraindicated for the treatment of a periodontal abscess?

Frequently the spectrum of a third-generation cephalosporin becomes so specific that it does not provide adequate antimicrobial coverage. Penicillins should be the first choice; erythromycin is used in penicillin-allergic patients.

76. What complication may occur with broad-spectrum antibiotics?

A major problem is the development of pseudomembranous colitis, which is caused by the overgrowth and toxin production of *Clostridium difficile*.

77. Why are tetracyclines used commonly in the treatment of periodontal disease?

Tetracycline is used primarily for antibiotic coverage, but it has advantages over other antibiotics because it concentrates at levels 2–4 times higher in the gingival crevicular fluid than in the serum, binds to the root surface and can be released over a prolonged time, prevents bacterial reattachment to the root surface, promotes reattachment of fibers to the root surface, and inhibits collagenolytic activity.

78. What are some of the common guidelines or precautions that should be given to a patient in prescribing tetracyclines?

Use of any antibiotic involves the potential to upset the natural bacterial flora. Gastrointestinal distress, including nausea, vomiting, and diarrhea, is possible. Women must be advised of the potential of yeast infections. Other side effects include tinnitus, vertigo, and photosensitivity.

79. Are tetracyclines safe and effective for women who are taking birth control pills?

In general, a woman who is taking birth control pills should avoid the use of tetracyclines. Clinical studies have shown that tetracyclines may cause abnormal breakthrough bleeding during the menstrual cycle.

80. If a patient is not sure whether she is pregnant, should tetracyclines be used to treat an acute periodontal infection?

Tetracyclines exert their bacteriostatic effect by inhibiting protein synthesis at the ribosome. They also cross the placenta and inhibit fetal protein synthesis. Avoid tetracyclines in pregnant patients.

81. What directions should be given to the patient in prescribing oral tetracyclines?

Tetracyclines should be taken between meals (on an empty stomach) with a tall glass of water. Foods and antacids containing relatively high concentration of calcium and iron should not be taken with tetracycline. Tetracycline acts as a chelator with these divalent cations, thereby interfering with its own intestinal absorption. Therapeutic dosages, therefore, are not achieved.

82. What are the major advantages and disadvantages of using doxycycline or minocycline in the treatment of periodontal disease?

The spectrum of doxycycline and minocycline may be slightly better, particularly in covering *P. gingivalis*. Other advantages include less photosensitivity, less chelating, and better patient compliance. Because both antibiotics are more fat-soluble, the dose is reduced to 50 or 100 mg bid. A big disadvantage is cost. Doxycycline and minocycline are much more expensive.

83. What is the major problem with the use of metronidazole?

When prescribing metronidazole, you should advise patients that they must refrain from alcohol or they may become violently ill from the combination (Antabuse effect). Patients should always be advised not to mix any medicine with alcohol.

84. Why is metronidazole effective in treating a periodontal infection?
Metronidazole is most effective in areas of low redox potential, making it ideal for the treatment of anaerobic infections. It is also effective in treating Montezuma's revenge that is caused by a parasite.

85. What is localized drug delivery? How does it apply to periodontal therapy?
Localized drug delivery is being developed to deliver the drug directly to the site of intended use—the periodontal sulcus. The great advantage of such systems is that because they are local, systemic side effects are almost nil. The best studied system involves a tetracycline fiber, but other systems exist. This method is the wave of the future with antibiotics, antiinflammatories, and growth factors.

86. What pathway do nonsteroidal, antiinflammatory drugs (NSAIDs) block?
NSAIDs block the cyclooxygenase metabolism of arachidonic acids.

87. Which mouth rinse appears to be most effective in the control of bacterial plaque?
Chlorhexidine gluconate is the most effective oral rinse for controlling bacterial plaque, particularly because it leaves the greatest residual concentration in the mouth after use.

88. What is sanguinaria? How is it used?
Sanguinaria, an extract from the blood root plant that exhibits antimicrobial properties, has been formulated into various dentifrices and mouthwashes. A major problem with sanguinaria is that it is easily washed from the oral cavity so that the antimicrobial effects are short-lived.

89. HIV-positive patients frequently manifest a condition called hairy leukoplakia in their oral cavity. What microbe is commonly associated with hairy leukoplakia? What is the treatment for this condition?
Candida albicans (yeast) is frequently associated with hairy leukoplakia and should be treated with antifungal medication, including nystatin or fluconazole. Chlorhexidine rinses should be included, because chlorhexidine is also effective against *C. albicans*.

90. What is the primary symptom of root sensitivity?
In general, the primary symptom is sensitivity to cold.

91. What is the cause of root sensitivity?
Root sensitivity is believed to be caused by the movement of fluid in the dentinal tubules, which stimulates the pain sensation (the hydrodynamic theory).

92. How is root sensitivity treated?
Treatment of root sensitivity usually involves seal-coating of the root. Substances routinely used are fluoride mouth rinses, fluoride toothpastes, desensitizing toothpaste, application of composite monomer, and iontophoresis.

93. What is iontophoresis? How is it used in periodontics?
Iontophoresis is analogous to electroplating. In periodontics it is used to treat dentinal sensitivity by electroplating fluoride to the root surface.

OCCLUSAL TREATMENT

94. What is the role of occlusion in periodontal disease?
As a primary player, occlusion has little significance in the etiology of periodontal disease, but it may act as a contributing factor.

95. What are primary and secondary occlusal trauma?
Primary occlusal trauma refers to excessive force applied to a tooth or teeth with normal supporting structures. Secondary occlusal trauma refers to excessive force applied to a tooth or teeth with inadequate support (periodontal disease).

96. When is a nightguard indicated?
A nightguard is indicated whenever the signs or symptoms of bruxism occur.

97. What are the clinical signs of bruxism?
Signs of bruxism may include faceting, TMJ symptoms, masticatory muscle soreness, fractured teeth or restorations, and widened periodontal ligament spaces (on radiographs). These signs may occur in various combinations.

98. What criteria should be followed in constructing a nightguard for the treatment of bruxism?
A nightguard should have four characteristics: (1) it should be made of hard acrylic; (2) it should snap gently over the occlusal surfaces of the maxillary teeth; (3) it should occlude evenly with the mandibular teeth; and (4) it should have even contacts in excursion and be comfortable so that the patient will wear it.

99. When should the splinting of teeth be considered?
Splinting of teeth is performed basically for patient comfort. Little evidence suggests that splinting improves the prognosis of periodontal mobile teeth. In fact, it may worsen the prognosis by limiting oral hygiene access.

100. What do widened periodontal ligament spaces indicate?
Widened periodontal ligament spaces are indicative of occlusal traumatism (no underlying medical problems).

101. What situation may be considered to be "controlled" occlusal trauma?
Orthodontic tooth movement may be considered to be controlled occlusal trauma.

NONSURGICAL TREATMENT OF PERIODONTAL DISEASE

102. What is scaling? root planing? curettage?
Scaling is the removal of hard and soft deposits (plaque and calculus) from tooth surfaces. Root planing is the smoothing of the root surfaces with a scaler or curet. The objective of root planing is to remove additional deposits as well as affected cementum in an attempt to achieve soft-tissue attachment. Curettage is the removal of the lining of the periodontal pocket. This procedure is frequently performed with root planing to promote soft-tissue attachment.

103. What is the treatment routinely used for acute necrotizing ulcerative gingivitis (ANUG)?
Treatment consists of debridement (scaling and root planing) with an antibiotic. Penicillin V/K, 260–500 mg qid for 7 days, should be sufficient. Pain relievers are prescribed if needed. Instructions for oral hygiene should be stressed.

104. What is the treatment for acute suppurating gingivitis?
The treatment is the same as that for ANUG. If the patient does not respond, you may consider changing the antibiotic. If the second antibiotic does not work, you may want to examine systemic factors; for example, diabetics are prone to this type of periodontal problem.

105. What is nonsurgical therapy for periodontal disease?
Nonsurgical treatment is centered on maintenance. Scaling and root planing are performed at greater frequency than in a normal recall schedule.

106. What is the Keyes technique?
The Keyes technique is a method of assessing bacterial plaque via microscopic means (wet-mount slides) and correlating periodontal infection, particularly the numbers of spirochetes and motile rods. This technique was in vogue during the past 10–20 years, but in my opinion additional validation studies are required.

SURGICAL TREATMENT OF PERIODONTAL DISEASE

107. What are the advantages of periodontal surgery over nonsurgical treatment?
The most important reason for performing periodontal surgery is access. It gives you the opportunity to visualize the roots so that calculus may be removed more completely.

108. Name the major complications that may be associated with periodontal surgery.
With any form of surgery, you run the risk of pain, fever, swelling, infection, and bleeding. In addition, other problems that may occur include gingival recession, root caries, and root sensitivity.

109. When is gingivectomy indicated?
Gingivectomies are indicated when there are copious amounts of attached tissue and no intrabony defects. The most common application is treatment of phenytoin hyperplasia.

110. What drugs may cause gingival hyperplasia?
Causative drugs include phenytoin, nifedipine, and cyclosporine A. These medications stimulate proliferation of gingival fibroblasts, causing an overgrowth of the gingiva.

111. What is a full-thickness periodontal flap? a partial-thickness periodontal flap?
After the incision is made, a full-thickness flap involves elevation of the entire soft tissue, whereas a partial-thickness flap involves the splitting (dissection) of the gingival flap, leaving the periosteum adherent to the bone.

112. What is an apically positioned flap? When is it most frequently performed?
The definition is in the name. After the flap has been elevated and the necessary treatment has been performed, the gingiva is positioned at the crest of bone. This procedure is most frequently performed after osseous surgery (e.g., positive architecture, crown lengthening) and usually requires vertical releasing components.

113. What is osteoplasty? What is ostectomy?
Osteoplasty is the reshaping or recontouring of nonsupportive bone. An example is the recontouring and ramping of interproximal bone. Ostectomy is the removal of supporting bone. This procedure is usually performed to create positive architecture or to increase the clinical crown length.

114. When is a crown-lengthening procedure indicated?
The procedure is indicated whenever clinical crown length is inadequate for the restoration. A general rule of thumb for a crown preparation is that you should have 4 mm between the margin of the preparation and the crest of bone to ensure adequate crown length. This measurement maintains a proper biologic width.

115. How are furcations routinely treated?
Formerly, as soon as a furcation became evident on the radiograph, the treatment was tincture of cold steel, better known as extraction. The treatment of furcations varies, depending on the type and the tooth. Treatment may range from simple management with scaling, root planing and curettage to tissue-guided regeneration with bone-grafting material.

116. What is a distal wedge procedure? Where is it commonly found clinically?
As the name implies, in a distal wedge procedure a block of tissue is removed from the distal aspect of a tooth to reduce the pocket depth. Distal wedge procedures are frequently the sequel to the extraction of a third molar. After the third molar is extracted, the bone fill is poor, leaving a periodontal defect.

117. What is a palatal/lingual curtain procedure? Where is it frequently used? Why?
The palatal/lingual curtain procedure is a surgical procedure commonly carried out in treating the maxillary anterior teeth. Deep, interproximal buccal incisions are made to free the palatal tissue; the buccal flap is not elevated. After the palatal/lingual flap is elevated, debridement and scaling/root planing are carried out from the palatal. The rationale behind this procedure is to maintain the buccal gingival architecture to minimize esthetic changes.

118. What is crestal anticipation?
This term is commonly used to describe flap design when surgery is performed, particularly when it would be extremely difficult to position the gingival flap apically at the crest of bone. (In palatal and lingual gingiva, vertical-releasing incisions are difficult or contraindicated.) Basically an inverse bevel gingivectomy to the crest is carried out.

119. When is a root amputation indicated?
Obviously the procedure applies only to multirooted teeth. In general, a root amputation may be performed when periodontal involvement of a single root is severe. Endodontic and prosthetic considerations also must be taken into account.

120. Which teeth are most frequently involved in root amputation procedures?
The requirement of multirooted teeth limits the number of candidates. A vast majority of root amputations involve the maxillary first and second molars.

121. Why are the maxillary first and second molars frequent candidates for root amputation?
Because of the convergence of the distobuccal root of the first molar and the mesiobuccal root of the second molar as the roots move apically, the first and second molars are commonly involved periodontal sites.

122. What are the major advantages of using a laser for periodontal procedures?
There are two major advantages of using a laser for periodontal surgery: (1) the incision is sterile, and (2) the laser cauterizes blood vessels during the procedure. It also has been reported that the postoperative period is less painful because of the desensitization of nerve endings.

123. Why may it be advantageous to use combination therapy (antibiotic and NSAID) in the treatment of periodontal disease?
Combination therapy attempts to kill two birds with one stone. It not only eliminates the etiologic agent but also attempts to control the resultant inflammation (hopefully to prevent bone loss).

124. What surgical procedure is performed as adjunctive therapy for orthodontic tooth rotation? How successful is it?
Routinely a fiberotomy is performed to prevent relapse of the tooth rotation. In general, a fiberotomy is not enough. The rotated tooth still requires some type of stabilization.

125. What medications may affect salivary flow? How may they affect the periodontal health?
Many medicines may influence salivary flow. Prime suspects are tricyclic antidepressants and antihypertensives. Decreased salivary flow diminishes the natural cleansing of the oral cavity, thus increasing the incidence of periodontal disease and caries. Watch for both supra- and subgingival root caries.

GINGIVAL AUGMENTATION AND MUCOGINGIVAL SURGERY

126. When should a soft-tissue graft be considered as an appropriate treatment of gingival recession?
A soft-tissue graft should be considered as soon as the mucogingival junction has been breached (i.e., probing extends beyond the mucogingival junction). Other factors also need consideration, such as location, frenum attachment, root sensitivity, root caries, and required restoration.

127. What is a free gingival graft? What other type of graft procedures may be used?
In a free gingival graft a section of attached gingiva is harvested from an area of the mouth. Routinely the hard palate is used, but any area with sufficient attached gingiva is appropriate. The graft is then sutured to the recipient site. Other grafting procedures include the pedicle or lateral sliding flap, in which the graft is lifted from an area adjacent to the recipient site, but the graft is not freed-up. This procedure maintains vascular supply to the graft.

128. How is bleeding controlled after the palate has been used as the donor site for a free gingival graft?
There are a number of ways to control bleeding at the donor site, including (1) pressure with a moistened gauze, (2) pressure with a tea bag, (3) vasoconstriction (epinephrine in the local anesthetic), (4) suturing (tie off the bleeders), (5) collagen with or without stent, and (6) topical thrombin. I am sure that there are more. If bleeding continues, it may not be a bad idea to assess prothrombin time (PT), partial thromboplastin time (PTT), and platelet count.

129. What is a primary reason for the failure of a free gingival graft?
The chief reason that a free gingival graft fails is disruption of the vascular supply before engraftment. The second most common reason is infection.

130. What is meant by the term necrotic slough of a free gingival graft?
After a free gingival graft has been placed, the healing involves revascularization of the graft. The superificial layers of the graft are the last to be revascularized; therefore, the layer dies off, producing a necrotic slough. Pedicle grafts take their vascular supply with them; hence, no necrotic slough.

131. What type of flap is used at the recipient site of a free gingival graft? Why?
Partial-thickness flaps are used so that the periosteum remains attached to the bone. The reason is that the periosteum is the blood supply for the graft.

132. Why is the bone/periosteum scored during a grafting procedure?
The bone is frequently scored during a free gingival graft to prevent the marsupialization of the graft. In other words, it helps to prevent the mucosa from covering over the graft. Additional methods to prevent this problem include suturing the base (apical) portion of the graft to the mucosa and tacking the mucosa to the periosteum.

133. Why is it difficult to place a free gingival graft in the buccal area of the mandibular premolars?
This procedure can be especially problematic when extensive recession has caused a mucogingival defect. The problem lies in the fact that you may encroach on the mental nerve/ vascular bundle with the graft and cause problems with these structures.

134. When is a frenectomy indicated?
In general, frenectomy is indicated whenever a frenum is causing a problem. For example, a high attachment of a frenum may cause the crestal gingiva to pull away during phonation (ankyloglossia) and mastication, thus opening the pocket for food impaction. This situation frequently arises in the premolar areas.

135. What procedure may be performed in conjunction with a frenectomy to prevent recurrence?
A frenum also may cause a problem in the area between the maxillary central incisors, thus contributing to a diastema. The fibers of the frenum cross the height of the maxilla to the incisive papilla. The papilla may blanch when the frenum is pulled. A free gingival graft is performed in conjunction with the frenectomy to prevent a recurrence of fiber attachment to the papilla.

136. What is a push-back procedure? Why was it used?
A push-back procedure was performed on a larger area of attached gingiva. As the name implies, an incision was made at the mucogingival junction, and the mucosa was pushed-back, leaving exposed bone. Ouch! The area would eventually granulate inward, followed by attached gingiva. Needless to say, the patient never spoke to you again because of the severe postoperative pain. As the question implies, this procedure is no longer in use.

REGENERATIVE PROCEDURES

137. What are the basic types of bone-grafting materials used in the treatment of periodontal defects?
Grafts may be broken down into three fundamental categories: (1) autografts (intraoral and extraoral), (2) allografts, and (3) alloplasts. The autografts may be bone harvested from the patient's hip (extraoral) or from a healing extraction socket or retromolar areas (intraoral). Allografts consist of freeze-dried bone and freeze-dried decalcified bone from another source (usually cadaver bone). Alloplasts are synthetic materials, most commonly used are tricalcium phosphate, calcium carbonate, and hydroxyapatite.

138. What is bone/blood coagulum? Where is it used?
Bone/blood coagulum is another type of grafting material, normally obtained with a chisel or file during osseous surgery. The bone/blood shavings are collected and then packed into the defect in an attempt to promote new bone formation. Because the bone is predominantly cortical, the results are not predictable.

139. What is bone swagging?
Swagging is the bending and breaking of the bony walls into the periodontal defect. It, too, has poor predictability and is not used with great frequency.

140. When should an intraoral autograft from an extraction site be harvested?
As a general guideline, the intraoral autograft should be harvested 6–8 weeks after extraction. This gives the extraction site enough time to become organized with osteogenic components.

141. Which bone-grafting material has the greatest osteogenic potential with the fewest sequelae in periodontal applications?
Osteogenic potential and sequelae are optimal with freeze-dried allografts (cadaver bone).

142. What sequelae may occur with autogenous bone grafts?
Possible sequelae include graft rejection, root resorption, and ankylosis.

143. What growth factors may potentially be used to stimulate osseous regeneration?
The purpose of this question is to inform you of one of the new hot spots in periodontal research. Some day, after the etiologic agents have been removed and the inflammation is under control, growth factors may be applied to regenerate the periodontium. Two growth factors that appear to have a great deal of potential are bone morphogenic protein, platelet-derived growth factor, and insulinlike growth factor. Surely others will emerge.

144. What is guided tissue regeneration (GTR)? Where is it most successful?

GTR involves the placement of a membrane (usually Gore-Tex) over a bony defect during periodontal surgery. A second surgical procedure is needed 6–8 weeks after initial surgery to retrieve the membrane. Defects amenable to this type of treatment are shallow furcations and narrow intrabony defects. GTR may also be applied to ridge augmentation procedures. A resorbable membrane is now commercially available. Therefore, no second surgery is needed to remove the membrane.

145. What are the two basic types of implant placement?

The two basic types of implant placement are submerged and nonsubmerged. Submerged implants require a second surgical procedure to uncover the fixture.

146. What is osseointegration?

Osseointegration is the same as ankylosis.

147. What bacteria are associated with peri-implantitis?

Many of the same species associated with peri-implantitis are also associated with adult periodontitis including *A. actinomycetemcomitans, P. gingivalis,* and *P. intermedia.* Other species frequently detected by cultural methods are *Capnocytophaga* species, *W. recta,* and *E. corrodens.*

148. How are implants maintained?

Implants require maintenance, much like crowns and bridges, and natural teeth. The same principle holds true: cleanliness is next to godliness. Implant systems may have different instruments associated with their maintenance. The instruments are usually plastic-tipped so that the surface of the implant is not scratched. Floss, superfloss, and braided floss are also handy.

BIBLIOGRAPHY

Classification of Periodontal Diseases and Etiologies

1. Haffajee AD, Socransky SS, Dzink JL, et al: Clinical, microbiological and immunological features of subjects with refractory periodontal diseases. J Clin Periodontol 15:390, 1988.
2. Kornman KS, Loesche WJ: Effects of estradiol and pregesterone on *Bacteroides melaningogenicus* and *Bacteroides gingivalis.* Infect Immun 35:256–263, 1982.
3. Listgarten MA: The role of dental plaque in gingivitis and periodontitis. J Clin Periodontol 15:485–487, 1988.
4. Mandell ID, Gaffar A: Calculus revisited. J Clin Periodontal 13:249–257, 1986.
5. Moore WEC, Moore LH, Ranney RR, et al: The microflora of periodontal sites showing active destruction progression. J Clin Periodontol 18:729–739, 1991.
6. Newman MN, Socransky SS: Predominant microbiota of periodontosis. J Periodontol Res 12:120–128, 1977.
7. Sooriyamoorthy M, Gower DB: Hormonal influences on gingival tissue: Relationship to periodontal disease. J Clin Periodontol 16:201–208, 1989.
8. Tanner ACR, Haffer C, Brathall GT, et al: A study of the bacteria associated with advancing periodontitis in man. J Clin Periodontol 6:278, 1979.
9. Zambon JJ, Reynolds HS, Genco RJ: Studies of the subgingival microflora in patients with acquired immunodeficiency syndrome. J Clin Periodontol 61:699–704, 1990.

Concept of Disease Activity

10. Jandinski JJ, Stashenko P, Feder LS, et al: Localization of interleukin 1-beta in human periodontal tissue. J Periodontol 62:36–43, 1991.
11. Lindhe J, Haffajee AD, Socransky SS: The progression of periodontal disease in the absence of periodontal therapy. J Clin Periodontol 10:433–442, 1983.
12. Rossomando EF, Kennedy JE, Handjmichael J: Tumor necrosis factor alpha in gingival crevicular fluid as a possible indicator of periodontal disease in humans. Arch Oral Biol 35:431–434, 1990.
13. Socransky SS, Haffajee AD, Goodson JM, Lindhe J: New concepts of destructive periodontal disease. J Clin Periodontol 11:21–32, 1984.

Periodontal Diagnosis

14. Cochran DL: Bacteriological monitoring of periodontal disease: Cultural, enzymatic, immunological, and nucleic acid studies. Curr Opin Dent 1:37–44, 1991.
15. Goultschin J, Cohen HDS, Donchin M, et al: Association of smoking with periodontal treatment needs. J Periodontol 61:364–367, 1990.
16. Grbic JT, Lamster IB, Celenti RS, Fine JB: Risk indicators for future clinical attachment loss in adult periodontitis: Patient variables. J Periodontol 62:322–329, 1991.
17. Savitt ED, Keville MW, Peros WJ: DNA probes in the diagnosis of periodontal microorganisms. Arch Oral Biol 35(Suppl):153S–159S, 1990.
18. Schlossman M, Knowler WC, Pettitt DT, Genco RJ: Type 2 diabetes mellitus and periodontal disease. J Am Dent Assoc 121:532–536, 1990.

Adjunctive Periodontal Therapy

19. Bonesville P: Oral pharmacology of chlorhexidine. J Clin Periodontol 4:49–65, 1977.
20. Ciancio SA: Antibiotics in periodontal care. In Newman MG, Kornman KS (eds): Antibiotic/Antimicrobial Use in Dental Practice. Carol Stream, IL, Quintessence, 1990, pp 136–147.
21. Goodson JM: Drug delivery. In Perspectives on Oral Antimicrobial Therapeutics. Chicago, IL, American Academy of Periodontology, 1987, pp 61–78.
22. Southard GL, Boulware RT, Walborn DR, et al: Sanguinarine: A new antiplaque agent. Compend Cont Educ Dent 5(Suppl):72–75, 1984.
23. Williams RC: Non-steroidal anti-inflammatory drugs in periodontal disease. In Lewis AJ, Furst DE (eds): Non-steroidal Anti-inflammatory Drugs. New York, Marcel Dekker, 1987, pp 143–155.

Nonsurgical Treatment of Periodontal Disease

24. Drisko CL, Killoy WJ: Scaling and root planing: Removal of calculus and subgingival organisms. Curr Opin Dent 1:74–80, 1991.
25. Hirshfeld L, Wasserman B: A long term survey of tooth loss in 600 treated periodontal patients. J Periodontol 49:225–237, 1978.
26. Pihlstrom B, McHugh RB, Oliphant TH, Ortiz-Campos C: Comparison of surgical and non-surgical treatment of periodontal disease. J Clin Periodontol 10:524–541, 1983.

Surgical Treatment of Periodontal Disease

27. Becker BE, Becker W, Caffesse R, et al: Three modalities of periodontal therapy: 5-year final results. J Dent Res 69:219, 1990.
28. Kalkwarf KL: Surgical treatment of periodontal diseases: Access flaps, bone resection techniques, root preparation, and flap closure. Curr Opin Dent 1:87–92, 1991.
29. Ramfjord SP, Morrison EC, Kerry GJ, et al: Four modalities of periodontal treatment compared over five years. J Clin Periodontol 14:445–452, 1987.
30. Ramfjord SP, Nissle RR, Shick RR, Cooper H: Subgingival curettage versus surgical elimination of periodontal pockets. J Periodontol 39:167–175, 1968.
31. Robertson PB: The residual calculus paradox. J Periodontol 61:65–66, 1990.
32. Tarnow DP, Fletcher P: Root resection vs. maintenance of furcated molars. NY State Dent J 55:34, 36, 39, 1989.

Gingival Augmentation and Mucogingival Surgery

33. Allen EP: Use of mucogingival surgery to enhance esthetics. Dent Clin North Am 32:307–330, 1988.
34. Lang NP, Loe H: The relationship between the width of keratinized gingiva and gingival health. J Periodontol 43:623–627, 1972.
35. Miller PD: Regenerative and reconstructive periodontal plastic surgery: Mucogingival surgery. Dent Clin North Am 32:287–306, 1988.
36. Prato GPP, De Sanctis M: Soft tissue plastic surgery. Curr Opin Dent 1:98–103, 1991.

Regenerative Procedures

37. Becker BE, Becker W: Regenerative procedures: Grafting materials, guided tissue regeneration, and growth factors. Curr Opin Dent 1:93–97, 1991.
38. Branemark PI, Zarb GA, Albrektsson T: Tissue-integrated prostheses. In Osseointegration in Clinical Dentistry. Carol Stream, IL, Quintessence, 1985.
39. Lynch SE, Williams RC, Polson AM, et al: A combination of platelet-derived growth factors enhances periodontal regeneration. J Clin Periodontol 16:545–548, 1989.
40. Magnusson I, Batch C, Collins BR: New attachment formation following controlled tissue regeneration using biodegradable membranes. J Periodontol 59:1–6, 1988.

7. ENDODONTICS

Steven P. Levine, D.M.D.

DIAGNOSIS

1. What is the proper role of the pulp tester in clinical diagnosis?
The pulp tester excites the nervous system of the pulp through electrical stimulation. However, the pulp tester only suggests whether the tooth is vital or nonvital; the crucial factor is the vascularity of the tooth. The pulp test alone is not sufficient to allow a diagnosis and must be combined with other tests.

2. What is the importance of percussion sensitivity in endodontic diagnosis?
Percussion sensitivity is a valuable diagnostic tool. Once the infection or inflammatory process has extended through the apical foramen into the periodontal ligament (PDL) space and apical tissues, pain is localizable with a percussion test. The PDL space is richly innervated by proprioceptive fibers, which make the percussion test a valuable tool.

3. Listening to a patient's complaint of pain is a valuable diagnostic aid. What differentiates reversible from irreversible pulpitis?
In general, with **reversible pulpitis** pain is elicited only on application of a stimulus (i.e., cold, sweets). The pain is sharp, quick, and disappears on removal of the stimulus. Spontaneous pain is absent. The pulp is generally noninflamed. Treatment usually is a sedative dressing or a new restoration with a base.

   Irreversible pulpitis is generally characterized by pain that is spontaneous and lingers for some time after stimulus removal. There are various forms of irreversible pulpitis, but all require endodontic intervention.

4. What are the clinical and radiographic signs of an acute apical abscess?
Clinically an acute apical abscess is characterized by acute pain of rapid onset. The affected tooth is exquisitely sensitive to percussion and may feel "elevated" because of apical suppuration. Radiographic examination may show a totally normal periapical complex or a slightly widened PDL space, because the infection has not had enough time to demineralize the cortical bone and reveal a radiolucency. Electric and thermal tests are negative.

5. Discuss the importance of inflammatory resorption.
Resorption after avulsion injuries depends on the thickness of cementum. When the PDL does not repair and the cementum is shallow, resorption penetrates to the dentinal tubules. If the tubules contain infected tissue, the toxic products pass into the surrounding alveolus to cause severe inflammatory resorption and potential loss of the tooth.

6. A patient presents with a "gumboil" or fistula. What steps do you take to diagnose the cause or to determine which tooth is involved?
All fistulas should be traced with a gutta percha cone, because the originating tooth may not be directly next to the fistula. Fistulas positioned high on the marginal gingiva, with concomitant deep probing and normal response of teeth to vitality testing, may have a periodontal etiology.

7. Why is it often quite difficult to find the source of pain in endodontic diagnosis when a patient complains of radiating pain without sensitivity to percussion or palpation?
Teeth are quite often the source of referred pain. Percussion or palpation pain may be lacking in a tooth in which the inflammatory process has not reached the proprioceptive fibers of the periodontal ligament. The pulp contains no proprioceptive fibers.

8. What is the anatomic reason that pain from pulpitis can be referred to all parts of the head and neck?
In brief, nerve endings of cranial nerves VII (facial), IX (glossopharyngeal), and X (vagus) are profusely and diffusely distributed within the subnucleus caudalis of the trigeminal (V) cranial nerve. A profuse intermingling of nerve fibers creates the potential for referral of dental pain to many sites.

9. Is there any correlation between the presence of symptoms and the histologic condition of the pulp?
No. Several studies have shown that the pulp may actually degenerate and necrose over a period of time without symptoms. Microabscess formation in the pulp may be totally asymptomatic.

10. Describe the process of internal resorption and the necessary treatment.
Internal resorption begins on the internal dentin surface and spreads laterally. It may or may not reach the external tooth surface. The process is often asymptomatic and becomes identifiable only after it has progressed enough to be seen radiographically.

The etiology is unknown. Trauma is often but not always implicated. Resorption that occurs in inflamed pulps is characterized histologically by dentinoclasts, which are specialized, multinucleated giant cells similar to osteoclasts.

Treatment is prompt endodontic therapy. However, once external perforation has caused a periodontal defect, the tooth is often lost.

11. How can one deduce a clinical impression of pulpal health by examining canal width on a radiograph?
Although not a definitive diagnostic tool, pulp chamber and root canal width on a radiograph may give a suggestion of pulp health. When compared with adjacent teeth, very narrowed root canals usually indicate pulpal pathology, such as degeneration due to prior trauma, capping, or pulpotomy or periodontal disease. Conversely, root canals that are very wide in comparison to adjacent teeth often indicate prior pulp damage that has led to pulpal necrosis.

12. What is the significance of the intact lamina dura in radiographic diagnosis?
The lamina dura is the cribriform plate or alveolar bone proper, a layer of compact bone lining the socket. Because of its thickness, an x-ray beam passing through it produces a white line around the root on the radiograph. Byproducts of pupal disease, passing from the apex or lateral canals, may degenerate the compact bone; its loss can be seen on a radiograph. However, this finding is not always diagnostic, because teeth with normal pulps may have no lamina dura.

13. Which radiographic technique produces the most accurate radiograph of the root and surrounding tissues?
The paralleling or right-angle technique is best for endodontics. The film is placed parallel to the long axis of the tooth and the beam at a right angle to the film. The technique allows for the most accurate representation of tooth size.

14. What is the definition of a true combined lesion?
A true combined lesion is due to both endodontic and periodontal disorders that progress independently. The lesions may join as the periodontal lesion progresses apically. Such lesions, if any chance of healing is to occur, require both endodontic therapy and aggressive periodontal therapy. Usually, the prognosis is determined more by the extent of the periodontal lesion.

15. What is the reason that radiographic examination does not show periapical radiolucencies in certain teeth with acute abscesses?
One study showed that 30–50% of bone calcium must be altered before radiographic evidence of periapical breakdown appears. Therefore, in acute infection apical radiolucencies may not appear until later, as treatment progresses.

16. Why do pulpal-periapical infections of mandibular second and third molars often involve the submandibular space?

Extension of any infection is closely tied to bone density, the proximity of root apices to cortical bone, and muscle attachments. The apices of the mandibular second and third molars are usually below the mylohyoid attachment; therefore infection usually spreads to the lingual and submandibular spaces; often the masticator space is also involved.

17. A patient presents with a large swelling involving her chin. Diagnostic tests reveal that the culprit is the lower right lateral incisor. What factor determines whether the swelling extends into the buccal fold or points facially?

A major determining factor in the spread of an apical abscess is the position of the root apex in relation to local muscle attachments. In this particular case, the apex of the lateral incisor is below the level of the attachment of the mentalis muscle; therefore, the abscess extends into the soft tissues of the chin.

CLINICAL ENDODONTICS (TREATMENT)

18. What is the current thinking on use of the rubber dam?

The dam is an absolute necessity for treatment. It ensures a surgically clean operating field that reduces chance of cross contamination of the root canal, retracts tissues, improves visibility, and improves efficiency. It protects the patient from aspiration of files, debris, irrigating solutions, and medicaments. From a medicolegal standpoint, use of the dam is considered the standard of care.

19. What basic principles should be kept in mind for proper access opening?

Proper access is a crucial and overlooked aspect of endodontic practice. The root canal system is usually a multicanaled configuration with fins, loops, and accessory foramina. When possible, the opening must be of sufficient size, position, and shape to allow straight-line access into the canals. Access of inadequate size and position invites inadequate removal of caries, compromises proper instrumentation, and inhibits proper obturation. However, overzealous access leads to perforation, weakening of tooth structure, and potential fracture.

20. What are the current concepts on irrigating solutions in endodontics?

The type of irrigant used is of minor importance in relation to the volume and frequency. The crucial factor is constant irrigation to remove dentinal debris, to prevent blockage, and to lessen the chance of apical introduction of debris. Several studies have shown the efficacy of saline, distilled water, sodium hypochlorite, hydrogen peroxide, combinations of the above, and many other agents. The results show no advantage to chemomechanical preparation of the root canal system.

21. Of what material are endodontic files currently made?

Hand-operated instruments, including broaches, H-type files, K-type files and reamers, K-flex files, and S-files, are made of stainless steel as opposed to carbon steel, which was used in the past. Stainless steel bends more easily, is not as brittle, is less likely to break compared with carbon steel, and can be autoclaved without dulling.

22. What types of hand-operated implements for root canal instrumentation are currently available?

A detailed discussion of the various properties and differences in file-reamer types is beyond the scope of this chapter. K-type files and reamers are still widely used because of their strength and flexibility. H-type Hedstrom files are quite popular because of their aggressive ability to cut dentin. S-files are very efficient for cutting dentin on the withdrawal stroke and for filing and reaming. Flex-R files are a new modification with a noncutting tip design. This design allows for guiding of the tip through curvatures and reduces the risk of ledging, perforation, and transportation of the apex.

For an excellent discussion of instrumentation devices and techniques, the reader is referred to Cohen S, Burns RC (eds): Pathways of the Pulp, 6th ed. St. Louis, Mosby, 1994.

23. What is the current status on acceptability of root canal obturation materials?
Gutta percha remains the most popular and accepted filling material for root canals. Numerous studies have demonstrated that it is the least tissue-irritating and most biocompatible material available. Although differences occur among manufacturers, gutta percha contains transpoly-isoprene, barium sulfate, and zinc oxide, which provide an inert, compactible, dimensionally stable material that can adapt to the root canal walls.

N-2 pastes and other paraformaldehyde-containing pastes are not approved drugs by the Food and Drug Administration (FDA). Several studies have shown conclusively that such root-filling pastes are highly cytotoxic in tissue culture; reactions to bone include chronic inflammation, necrosis, and bone sequestration. Compared with gutta percha, the pastes are highly antigenic and perpetuate inflammatory lesions. For these reasons they are not considered the standard of endodontic care.

24. What is the proper apical extension of a root canal filling?
The proper apical extension of a root canal filling has been discussed extensively for years, and the debate continues. For years recommendations were made to fill a root canal to the radiographic apex in teeth that exhibited necrosis or areas of periapical breakdown and to stop slightly short of this point in vital teeth. Currently, however, it is generally recommended that a root canal be filled to the dentinocementum junction, which is 0.5–2 mm from the radiographic apex. Filling to the radiographic apex is usually overfilling or overextending and increases the chance of chronic irritation of periapical tissues.

25. Describe the walking bleach technique.
The walking bleach technique is used to bleach nonvital teeth with roots that have been filled. The technique involves the placement of a thick white paste composed of sodium perborate and Superoxol in the tooth chamber with a temporary restoration. Several repetitions of this procedure, along with the in-office application of heat to Superoxol-saturated cotton pellets in the tooth chamber, work quite well.

26. List four useful tools in the diagnosis of a vertical crown-root fracture.
1. Transillumination with fiberoptic light
2. Persistent periodontal defects in otherwise healthy teeth
3. Wedging and staining of defects
4. Radiographs rarely show vertical fractures but do show a radiolucent defect laterally from sulcus to apex (which can be probed).

27. Describe the crown-down pressureless technique of root canal instrumentation.
With the crown-down pressureless technique the canal is prepared in a coronal to apical direction by initially instrumenting the coronal two-thirds of the canal before any apical preparation. This technique, popularized by Marshall-Pappin, minimizes apically extruded debris and eliminates binding of instruments coronally, thereby making apical preparation more difficult.

28. What is the balanced-force concept of root canal instrumentation and preparation?
The balanced-force concept, proposed by Roane and Sabala, is based on the idea of balancing the cutting forces over a greater area of the canal and focusing less force on the area where the file tip engages the dentin. The technique is done with the Flex-R file with a noncutting tip and a triangular cross-section. By using this type of file in a counterclockwise reaming motion, ledging is minimized, more inner canal curvature is accomplished, and less zipping of the apex occurs.

Roane JB, Sabala C, Duncanson M: The "balanced force" concept for instrumentation of curved canals. J Endod 11:203, 1985.

29. What is the frequency of fourth canals in mesial roots of maxillary first molars?

In an extensive study of maxillary first molars, 51% of the mesiobuccal roots contained either a larger buccal and smaller lingual canal or two separate canals and foramina. This finding shows the importance of searching for a fourth canal to ensure clinical success.

30. What is the current guideline for the length of time to splint an avulsed tooth (without alveolar fracture)?

It is currently recommended to splint an avulsed tooth for 7–14 days (3–5 weeks with alveolar fracture). If an avulsed tooth is replanted fairly quickly (within 1 hour) and some of the fibroblasts of the periodontal ligament (PDL) and cementoblasts of the root surface remain viable, initial PDL repair may occur in 7–14 days.

31. What is the physiologic basis for the use of calcium hydroxide pastes for resorptive defects or avulsed teeth?

The theory behind the use of calcium hydroxide pastes is that areas of resorption have an acidic pH of approximately 4.5–5. Such areas are more acidic than normal tissue because of the effects of inflammatory mediators and tissue breakdown products. The basic pH of calcium hydroxide neutralizes the acidic pH of the area, thereby inhibiting the resorptive process of osteoclastic hydrolases.

Tronstad L, et al: pH changes in dental tissues after root canal with calcium hydroxide. J Endod 7:17, 1981.

32. What is the current thinking on the use of medicaments in endodontic practice?

Formerly, medicaments were in wide use in endodontics to kill bacteria in the canal. However, current thinking stresses thorough debridement of canals and the use of irrigating solutions to clean canals. Medicaments are not stressed, because all have been shown to be cytotoxic in tissue culture. In addition, several medicaments have been shown to elicit immunologic reactions in animal studies. Mechanical canal cleaning sufficiently lowers microbial levels to allow the local defense mechanisms to heal endodontic periapical lesions.

33. Discuss the variations of postoperative pain in one-visit vs. two-visit endodontic procedures.

Several studies show no difference in postoperative pain in one-visit vs. two-visit endodontic procedures. In fact, one study found that single-visit therapy resulted in postoperative pain approximately one-half as often as multiple-visit therapy.

34. What is the treatment of choice for an intruded maxillary central incisor with a fully formed apex?

Repositioning or surgical extrusion should be done immediately with splinting for 7–10 days. Because pupal necrosis is the usual outcome, pulpectomy within 2 weeks and placement of calcium hydroxide are recommended. Close observation every few months is needed.

35. What is the desired shape of the endodontic cavity (root canal) for obturation in both lateral and vertical condensation techniques?

The canal should be instrumented and shaped so that it has a continuously tapering funnel shape. The narrowest diameter should be at the dentinocemental junction (0.5–1 mm from apex) and the widest at the canal opening.

36. Are electronic measuring devices for root canal of any clinical value in everyday endodontic practice?

Yes. Electronic measuring devices have been shown by several investigators to be quite accurate. In general, they work by measuring gradients in electrical resistance when a file passes from dentin (insulator) to conductive apical tissues. They are quite useful when the apex is obscured on a radiograph by sinus superimposition, other roots, or osseous structures.

37. What is the accepted material of choice for pulp-capping procedures?
The literature has reports of many drugs, medicaments, and antiinflammatory agents used for pulp capping, but the material of choice remains calcium hydroxide. Calcium hydroxide, applied to the pulp tissue, seems to cause necrosis of the underlying tissue, but the continuous tissue often forms calcific bridges.

38. Describe the process of apexification.
Apexification involves the placement of agents in the pulpless permanent tooth, with an incompletely formed apex, to stimulate continued apical closure. Calcium hydroxide pastes are the accepted agents for use in the canals.

39. What is the accepted treatment for carious exposures in primary teeth?
For carious exposures in primary teeth in which the tissue appears vital and the inflammation is only in the coronal pulp, the formocresol pulpotomy is still widely accepted. When a carious exposure shows total pulpal degeneration (necrosis), full pulpectomy is indicated with placement of a resorbable zinc oxide-eugenol (ZOE) paste.

40. What is the role of sealer-cements in root canal obturation?
Sealer-cements are still widely recommended for use with a semisolid obturating material (gutta percha). The sealers fill discrepancies between the root filling and canal wall, act as a lubricant, help to seat cones of gutta percha, and fill accessory canals and/or foramina apically.

41. What biologic property is shared by all sealer-cements used in endodontics?
Studies of biocompatability have shown that all sealer-cements are highly toxic when freshly mixed, but the toxicity is reduced on setting. Chronic inflammatory responses, which usually persist for several days, are often cited as a reason not to avoid apical over-extension of the sealer. Several studies have recommended the use of sealers that are more biocompatible, such as AH-26 and the newer calcium hydroxide-based sealers (Sealapex and CRCS).

42. In using Cavit as an interappointment temporary seal, what precautions must be taken?
Cavit, which is a hygroscopic single paste containing zinc oxide, calcium and zinc phosphate, polyvinyl and chloride acetate, and triethanolamine, requires placement of at least 3 mm of material to ensure a proper seal and fracture resistance.

43. What materials or devices are of use in removing gutta percha for retreatment?
Initial removal should be done with endodontic drills (Gates-Glidden or Peezo) or by using a heated plugger to remove the coronal portion of the gutta percha. This procedure allows space in the canal for placement of solvents to dissolve remaining material. Solvents include chloroform, xylene, methyl chlororform and eucalyptol. Chloroform is the most effective, although it has been used less because of reported carcinogenic potential. Xylene and eucalyptol are the least effective. Once the remaining gutta percha has been softened, it often can be removed by files or reamers.

Wennberg A, Orstavik D: Evaluation of alternatives to chloroform in endodontic practice. Endod Dent Traumatol. 5:234,1989.

44. What are the etiology, histologic characteristics, and treatment for internal resorption?
The exact etiology is unknown, but internal resorption is often seen after trauma that results in hemorrhage of vessels in the pulp and chronic inflammatory cells. Macrophages have been shown to differentiate into dentinoclastic-type cells. With this proliferation of granulation tissue, resorption can occur. Treatment is to remove the pulpal tissues as soon as possible so that tooth structure is not perforated.

45. Does preparation of the post immediately on obturation have a different effect on the apical seal of a root canal filling from delayed preparation?
Research with dye leakage studies has shown no difference and no effect on the apical seal whether post preparation is immediate or delayed.

Madison S, Zakariasen K: Linear and volumetric analysis of apical leakage in teeth prepared for posts. J Endod 10:422–427, 1984.

46. What temperature and immersion time are needed to sterilize endodontic files in a bead sterilizer?
At the proper temperature of 220° C (428° F) in the bead sterilizer, an endodontic file should be immersed for 15 seconds. However, because of the potential for a wide variation of temperatures in the transfer medium (beads or salt), this technique should be secondary to other, more reliable techniques of sterilization.

47. What is the best and easiest technique for sterilization of gutta percha cones?
Immersion of the cone in a 5.25% solution of sodium hypochlorite for 1 minute is quite effective in killing spores and vegetative organisms.

Senia SE, et al: Rapid sterilization of gutta percha cones with 5.25% sodium hypochlorite. J Endod 1:136, 1975.

48. What simple techniques should be used to avoid apical ledging and perforation?
Overly aggressive force should not be used in the apical area. A light touch with a precurved file used to negotiate apical curvature is necessary to maintain proper canal curvature.

49. Which type of file is the strongest of all files and cuts least aggressively?
K-files are the strongest of all files, and because they cut the least aggressively, they can be used with quarter-turn pulling motion, rasping, or clockwise-counterclockwise motions.

50. List four criteria that must be met before obturation of a canal.
　　1. The patient must be asymptomatic; the tooth in question must not be sensitive to percussion or palpation.
　　2. No foul odor should emanate from the tooth.
　　3. The canal should not produce exudate.
　　4. The temporary restoration should be intact, i.e., no leakage has contaminated the canal.

51. How does preparation of the canal for filling techniques that use injection of gutta percha differ from that for conventional techniques?
All injection techniques require a more flared canal body and a definite apical constriction to prevent flow of softened gutta percha into periapical tissues.

52. What is the treatment of choice for a primary endodontic lesion in a mandibular molar with secondary periodontal involvement (including furcation lucency) in a periodontally healthy mouth?
Treatment generally consists solely of endodontic therapy. Necrotic pulpal tissue that causes furcation and lateral root or apical breakdown also may cause periodontal pockets through the sulcus, but these are actually fistulas rather than true pockets. Endodontic therapy alone often heals this secondary periodontal involvement.

53. What is the current thinking on the prognosis of pulp capping and partial pulpectomy procedures on traumatically exposed pulps?
In a study of traumatically exposed pulps, including both mature teeth and teeth with immature apices, Cvek found that pulp capping or partial pulpectomy procedures were

successful in 96% of cases. In all teeth the superficial pulp in the traumatized area was carefully excised. Cvek and others agree that such procedures are generally more successful in vital teeth with immature root formation.

Cvek M, Lundberg M: et al: Histological appearance of pulps after exposure by a crown fracture: Partial pulpotomy and clinical diagnosis of healing. J Endod 9:8–11, 1983.

54. What is the current thinking on ideal treatment for carious exposure of a mature permanent tooth?

There is general agreement that carious exposure of a mature permanent tooth generally requires endodontic therapy. Carious exposure generally implies bacterial invasion of the pulp, with toxic products involving much of the pulp. However, partial pulpotomy and pulp capping of a carious exposure in a tooth with an immature apex have a higher chance of working.

55. You have elected to perform partial pulpotomy and to place a calcium hydroxide cap on a maxillary permanent central incisor with blunderbuss apex in a young boy. What follow-up is necessary?

Close monitoring of the tooth is necessary. First, it is important to see whether any pathology develops. If necrosis occurs with apical pathology, extirpation with apexification is needed. On the other hand, if vitality is maintained in such teeth, root formation continues, along with dystrophic calcification.

56. What is the recommended technique for the access opening in endodontic therapy for maxillary primary incisors?

A facial approach is generally recommended for such teeth, which need pulpectomy with a filling of zinc oxide-eugenol paste. Because of esthetic problems and the difficulty in bleaching, endodontic therapy is followed by composite facial restoration.

57. Can infections of deciduous teeth cause odontogenesis of the permanent teeth?

In one study, local infections of deciduous teeth for up to 6 weeks did not influence odontogenesis of the permanent central incisors. However, longstanding infections may have a profound effect on permanent teeth buds because of direct communication between the pulpal and periodontal vasculature of the deciduous tooth and the plexus surrounding the developing permanent tooth.

58. Thermafil endodontic obturators are now widely used. What is the basic methodology?

Prenotched stainless steel files coated with alpha-phase gutta percha are used to obturate the canal. Selection of the Thermafil device depends on the last carrier and condenser for the thermally plasticized alpha-phase gutta percha. Alpha-phase rather than the more common beta-phase gutta percha is used, because, when heated, it has superior flow properties and adheres well to the metal carrier.

59. What is the major difference between the two main thermoplasticized gutta percha techniques on the market?

In the Obtara II system, gutta percha heated to 160°C is injected through a silver needle tip at a temperature of about 65°C. The Ultrafil system is a low-temperature technique that heats the gutta percha to 70°C for injection. Both techniques stress the importance of maintaining constriction at the cementodential junction to prevent flow of gutta percha beyond the apex.

60. What is the "dentin-chips apical-plug filling technique"?

This technique consists of filling the last 1–2 mm of the apex of the canal with dentin chips to seal the apical foramen. Above this is placed a seal of gutta percha. This so-called biologic seal of dentin chips should be made only after proper debridement of the canal to avoid apical placement of infected chips. The efficacy of this technique is controversial.

61. What are the characteristics of the recently introduced Lee Endo-fill technique?
This injectable silicone resin can be used by itself or in conjunction with gutta percha. It consists of a silicone monomer and silicone-based catalyst with bismuth subnitrate filler. The resin adapts well to tooth structure, penetrates accessory canals and has low tissue toxicity.

62. In treating a maxillary lateral incisor, what particular care must be taken in instrumenting the apical portion?
The apical root portion usually curves toward the distal palatal space; this configuration must be negotiated carefully.

63. Should the smeared layer of dentinal debris be removed from canal walls?
Yes. Removal of the smeared layer is recommended because of the possibility that it harbors bacteria.

64. What is considered the most reliable technique to remove the smeared layer of organic and inorganic dentinal debris from canal walls?
The recommended technique is the use of a chelating agent, such as EDTA with sodium hypochlorite, during instrumentation.

65. What are the ideal storage media for avulsed teeth?
If possible, an avulsed tooth should be left in the socket or in the oral fluids (for example, in the vestibule). If this is not possible, milk is a suitable storage medium. Milk and saliva are equally suitable storage media because of their osmotic properties and ability to preserve viability of cells in the periodontal ligament. Because of its hypotonicity, water is not a suitable medium.

66. When an avulsed tooth is replanted, what are the current recommendations concerning rigid or functional splinting?
Recent studies show that early functional stimulus may improve the healing of luxated teeth. It is advantageous to reduce the time of fixation to the time necessary for clinical healing of the periodontium, which may take place in a few weeks. Andreasen has shown that prolonged rigid immobilization increases the risk of ankylosis; thus the splint should allow some vertical movement of the involved teeth.

> Andreasen J: Effect of masticatory stimulation on dentoalveolar ankylosis after experimental tooth replantation. Endod Dent Traumatol 1:13–16, 1985.
> Andreasen J: Periodontal healing after replantation of traumatically avulsed human teeth: Assessment by mobility testing and radiography. Acta Odontol Scand 33:325–335, 1975.

67. What is the single most important factor in determining the degree and severity of the pulpal response to a tooth preparation (cutting) procedure?
Research has shown that the remaining dentin thickness between the floor of the cavity preparation and the pulp chamber is the most crucial determinant of the pulpal response. In general, a 2-mm thickness of dentin provides a sufficient degree of protection from the trauma of high-speed drills and restorative materials. With a thickness less than 2 mm, the inflammatory response in the pulp seems to increase dramatically. Neither age nor tooth size has as significant an effect.

> Swerdlow H, Stanley HR: Reaction of human dental pulp to cavity preparation. J Prosthet Dent 9:121, 1959.

68. In restoring a tooth with a deep carious lesion, clinicians often excavate the caries and place a temporary sedative restoration to allow symptoms to subside. What is the rationale behind this procedure in relation to pulpal physiology?
A deep carious lesion produces an inflammatory response in the pulp tissue adjacent to the dentinal tubules in the area of the caries. Removal of the irritation to the pulp and placement

of a sedative filling allow new odontoblasts to differentiate and to produce a reparative dentin in the involved area. This process usually requires approximately 20 days for odontoplastic regeneration and 80 days for reparative dentin formation.

Stanley HR: The rate of tertiary dentin formation in the human tooth. Oral Surg 21:100, 1966.

69. What is the most common reason for failure of root canals?

Although an endodontically treated tooth may fail for various reasons, including fracture, periodontal disease, or prosthetic complication leading to one of the above, the most common cause of failure is incompletely and inadequately debrided and disinfected root canals. The time-honored saying that what you take out of the canal is not as important as what you put in has much merit. The chemomechanical debridement of the root canal system, which is necessary to remove all irritants to the surrounding apical and periodontal tissues, is still the crucial aspect of root canal treatment.

PULP AND PERIAPICAL BIOLOGY

70. What is the dental pulp? Describe in a brief paragraph the ultrastructural characteristics of this remarkable tissue.

The dental pulp is a matrix composed of ground substance, connective cells and fibers, nerves, a microcirculatory system, and a highly specialized and differentiated cell called the odontoblast. The dental pulp is similar to other connective tissues in the body, but its ability to deal with injury and inflammatory reactions is severely limited by the mineralized walls that surround it. Therefore, its ability to increase blood supply during vasodilation is impaired.

71. Give a brief description of the most accepted theory about the mechanism of dentin sensitivity.

Several ideas have been postulated, but the most plausible theories are based on the fact that the dentinal tubule acts as a capillary tube. The tubule contains fluid, or a pulpal transudate, that is displaced easily by air, heat, cold, and explorer tips. This rapid inward or outward movement of fluid in tubules may excite odontoblastic processes, which have been shown to travel within the tubules, or sensory receptors in the underlying pulp.

Brannstrom M, Astrom A: The hydrodynamics of the dentine: Its possible relationship to dentinal pain. Int Dent J 22:219–227, 1972.

72. A 45-year-old woman presents for consultation. She is asymptomatic. Radiographs reveal a radiolucent lesion apical to teeth 24 and 25 with no swelling or buccal plate expansion. The dentist diagnosed periapical cemental dysplasia. How is this diagnosis confirmed?

Periapical cemental dysplasia or cementoma presents as a radiolucent lesion in its early stages. It is a fibroosseous lesion developing from cells in the periodontal ligament space. The teeth involved respond normally to vitality testing.

73. What is the effect of orthodontic tooth movement on the pulp?

In progressive, slow orthodontic movement, the minor circulatory changes and inflammatory reactions are reversible. However, with excessively severe orthodontic forces, disruption of pulpal vascularity may be irreversible, leading to disruption of odontoblasts and fibroblasts and possible pulpal necrosis. Rupture of blood vessels in the periodontal ligament also may affect pulpal vascularity. In addition, orthodontic tooth movement is associated with excessive root resorption and blunted roots, both of which may occur with continued vitality.

74. Inflammatory mediators cause vasodilation of blood vessels. How does vasodilation in the pulp differ from that in other tissues?

Vasodilation in all tissues is a defense mechanism, controlled by various inflammatory mediators, to allow tissue survival during inflammation. The pulp responds differently, with an initial increase in blood flow followed by a sustained decrease. This secondary vasoconstriction often leads to the demise of the pulp.

Kim S: Regulation of blood flow of the dental pulp. J Endod 15(9):1989.

75. Is it possible to differentiate a periapical cyst from a periapical granuloma on the basis of radiographic appearance alone?

No. Radiographic appearance is not diagnostic. Often a sclerotic border may be present, but its absence does not preclude cystic formation. An exhaustive study indicates that lesions greater than 200 mm^3 are usually cystic in nature.

Natkin E, Oswald RJ, Carnes LI: The relationship of lesion size to diagnosis, incidence and treatment of periapical cysts and granulomas. Oral Surg Oral Med Oral Pathol 57:82–94, 1984.

76. A patient presents for diagnosis and treatment. A maxillary central incisor has a prior history of trauma. The patient is asymptomatic, and the radiograph is normal. Because the tooth gives no response to electric pulp tester, you elect to do endodontic therapy without anesthesia. However, with access and instrumentation the patient feels everything. Explain the inconsistency.

The electric pulp tester excites the A8 fibers in the tooth. The pulp contains A8 and C nociceptive fibers; the A8 fibers have a lower stimulation threshold than the C fibers. The C fibers are more resistant to hypoxia and can function long after the A8 fibers are inactivated by injury to pulp tissue. The electric pulp tester does not stimulate C fibers.

77. List six normal changes in pulp tissue due to age.

(1) Decrease in size and volume of pulp, (2) increase in number of collagen fibers, (3) decreased number of odontoblasts (4) decrease in number and quality of nerves, (5) decreased vascularity, and (6) overall increase in cellularity.

Bernick S: Effect of aging on the nerve supply to human teeth. J Dent Res 46:694, 1967.

78. What is the meaning of the term dentinal pain?

Dentinal pain is due to the outflow of fluid in dentinal tubules that stimulates free nerve endings, most likely A8 fibers. Dentinal pain is usually associated with cracked teeth (into the dentin), defective fillings, or hypersensitive dentin. The pain produced by such stimulation does not usually signify that the pulp is inflamed or the tissue injured, whereas pulpal pain is due to true tissue injury associated with stimulation of C fibers.

79. Do the odontoblastic processes extend all the way through the dentin?

This controversial topic has been studied extensively by several investigators. The process is basically an extension of the cell body of the odontoblast. It is the secretory portion of the odontoblast and contains large amounts of microtubules and microfilaments. Light microscopic studies have generally shown odontoblastic processes only in the inner one-third of dentin; this finding agrees with scanning electron microscope studies and transmission electron microscope studies, which showed processes mainly in the inner one-third of dentin. However, one series of studies suggested that processes go all the way through dentin. More elaborate techniques with immunofluorescent antibody labeling against microtubules also showed staining the entire length of the dentin, suggesting that the processes extend the entire length of the dentinal tubule.

Brannstrom M: The dentinal tubules and the odontoblast processes. Acta Odontol Scand 30:291, 1972.

Gunji T, et al: Distribution and organization of odontoblast processes in human dentin. Arch Histol Jpn 46:213, 1983.

Sigal MJ: The odontoblast process extends to the dentinoenamel junction: An immunocytochemical study of rat dentine. J Histochem Cytochem 32:872, 1984.

Thomas HF: The extent of the odontoblast process in human dentin. J Dent Res 58:2207, 1979.

80. Describe briefly the circulatory system of the dental pulp.

The pulp contains a true microcirculatory system. The major vessels are arterioles, venules, and capillaries. The capillary network in the pulp is extensive, especially in the subodontoblastic region, where the important functions of transporting nutrients and oxygen to pulpal cells occurs and waste products are removed. The pulpal microcirculation is under neural control and also under the influence of chemical agents, such as catecholamines, that exert their effects at the alpha and beta receptors found in pulpal arterioles.

Cohen S, Burns RC (eds): Pathways of the Pulp, 6th ed. St. Louis, Mosby, 1994.

81. Have immunoglobulins and immunocompetent cells been found in the dental pulp?

Yes. Numerous studies have demonstrated that the pulp and periapical tissues are able to mount an immune response against injury to the pulp and apical tissues. All classes of immunoglobulins have been identified in the dental pulp, and microscopic examination of damaged pulpal tissue reveals the presence of leukocytes, macrophages, plasma cells, lymphocytes, giant cells, and mast cells.

MICROBIOLOGY AND PHARMACOLOGY

82. What types of bacteria are the predominant pathogens in endodontic-periapical infections?

Many well-done studies have shown definitively the predominant role of gram-negative obligate anaerobic bacteria in endodontic-periapical infections. Earlier studies generally implicated facultative organisms (streptococci, enterococci, lactobacilli), but improved culturing techniques established the predominance of obligate anaerobes. A recent study further demonstrated the important role of *Porphyromonas endodontalis* (formerly *Bacteroides endodontalis*) in endodontic infections.

Van Winkelhoff, et al: *Porphyromonas endodontalis:* Its role in endodontic infections. J Endod 18:431, 1992.

83. What is considered the antibiotic of choice in treatment of orofacial infections of endodontic origin?

In light of all the new microbiologic research implicating the predominance of obligate anaerobes, drug sensitivity tests still show the penicillins to be the drugs of choice. Penicillin is highly effective against most of the obligate anaerobes in endodontic infections, and because the infections are of a mixed nature with strict substrate interrelationships among various bacteria, the death of several strains has a profound effect on the overall population of an endodontic-periapical infection.

84. What antibiotics are considered most effective in treatment of orofacial infections of endodontic origin that do not respond to the penicillins?

For infections not responding to the penicillins, clindamycin is often recommended. It produces high bone levels and is highly effective against anaerobic bacteria, but it must be used with caution because of the potential for pseudomembranous colitis. A second choice is metronidazole, which also is quite effective against gram-negative obligate anaerobes.

85. What is the current status of culturing and sensitivity testing for endodontic-periapical infections?

Culturing and sensitivity testing have been a controversial topic in endodontic practice for years. According to current thinking, if the proper clinical guidelines are followed, including use of rubber dam, proper chemomechanical cleaning of the root canal system, and proper use of correct antibiotics as indicated, culturing and sensitivity testing are not required. Proper culturing for both facultative and anaerobic bacteria is expensive, time-consuming, and not cost-effective, given the high success rate of properly done endodontic therapy.

86. The role of gram-negative anaerobic bacteria is an established fact in the pathogenesis of endodontic lesions. What role does the bacterial endotoxin play?

Endotoxins are highly potent lipopolysaccharides released from the cell walls of gram-negative bacteria. They are able to resorb bone via stimulation of osteoclastic activity, activation of complement cascades, and stimulation of lymphocytes and macrophages. Various studies have demonstrated their presence in pulpless teeth (with necrotic tissue) and apical lesions.

87. What roles do nonsteroidal anti-inflammatory drugs (NSAIDs) have in endodontic practice?

NSAIDs have a significant role in endodontic practice. In many clinical cases the patient requires postoperative medication to control pericementitis, which can be quite painful after pulpectomy and may persist for several days. The NSAIDs are quite effective; their mechanism of action is to inhibit synthesis of prostaglandins. One study showed that ibuprofen, when given preoperatively to symptomatic and asymptomatic patients, significantly reduces postoperative pericementitis.

Dionne RA, et al: Suppression of postoperative pain by preoperative administration of ibuprofen in comparison to placebo, acetaminophen and acetominophen plus codeine. J Clin Pharmacol 23:37–43, 1983.

88. What is the latest thinking on the role of black-pigmented anaerobic rods in the etiology of infected root canals and periapical infection?

Black-pigmented anaerobic rods have been shown to play an essential role in the etiology of endodontic infections when present in anaerobic mixed infections. The most strongly implicated organism is *Porphyromonas endodontalis*, which, because of its need for various growth factors, is directly related to the presence of acute periapical inflammation, pain, and exudation.

89. A patient presents with swelling, in obvious need of endodontic therapy. His medical history is significant for penicillin allergy and asthma, for which he is taking Theo-Dur. What precautions should you exercise?

By no means should erythromycin be used as an alternative to penicillin. Theo-Dur is a form of theophylline used for chronic reversible bronchospasm associated with bronchial asthma, and erythromycin has been shown to elevate significantly serum levels of theophylline.

90. For years it was taught that any bacteria left behind in an obturated canal would die and therefore cause no problems. What are the latest findings about this controversy?

The most recent electron micrograph studies have shown persistence of bacteria in the apical portion of roots in therapy-resistant lesions. The result is persistent periapical pathosis.

91. What efficacy do the cephalosporins have in treating acute pulpal-periapical infections?

Although the cephalosporins are broad-spectrum antibiotics, their activity is limited in pulpal-periapical infections, which are mixed infections predominantly due to obligate anaerobic bacteria. The cephalosporins are not highly effective against such bacteria and actually have less activity against many anaerobes than penicillin. For serious infections that are penicillin- or erythromycin-resistant, clindamycin is much more effective because of its activity against the obligate and facultative organisms in pulpal-periapical infections.

ANESTHESIA

92. What is the physiologic basis of the difficulty in achieving proper pulpal anesthesia in the presence of inflammation or infection?

Attaining effective pulpal anesthesia in the presence of pulpal-alveolar infection or inflammation is often quite difficult because of changes in tissue pH. The normal tissue pH of 7.4 decreases to 4.5–5.5. This change in pH due to pulpal-periapical pathology favors a shift to a cationic form of the local anesthesia molecule, which cannot diffuse through the lipoprotein neural sheath. Therefore, anesthesia is ineffective.

93. What is the significance of the mylohyoid nerve in successful anesthesia of the mandibular first molar?

The mylohyoid nerve is often implicated in unsuccessful anesthesia of the first molar. This nerve branches off the inferior alveolar nerve above its entry into the mandibular foramen. The mylohyoid nerve then travels in the mylohyoid groove in the lingual border of the mandible to the digastric and mylohyoid muscles. However, because it often carries sensory fibers to the mesial root of the first molar, lingual anesthetic infiltration may be required to block it.

94. What is the method of action of injection into the periodontal ligament?

Injection into the periodontal ligament is not a pressure-dependent technique. The local anesthetic works by traveling down the periodontal ligament space and shutting off the pulpal microcirculation. To be effective, this technique requires the use of a local anesthetic with a vasoconstrictor.

95. The Gow-Gates block is an effective alternative to the inferior alveolar block. When is it indicated? Briefly describe how it works.

In patients in whom the traditional inferior alveolar block is ineffective or impossible to perform because of infection or inflammation, the Gow-Gates block has a high success rate. It is a true mandibular block that anesthetizes all the sensory portions of the mandibular nerve. The injection site is the lateral side of the neck of the mandibular condyle; thus it is effective when intraoral swelling contraindicates the inferior alveolar block.

96. What is the reason for attempting to anesthetize the mylohyoid nerve for endodontic treatment of a symptomatic lower first molar?

The mylohyoid nerve has been shown to supply sensory innervation to mandibular molars, especially the mesial root of first molars. Infiltration of this nerve as it courses along the medial surface of the mandible is often helpful.

97. A drug salesman has convinced you to use propoxycaine hydrochloride as a local anesthetic. Is there any true or absolute contraindication to use of an ester anesthetic?

Yes. Patients who have a hereditary trait known as atypical pseudocholinesterase have an inability to hydrolyze ester-type local anesthetics. Therefore, toxic reactions may result. Only amide anesthetics should be used.

98. A patient presents with an extremely painful lower molar requiring endodontic therapy. You have already used six cartridges of lidocaine with epinephrine to achieve anesthesia. The patient begins to react differently. In brief, what are the signs of local anesthetic toxicity?

Local anesthetic toxicity depends on the blood level and the patient's status. In general, a mild toxic reaction manifests as agitation, talkativeness, and increased vital parameters (blood pressure, heart rate, and respiration). A massive reaction manifests as seizures, generalized collapse of the central nervous system, and possible myocardial depression and vasodilation.

SURGICAL ENDODONTICS

99. What is the purpose of the apicoectomy procedure in surgical endodontics?

Perpetuation of apical inflammation or infection often is due to poorly obturated canals, tissue left in the canal, or quite often an apical delta of accessory foramina containing remnants of necrotic tissue. The removal of this apical segment via apicoectomy usually removes the nidus of infection.

100. A patient presents for apicoectomy on a maxillary central incisor with failed endodontic therapy. A well-done porcelain-to-gold crown is present, with the gold margin placed in the gingival sulcus for esthetic purposes. What flap design is most appropriate?

A full mucoperiosteal flap involving the marginal and interdental gingival tissues may potentially cause loss of soft-tissue attachments and crestal bone height, thereby causing an esthetic problem with the gold margin of the crown. Instead, a submarginal rectangular (Luebke-Ochsenbein) flap, preserving the marginal and interdental gingiva, is recommended.

101. What is the material of choice for root end fillings in surgical endodontics?

Histologic studies have compared several materials, including amalgam, EBA cement, resins, polycarboxylate cements, glass ionomers, and gold foils. Although no study has shown a definitive superiority of one over another, the most commonly used today are amalgam and EBA cements. The type of material is properly secondary in importance to the root resection technique, apical preparation, curettage of the lesion, and technique in placement.

102. What type of scalpel is best used for intraoral incision and drainage of an endodontic abscess?

A pointed no. 11 or no. 12 blade is preferred over a rounded no. 15 blade.

103. In performing apical surgery on the mesial root of maxillary molars, what mistake is commonly made?

It is important to look for unfilled mesiolingual canals in such roots. Therefore, a proper long bevel is necessary to expose this commonly unfilled fourth canal.

104. Numerous studies have addressed the success rates of endodontic surgery. Most agree, however, on certain basic conclusions. Can you name the most common conclusions?

All the success studies share cetain basic conclusions. First, the success of endodontic surgery is closely related to the standard of treatment of the root canal. Second, orthograde (conventional) root fills are preferred, if possible. Thirdly, the success rate is about 20% lower for retrograde fills than for properly done orthograde fills.

Andreasen JO, Rud J: A multivariate analysis of various factors upon healing after endodontic surgery. Int J Oral Surg 1:258–271, 1972.

Rud J, Andreasen JO: Radiographic criteria for the assessment of healing after endodontic surgery. Int J Oral Surg 1:195–214, 1972.

105. What is the recommended surgical approach for apical surgery on palatal roots of maxillary molars?

The palatal approach is recommended; with proper flap design, size of flap and proper reflection are not difficult procedures. The buccal approach is potentially too damaging to supporting bone of the molar and may actually cause more risk of postoperative sinus problems.

106. Why is a "slot preparation" often recommended in preparation of root end filling for mesial roots of maxillary or mandibular roots?

The slot preparation is a trough-type preparation that extends from one canal orifice to another canal orifice in the same root. This procedure is accomplished with undercuts in the adjacent walls. The slot preparation allows not only sealing of the canal orifices but also small anastomoses between the main canals.

107. Has the ideal retrosurgical material been developed?

No. Many research studies have been published about a myriad of materials. However, the ideal is not yet determined. Most likely the material itself is not as important as the surgical preparation, the depth of the preparation, and how it is placed.

108. After root end resection during endodontic surgery, many practitioners apply citric acid to the exposed dentin surface. What is the rationale behind this practice?

A desired result of root end surgery (apicoectomy) is to achieve, if possible, a functional apical dentoalveolar apparatus with cementum deposition on the root end. However, the resected root end is covered with a smeared layer of dentin from the high-speed bur, which does not allow reattachment of newly deposited cementum. Applying citric acid for 2 or 3 minutes dissolves the smear layer and causes a small degree of demineralization of dentin. This, in turn, exposes collagen fibrils of the dentinal organic matrix and allows a proper area for attachment of collagen fibrils from newly formed cementum.

Polson AM, et al: The production of a root surface smear layer by instrumentation and its removal by citric acid. J Periodontol 55:443–446, 1984.

109. Several studies have shown that resected mandibular molars fail twice as often as resected maxillary molars. What are the major etiologic reasons for failure?

The most common cause of failure is root fracture, followed in order by cement washouts around restorations, undermining caries, and recurrent periodontal pathoses around remaining roots.

Langer, Wagenberg: An evaluation of root resections: A ten-year study. J Periodontol 52:719–722, 1981.

Erpensten: A 3-year study of hemisectioned molars. J Clin Periodontol 10:1–10, 1983.

BIBLIOGRAPHY

1. Cohen S, Burns RC (eds): Pathways of the Pulp, 6th ed. St. Louis, Mosby, 1994.
2. Guttman J, Harrison J: Surgical Endodontics. Cambridge, MA, Blackwell Scientific Publications, 1991.
3. Journal of Endodontics.

8. RESTORATIVE DENTISTRY

Elliot V. Feldbau, D.M.D., and Steven Migliorini, D.M.D.

1. How is a fractured porcelain restoration repaired?

The first step is to determine the cause. Is it a structural weakness or perhaps an occlusal stress-related fracture? Try to resolve any causative factors first. The next step is to create some mechanical hold wherever possible. Roughen and bevel around the defect, because the restorative cannot bond to a glazed surface. Microetch when possible with a microetcher or a porcelain acid etchant such as 10–12% hydrofluoric acid gel. Then silenate and apply bonding resin, opaquers, and finally the appropriate color of composite restorative.

2. How does bonding to a metal surface differ from the porcelain repair?

The principal steps of bonding are similar, but the preparation of the metal surface may include air abrasion of the nonprecious metal (with a microetcher) and tin-plating of the precious metal. The bond strengths of resin cements are greatly enhanced.

3. What are helpful aids in choosing colors for anterior restorations?

Choose the color with color-corrected or natural light. Match teeth that are moist. Liquid coatings (saliva) alter reflected light. Place a cotton roll behind the adjacent tooth to study changes in color and note incisal shade changes that occur with light and dark backgrounds.

4. What is the under 30, over 50 rule for choice of anterior restorations?

If <30% of tooth structure is missing and no major color change is necessary, then a direct-bonded resin restoration is indicated. If >50% of tooth structure is missing, then full coverage is indicated. When 30–50% of the tooth structure is missing, there is a choice of porcelain laminates with resin buildup.

5. What is the single most important preparation parameter for successful bonding?

A clean surface cannot be overestimated. Any adhesive debris on interproximal or other surfaces will interfere with etching and weaken the strength of the bond.

6. How may vital teeth be lightened?

The most conservative approach is bleaching, either done in-office or by the patient at home. In-office systems are generally rapid and require isolation of teeth with rubber dam (paint-on or sheet material). An example is Shufu Hi Light, which uses a light-activated solution of 35% peroxide in 4–10 minute cycles. Home bleaching systems with custom trays incorporating spacers at each tooth position generally use a 10% carbamide peroxide solution in a viscous medium. One to two hours per day for 2–3 weeks can achieve a 2–3-point shade lightening on the Vita Shade scale.

Direct composite or laboratory-fabricated porcelain veneers would be the next most conservative approach and are useful in cases of tetracycline discoloration, which tends not to respond as well to bleaching. Veneers are also useful when the shape, size and arrangement of teeth are esthetically unacceptable. Lastly, full-coverage crowns are the most invasive and generally costly way to change the appearance of the teeth and may be all-ceramic or porcelain fused to gold.

7. What variables affect vital bleaching results?

Type of stain and intensity, bleach contact times, and concentration of active reagent.

8. What type of tooth colors respond best to vital bleaching?

Extrinsic stains respond best, whereas intrinsic stain and discoloration may show no change. In general, yellow stains are much easier to correct than brown/orange, which are easier to correct than gray shades. Tetracycline intrinsic stain generally does not benefit if the dentin is dark. Fluorosis and certain enamel defects will change somewhat but are not predictable on a case-by-case basis.

9. What is a good maintenance material for bleached teeth or composite restorations?
Toothpastes such as Rembrandt (Den-Mat) are effective in lightening teeth and removing stains.

10. How long will bleached teeth stay light?
The answer is unknown. Variables such as dietary choices, smoking habits, and oral hygiene in general can affect longevity. The procedure is cosmetic and thus requires maintenance, just as the coloring of hair. Rebleaching is easy, however, and cases have remained stable for as long as 6–12 months.

11. Are there any side effects to bleaching?
Dentist-supervised systems with neutral pH are considered safest. Tooth sensitivity, soft-tissue irritation or sloughing, or nausea from swallowing the bleach have been reported in some patients but are considered rare.

12. Should teeth be etched before bleaching?
Etching removes tooth enamel. Repeated use of acidic solutions is contraindicated.

13. When is the optimal time to bleach in the treatment-planning sequence?
In general, the optimal time is before beginning the final restorative procedures. Bleaching may lighten teeth so that subsequent matching of colors is accurate. This is necessary because composite and porcelain restorations do not change color and will be mismatched if subsequent bleaching is performed.

14. What are the requirements of the ideal bonding system?
  1. High bonding strength in minimal time to enamel, dentin, porcelain, and metal surfaces
  2. Clinical ability to form gap-free restorative margins
  3. Biocompatibility
  4. Bonding to moist tooth surfaces
  5. Simultaneous treatment of dentin and enamel

15. List the major indications for bonding anterior teeth.
  Small chips, fractures, cracks, or caries of a single tooth
  Closing of small spaces between teeth and correction of minor malpositions
  Color correction of small spots and enamel dysplasias
  Correction of esthetic problems in children and young adults

16. Which clinical variables determine the choice among direct bonding with composite resins, porcelain veneers, or full-coverage crowns?
  1. **Amount of remaining tooth structure:** >50% tooth loss requires full coverage. Small discrepancies and small losses of tooth structure are bondable with composite resins.
  2. **Financial considerations:** In general, full coverage is the most expensive and bonding with composite resins the least expensive. Porcelain veneers are moderately priced.
  3. **Age of the patient:** Bonding, which is flexible and easy to change as the situation may require, may be best for the younger patient.
  4. **Occlusal variables:** Full-coverage crowns have greater strength.
  5. **Periodontal considerations:** Unstable periodontal maintenance and unknown outcomes or prognosis generally suggest provisional reconstruction.
  6. **Correction of color discrepancy:** Darkly stained teeth are best masked with porcelain. Tooth reduction is necessary to allow room for opaquers and to mask stain properly without overcontouring.

7. **Maintenance requirements:** Bonding requires the most maintenance, porcelain the least. Porcelain is more color-stable in heavy smokers and in drinkers of alcohol, coffee, and tea.

8. **Tooth reduction issues:** With porcelain tooth reduction is always needed. Bonding may need little to no reduction.

9. **Esthetic color issues:** For single or few color changes, bonding is esthetic in low-light conditions and with flash photography. Porcelain has poor metamerism (reflection characteristics) when mixed with natural teeth or composites.

10. **Correction of failures:** Porcelain can fracture or debond. When the natural life expectancy expires, more aggressive treatment is necessary. Bonding is relatively easy to correct.

17. What are dentin-bonding agents?
Hydrophilic wetting agents coupled with alteration or removal of the smear layer represent the current generation of dentin-bonding agents. Often called dentin primers, these agents are generally oxalates, phosphate ester, polyacids, or dimethacrylates. They are applied in multiple coatings and air-dried before placement of bonding resins. Representative products are ALL Bond II (Bisco), Power Bond (Cosmedent), Tenure (Den-Mat), and Multibond (3M).

18. What are dentin conditioners?
Before direct dentin bonding, treatment with dilute acids of phosphoric, citric, maleic, or polyacrylic compounds is recommended to clean the dentin surface and tubules and to allow permeation by the bonding system, thus increasing bond strengths.

19. What are typical etch times for enamel and dentin?
10% etchants	30 sec
32% etchants	20 sec
37% etchants	15 sec

20. What are metal-bonding cements?
They are self-curing luting cements that bond to metal and to dentin-bonded materials. Air-abrading with a microetcher of nonprecious and tin-plating of precious metal surfaces increase the bond strength of resin cements such as Panavia (J. Morita) and C & B Metabond (Parkell).

21. What are silane-coupling agents?
Silane-coupling agents are compounds that enhance the micromechanical bond strength of unfilled resin to etched or abraded porcelain by chemical means. Representative products are Scotchprime (3M), Silanator (Cosmedent), and Clearfill Porcelain Bond (J. Morita).

22. What are the advantages of all-purpose resin liners?
Products such as Geristore (Den-Mat) and Bis Fil 2B (Bisco) are generally multipurpose products. They are self- or dual-curing and have high compressive strengths and low viscosity. They have applications as cements, as fluoride-releasing glass ionomers, as bases and liners, or as pediatric restoratives. They bond to dentin, enamel porcelain, amalgam, precious and semiprecious metals, and moist surfaces. They function as luting materials for crowns (with dentin-bonding systems) and are suitable for Maryland Bridge bonding.

23. What are the desirable components and properties of resin luting cements for the porcelain veneer?
The luting cement should be matched to the Vita Shade system. Opaquing shades and try-in gels that match the color of the luting cement but do not cure allow color assessment before final placement. Color modifiers are also helpful. Water solubility of the try-in pastes is beneficial for easy cleaning of the veneer before bonding. Finally, a dual-cure system allows light-curing for anterior veneers and self-curing for posterior ceramic restorations. Representative products are Insure (Cosmedent), UltraBond (Den-Mat), Porcelite (Kerr), and Choice (Bisco).

24. What are the major differences between bonding to enamel and bonding to dentin?
Both enamel and dentin bonding involve micromechanical retention. The conditioned or acid-treated surface has porosities to receive the low-viscosity resins that interlock as they solidify. Acid-etched enamel, however, is more uniform, and bonding strengths are more predictable than with dentin bonding. This is due in part to the varying composition of different types of dentin, i.e., normal or sclerotic, primary or secondary, coronal or root dentin. The higher water and protein content of this vital tissue make the bonding process much more complex.

25. What is the structural nature of dentinal tubules?
Dentinal tubules resemble inverted cones. The smallest diameter is at the outer surface or at the dentinoenamel junction (DEJ), and the tubule increases in diameter as it progresses to the pulp. At the enamel junction the surface area of dentin is only about 1%, whereas at the pulp it increases to about 22%. Dentin-bonding systems may vary according to the depth of the dentin: the greater the water content in the tubules, the deeper the dentin. The most successful bonding systems bond equally well to wet and dry dentin.

26. What are the bond strengths of resins to dentin and enamel?
Bond strengths are measured in megapascals (MPa). Acid-etched enamel has bond strengths of 18–22 MPa. The adhesion of the smear layer is about 6 MPa. Some of the newer dentin-bonding systems can equal enamel strengths, especially if the dentin surface is purposely rewetted with water. There is, however, a great deal of variation in reported bonding strengths. Further research should define bonding strengths more precisely.

27. Can acid-etching of dentin increase bond strengths?
This is a hot issue about which current opinions are varied. The need for calcium hydroxide liners and the amount of dentin required to protect the pulp are debated. Most bonding systems use acid-etching with exposure times of <30 seconds. The larger the layer of calcium hydroxide that is applied, the smaller the amount of dentin surface that is available for bonding. Thus one must determine how much bond strength is required in each situation. In general, if pulp is exposed or nearly exposed, hard-setting calcium hydroxide is recommended. If the dentin thickness is 0.5–1.0 mm, there is probably enough dentin to protect the pulp. Removal of the smear layer in such cases allows the most recent generation of dentin-bonding agents to seal the dentin tubules and to prevent bacterial invasion. Some agents use the smear layer and may show less leakage because of the protective barrier that the smear layer provides, although bond strengths will be lower.

28. What physical property of composite resins complicates and may limit their use?
During polymerization, most composites exhibit a volumetric shrinkage. This applies a considerable amount of stress to the resin-dentin interface and may actually exceed the bond strength, creating gaps and leakage of restoration with resultant dentin sensitivity and pupal irritation. This is especially problematic at the gingival floor of the proximal box of class II posterior preparations, where there may not be any enamel for bonding.

29. What techniques are used to deal with composite shrinkage?
Avoidance of bulk packing limits the total amount of shrinkage. Inserting composites in multiple laminate layers minimizes the volumetric shrinkage. Using flexible or resilient liners, such as glass ionomers, in a sandwich may also help.

30. What is the composition of dental amalgam?
Dental amalgam is an alloy composed of silver, tin, copper, and mercury. The basic setting reaction involves the mixing of the alloy complex of silver (Ag) and tin (Sn) with mercury (Hg) to form the so-called gamma phase alloy (original silver/tin), surrounded by secondary phases

called gamma-1 (silver/mercury) and gamma-2 (tin/mercury). The weakest component is the gamma-2 phase, which is less resistant to corrosion.

$$Ag_2Sn + Hg \quad \rightarrow \quad \underset{\text{gamma}}{Ag_3Sn} \quad + \quad \underset{\text{gamma-1}}{Ag_2Hg_3} \quad + \quad \underset{\text{gamma-2}}{Sn_3Hg}$$

Alloys are manufactured as either filings or spherical particles; dispersed alloys are mixtures of both. Smaller particle size results in higher strength, lower flow, and better carvability. Spherical amalgams high in copper usually have the best tensile and compressive characteristics.

31. What is the functional advantage of a high copper content in dental amalgam?
Copper contents over 6% eliminate the gamma-2 phase and result in alloys of much better marginal stability.

32. How can one tell when an amalgam is properly triturated?
A properly triturated amalgam mix appears smooth and homogenous. No granular appearance or porosities should be evident. An overtriturated mix is preferable to an undertriturated mix.

33. What are the common types of alloys used today?
The blended alloy is a mixture of fine-cut and spherical particles (Dispersalloy, J&J). Because spherical alloys (Tytin, Kerr) are very fast setting, they are particularly suitable for core buildups and impression-taking in one visit.

34. List the major guidelines for the use of pins to retain dental amalgams.
1. Pins should extend 2 mm into tooth structure.
2. Pins should be placed fully in dentin; if they are too close to the dentinoenamel junction, the enamel may fracture from the tooth.
3. Pins should extend 2 mm into amalgam; further extension only weakens the tensile and shear strength of the amalgam.
4. Pins should be aligned parallel to the radicular emergence profile or to the nearest external enamel wall.
5. Additional angulations may be used when there is no danger of pupal or periodontal ligament perforation.
6. Larger cement bases under pin-retained amalgams tend to weaken the restoration and should be avoided.
7. If the tooth structure is flat, the use of small retentive channels cut into the tooth structue prevents potential torsional and lateral stress.

35. What are the disadvantages of using pins in amalgam retention?
Pin placement can result in pulpal exposure, perforation, and fracture of the tooth. Additionally, pins make amalgam more subject to fracture under compressive forces by interrupting the continuity of the restorative material. Pins cannot be used in areas of limited occlusal clearance, as there will be an insufficient bulk of amalgam over the pin to resist fracture.

36. What should be done if accidental exposure of the pulp or perforation of the periodontal ligament occurs during pin placement?
If the pulp is exposed by the pinhole, allow the bleeding to stop, dry with a sterile paper point, and place calcium hydroxide in the hole. Do not place a pin in the hole. Usually the pulp will heal. If a penetration of the gingival sulcus or periodontal ligament space occurs, clean, dry, and place the pin to the measured depth of the external tooth surface to seal the opening.

37. When should freshly placed amalgam be carved?
It is best to start carving once the mix has begun to set and a clear scraping sound is heard. This necessitates sharp instruments. At this time cavosurface margins can be exposed and the proper anatomy created.

38. What is the purpose of finishing and polishing amalgam restorations? Describe the sequence for polishing.

They should be finished and polished for three major reasons: (1) to reduce marginal discrepancies and to create a more hygienic restoration; (2) to reduce marginal breakdown and recurrent decay; and (3) to prevent tarnishing and to increase the quality of appearance of the restoration. Polishing is often a neglected part of treatment, either from lack of opportunity to recall the patient or from the feeling of not being compensated for the added service. However, polishing a restoration or two at each recall defines the state-of-the-art dental practice.

Begin gross contouring with multifluted finishing burs, usually at least 1 day after insertion. Burs, which come in a variety of round, pear, flame, and bullet-nosed shapes, allow anatomic contouring. Then Shufu-type brownie and greenie points can be used to create a high luster. Final pumicing and rubber cups complete the finishing.

39. What is the function of a pin in retained restorations?

The foremost function is to retain the restorative material that replaces tooth structure lost to decay or fracture. Pins also function to resist dislodgment from laterally directed forces.

40. What are the most commonly used pin systems?

Stainless steel pins are placed in sized holes that allow a passive fit and then cemented in place. More commonly, **self-threaded pin systems** (TMS, Whaledent) use holes sized just under the screw diameter. The elasticity of dentin functions to retain the screwed pin. The system comes with a self-limiting drill of the optimal 2-mm depth and self-shearing pins that guard against overtightening. Finally, an **amalgapin concept** described by Shavell uses a channel cut 3 mm into the dentin with an undercut established by an inverted cone bur to retain the amalgam. Use is limited by the amount of remaining tooth structure. The amalgapin concept can be combined with traditional pins for added retention to amalgam restorations.

41. What other means are used to retain amalgam in tooth structure?

State-of-the-art systems are now available for bonding amalgam to dentin and enamel. Products such as Amalgambond (Parkell) and All Bond 2 (Bisco) allow adhesion to preconditioned substrate with the added benefits of retention and sealing of the restoration and a stronger total cohesive mass to support all remaining cuspal segments of the tooth.

42. What is the effect of pins on the properties of the amalgam core?

Pins retain but do not increase the strength of the amalgam core. Tensile strength and transverse strength are actually lowered. Pins should extend only 2 mm into the amalgam core.

43. Where should pins be placed in teeth?

Usually the optimal placement is at the line angles or corners of the tooth, where the tooth/root mass is greatest and the risks of perforation to pulp or furcation are minimal.

44. Is amalgam a safe restorative material? Discuss the mercury issue.

Dental amalgam, a mixture of 40–45% mercury (Hg) and elements of silver, tin and copper, has been used in dentistry for over 150 years. In recent years, the mercury content has come under closer scrutiny because of possible adverse biologic effects from the adsorption of free mercury by human tissues. In response to the media, "antiamalgam" advocates have created a scare without the benefit of scientific evidence. To explore this matter fully is beyond the scope of this chapter, but the dentist should be familiar with questions commonly asked by patients about the safety of amalgam.

First, the amalgam reaction of silver and tin alloy with mercury results in an equilibrium in which only minute amounts of the reactants are evident after the reaction is complete.

Highly sensitive instrumentation can now measure Hg vapor after abrasion of the restoration. The scientific interpretation of such data has caused much sensationalism and controversy and placed many a dental practitioner in a difficult position when confronted by a patient. Some crucial questions and answers follow:

1. **Are certain people hypersensitive to mercury?**

Yes. But according to the North American Contact Dermatitis Group, true sensitivity to mercury appears to be very rare. Studies show that 3% of people will respond to a 1% mercury patch test. Of these, <0.6% will have any clinical manifestations of mercury sensitivity allergy. This equals 1.8 per 100 people.

2. **What about measurements of mercury in the mouth over fillings?**

Mercury vapor detectors commonly used by dentists and other researchers to measure the mercury vapor over an amalgam are grossly uncalibrated for the actual Hg level in inspired air (as measured in the trachea). Values inflated by over 16-fold have resulted because the rate of air sampling by the intake manifold of the vapor analyzer is much larger than the rate of inspiration and air exchange calculated for humans. Hence, the use of a sensitive measuring device alone, with no understanding of the dynamics of air exchange and vapor release, may lead to erroneous conclusions.

3. **How much mercury is ingested from dental amalgams?**

The daily intake of mercury attributable to dental amalgams, as measured by blood levels of Hg, is reported to be only one-seventh of that measured from eating one seafood meal per week. The total daily intake from 8–12 amalgam surfaces is about 1–2 μg. This again is 7 times lower than the intake from one seafood meal per week and only about 10–20% of the average total exposure from all environmental sources.

4. **How valid is extrapolation of animal model experiments to humans?**

Differences are observed in the absorption of elemental Hg in various species. When sheep, monkeys, and humans are compared, sheep absorb the greatest amount, followed by monkeys and then by humans. Sheep absorb 18–25 times more Hg than humans. This fact must be taken into account in comparing animal and human data.

5. **Is there any evidence of biologic injury from the use of dental amalgams?**

Repeated studies on humans with and without amalgam restorations show no significant differences in any organ system. Comparisons of immune cells show no differences in function. Furthermore, no recoveries or remissions of any chronic illness after the removal of amalgams have been scientifically demonstrated.

In conclusion, the contribution of mercury from dental amalgams is minor. No adverse health effects can be attributed to dental amalgams.

45. What are the major uses of the stainless steel crown (SSC) in adult dentition?

1. Extensive decay in the dentition of young adults may leave a vital tooth with limited structure that requires a crown. If a permanent cast or ceramic restoration is not feasible, one may use the SSC in conjunction with a pin composite core buildup to stabilize the tooth until a permanent crown is constructed.

A typical restoration involves the following steps: (1) complete excavation; (2) application of a glass ionomer liner or dentin bonding; (3) placement of pins at the four corner line angles; (4) beveling of the cervical enamel or dentin margin; (5) trial fitting of the SSC with careful adaptation of the cervical margins and checking for occlusal clearance; (6) etching of the cervical bevel; (7) application of an unfilled resin; (8) filling of a well-adapted SSC with self-curing composite core material, and (9) seating of the crown. Removal of excess and expressed composite leaves a well-sealed restoration that may serve for many years. When it is time to prepare the tooth for the permanent crown, slitting the SSC leaves the core buildup ready for final preparation.

2. SSCs may be used to stabilize rampant decay at any age.

3. SSCs may be used as a substitute for the copper band to stabilize a tooth before endodontic treatment. The SSC is more hygienic and kinder to the periodontium when it has been well adapted. Traditional access is through the occlusal dimension.

46. What is the "tunnel preparation"?

The tunnel preparation is a conservative approach to restoring class II caries in teeth with relatively small interproximal lesions. It conserves the proximal marginal enamel by using only the occlusal access and then angulating either mesially or distally until the external tooth enamel is perforated. Usually prior application of a matrix band protects the adjacent tooth wall. The tooth cavity is then packed from the occlusal dimension.

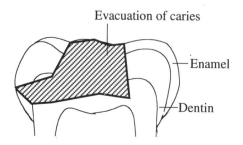

Evacuation of caries

Enamel

Dentin

47. What is the purpose of a cavity varnish?

Typically cavity varnishes, such as Copalite, are used to seal dentin tubules without adding bulk and to protect pupal tissue from the phosphoric acid in zinc phosphate cements.

Formerly cavity varnishes were believed to be effective in reducing microleakage at the cavosurface interface of amalgam restorations until the corrosive products filled the gap. But current high-copper restorations limit the corrosion products of the gamma-2 phase, and varnishes have been shown to wash out. Thus their continued use for this purpose is questionable.

48. What is a cavity liner? What are the indications for use?

A cavity liner is a relatively thin coating over exposed dentin. It may be self-hardening or light-cured, and it is usually nonirritating to pulpal tissues. The purpose is to create a barrier between dentin and pulpally irritating agents, such as acids from etchants or cements, composite restorative materials, or stimulants to the formation of reparative, secondary dentin. Calcium hydroxide has traditionally been placed on dentin with a thickness ≤ 0.5 mm as a pulpal protective agent. Contemporary practice uses newer dentin-bonding agents for liner materials. These not only provide a barrier to pulpally toxic agents but also seal the dentin tubules from bacterial microleakage and provide a bondable surface to increase retention of the restoration. Glass ionomer cements and dentin-bonding systems may become the standard liner materials in restorative dentistry.

49. What is a base? What are the indications for use?

In general, cements that are thicker than 2–4 mm are termed bases and as such function to replace lost dentin structure beneath restorations. A base may be used to provide thermal protection under metallic restorations, to increase the resistance to forces of condensation of amalgam, or to block out undercuts in taking impressions for cast restorations. A base should not be used unnecessarily. Pulpal thermal protection requires a thickness of at least 1 mm, but covering the entire dentin floor with a base is not thought to be necessary. In general, the following guidelines may be used:

1. For deep caries with frank or near exposures or with <0.5 mm of dentin, apply calcium hydroxide.

2. Under a metal restoration, a hard base may be applied (over the calcium hydroxide) up to 2.0 mm in thickness to increase resistance to forces of condensation.

3. If >2 mm of dentin is present, usually no base is needed under amalgam, and a liner may be used under composite.

4. Use of a dentin-bonding agent that seals the dentin tubules and bonds to the restorative material is desirable.

50. What are the compressive strengths of representative base materials?

Zinc phosphate	25,000 lbs/in^2
Glass ionomer	17–20,000 lbs/in^2
Dycal	1500–4000 lbs/in^2

51. What are glass ionomer cements (GICs)?
GICs are mixed powder-liquid component systems. The powder consists of a calcium-aluminofluorosilicate glass that reacts with polyacrylic acid to form a cement of glass particles surrounded by a matrix of fluoride elements.

52. How are GICs classified?
   1. **Hydrous types:** a slower-setting material characterized by a viscous liquid of polyacrylic acid, tartaric acid, itaconic acid, and water plus fluoroaluminosilicate glass powder. Examples: GC Lining cement (GC America), Chelon-Silver (Espe-America).
   2. **Anhydrous types:** flouroaluminosilicate glass, vacuum-dried polyacrylic acid, itaconic acid powder, and a water and tartaric acid solution. These materials have better shelf life. Example: Ketac Chem (Espe-Premiere).
   3. **Hybrid forms:** combination of anhydrous and hydrous forms of glass ionomer powder and liquid. Example: Fuji II (GC America).
   4. **Light-cured glass ionomers:** an acid-base setting material in a photo-initiated liquid. These materials offer extended working times and rapid on-demand set-up and are less technique-sensitive on mixing. Examples: Vitrabond (3M) and XR Ionomer (Kerr).

53. What physical properties of GICs make them so attractive for use in dentistry?
   1. All GICs release fluoride as a sodium salt during the setting reaction and thereafter when moisture is present. This property has the potential to make GICs anticariogenic.
   2. GICs form a molecular bond to enamel, dentin, and certain metals. The dentin surface is pretreated with polyacrylic acid to remove the smear layer for some products, whereas others alter the smear layer that remains. Enamel is best etched to enhance bond strength. GICs bond to base metals but less so to precious metals.
   3. GICs form a micromechanical bond to composite resins and thus make an effective sandwich layer for retaining composites to dentin.
   4. The biocompatability of GICs is high. When there is 0.5–1 mm of dentin, no calcium hydroxide is necessary. GICs are considered only mildly irritating to the dental pulp, and although the pulp inflammatory response resolves within 30 days, they do not stimulate secondary dentin formation.
   5. The thermal insulation of GICs is equal to that of natural dentin.
   6. Because the thermal expansion of GICs is similar to that of tooth structure, one can achieve improved marginal integrity by combining GICs with composite or amalgam restorations.
   7. After setting, GICs have low solubility in the oral environment.

54. What are the major limitations for the use of GICs?
   1. As a sole restorative, GICs are esthetic but do not polish as well as composites.
   2. Compressive strength, tensile strength, and hardness are less for GICs than for composites.
   3. GICs generally are technique-sensitive because of their high solubility when first mixed. Extraneous moisture will cause failures. It is necessary to protect the cement for at least 24 hours with varnish or light-cured resin before finishing.
   4. GICs can be damaged by desiccation.
   Light-cured GICs overcome most of these problems, but we recommend that they be used under composite restorations rather than as the sole restorative material.

55. What are metal-reinforced GICs?
Metallic silver particles of up to 40% of weight are added to GICs to increase the strength and to speed the setting time. Metal-reinforced GICs may be used for (1) core buildups when

at least 50% of tooth structure remains (GICs alone do not have the strength to be a total core); (2) repair of crown margins; and (3) repair of small occlusal lesions with no occlusal function.

56. Discuss the use of GICs as a base or liner material.

GICs are generally considered the nearly ideal base/liner material because of their adhesive bond to tooth structure. Their snap-set in the light-cured form and their cariostatic properties enhance their benefit. Because GICs bond to composite, they are excellent liners for class V root caries restorations. When there is less than 0.5 mm of dentin in deep preparations, we recommend application of calcium hydroxide to the immediate area.

57. Compare amalgam, composites, and GICs as core buildup materials.

Amalgam is the standard of core buildup materials. Used with pins, posts, channel preparations, and dentin-bonding systems, it has the longest clinical track record, approaching the cast core.

Composite core buildups in posterior teeth generally are not recommended because of marginal microleakage, pulpal irritation without liners, and the general superiority of amalgam. Newer dentin-bonding systems may in time alter this. In anterior teeth with a cavity that has minimal endodontic access or in teeth with >50% of the crown remaining, a bonded composite buildup is suitable. **GICs** are appropriate when at least 50% of the tooth structure is present in posterior or anterior teeth.

58. Why is the combined use of GICs and composite resins so advantageous for cervical restorations?

In the so-called sandwich technique, GICs are used to overcome the limitations of composites. GICs bond to both dentin and composite with negligible shrinkage on setting and a thermal expansion rate closely matched to that of tooth structure. Hence their marginal seal properties are superior to those of composite resin. Finally, the slow release of fluoride contributes to their anticariogenic potential. When dentin bonding is involved, as in the class V restoration of the cementoenamel junction, the overlaying of composite on a glass ionomer liner achieves all the benefits of the GIC plus the high polishability, surface hardness, and strong bond to enamel of the composite resin. Composite shrinkage and marginal microleakage are greatly reduced.

59. Outline the clinical technique for class V restorations with the combination of GICs and composite resins.

1. Place the rubber dam, retract the gingival tissues, and establish moisture control.
2. Excavate the caries and establish a conservative outline form. Adding axial retention at the axial gingival-line angles does no harm. Bevel the enamel cavosurface margin, and butt the dentin/cementum cavosurface margin. Pumice and wash well the entire area.
3. In deeply excavated areas, where estimated dentin may be less than 0.5 mm, apply hard-setting calcium hydroxide. Limit the covered dentin to the thin areas.
4. If the glass ionomer product so indicates, treat or leave intact the smear layer. Usually a dentin conditioner of polyacrylic acid is applied for 10–15 seconds to remove the layer if indicated. Again wash, but do not desiccate the dentin. Leave a moist layer.
5. Apply the GIC over all dentin, and allow it to set or light-cure.
6. Etch enamel for 15 seconds with a solution of 37% phosphoric acid. Wash and dry. Do not purposely etch the glass ionomer.
7. Apply bonding agent over the entire preparation and cure for 20 seconds.
8. Apply incremental layers of composite and cure. Shrinkage due to polymerization is proportional to the volume of composite; thus small increments minimize shrinkage.
9. Finish and polish. The enamel junction is feather-edged 2–3 mm and the gingival margin is butted.

60. Describe dentin-bonding systems.

Dentin-bonding agents are complex and multistep systems. Some products remove the smear layer, whereas others do not. Examples of products are Tenure/Den-Mat, Multibond (3M), and ProBond (L.D. Caulk). The components of each system include:

1. The etchant: maleic acid, phosphoric acid, nitric acid, or another agent is used to etch the enamel and/or to precondition the dentin. Other dentin conditioners, such as EDTA, may be used to remove the smear layer.

2. The primer: a hydrophylic monomer in solvent, such as hydroxymethylmethacrylate (HEMA), is applied in several coatings and air-dried. This wetting agent provides micromechanical and chemical bonding to dentin.

3. The resin: the unfilled resin is then applied and light- or dual-cured. This layer can now bond to composite, pretreated porcelain luted with composite, or amalgam.

61. What is accomplished by enamel etching prior to the placement of composite resins?

Etching of enamel with phosphoric acid predictably creates surface microporosities into which resin liquid can flow, thereby achieving micromechanical retention and margin sealing.

62. When are posterior composite restorations most successful?

Posterior composite restorations are most successful when placed in small cavity preparations, such as premolars, where occlusal wear is not a factor. Criteria are (1) noninvolvement of cusps; (2) no occlusal contact; (3) no excessive wear; (4) isthmus no wider than one-third of intercuspal distance; (5) gingival extension in sound enamel; and (6) moisture control. Further uses may be as a temporary restoration, as pit-and-fissure sealants, and for class I and II restorations in primary teeth. These restorations are technique-sensitive. How well the procedure is executed ultimately determines the longevity of posterior composites.

63. What is the most serious limitation of the posterior composite restoration?

The polymerization shrinkage of visible light-cured composites (up to 2% by volume) can cause internal stresses and gap formations at butt-joint interfaces, as at the gingival floor of class II and V restorations. Composites do best when they overlap onto an etched enamel surface in the restoration design.

64. What are the likely causes of postoperative sensitivity in posterior composite restorations?

1. Hyperocclusion (Carefully check and adjust; close color matches can make this more difficult.)
2. Marginal leakage due to polymerization shrinkage
3. Contact of the composite to the tooth dentin

65. How can one best manage postoperative sensitivity after a restoration?

Try to determine the cause from the symptoms. **Pain on biting** suggests that the occlusion needs adjustment. For **cold thermal sensitivity** wait 1–2 weeks. It may be necessary to remove the restoration and place a sedative filling until the sensitivity subsides and then try the restoration again. For **hot thermal sensitivity**, rule out the possibility of endodontic pathology. Place a sedative filling and observe for 2–3 weeks. If symptoms are severe, initiate endodontic treatment.

66. List the liners suitable for amalgam and composite restorations.

Amalgams:	<0.5 mm of dentin	Hard-setting calcium hydroxide
	0.5–1 mm or greater	Glass ionomer/visible light-cured
	>1.0–2.0 mm	Not needed

Composites: Always cover dentin with suitable liner or protective dentin-bonding system, because composites are toxic to pulpal tissues. Use calcium hydroxide on the deepest areas (dentin≤0.5 mm) and GIC on the remaining exposed dentin. Copal liners and varnishes are contraindicated for composites and no longer useful for amalgams.

67. What are the advantages of light-cured GICs?
1. Extended working times
2. Short on-demand setting times
3. Stronger, more adhesive, and more resistant to desiccation than self-cure GICs

68. How are pulpal tissues affected by zinc phosphate, zinc oxide, polyacrylate, and glass ionomer cements?
When a luting agent of **zinc phosphate** is used to cement a crown, the pressure of seating causes phosphoric acid to leak into dentin tubules of an *unprotected* crown preparation. The result is a high level of pulpal inflammation. Using two coats of copal varnish blocks about 90% of the phosphoric acid. **Zinc oxide** eugenol cement and **polyacrylate** cements cause no pulpal inflammatory response. As a luting cement **glass ionomer** may cause a pulpal inflammation that becomes progressively worse. Some have argued that this occurs only if the preparation is desiccated; if left moist, no irreversible effects are experienced.

69. What techniques can be used to achieve marginal exposure and to control hemorrhage in a class V cavity preparation?
If the preparation is <2 mm below the gingival sulcus, an impregnated retraction cord with a gingival retraction rubber-dam clamp may be effective. If the defect approaches 3 mm or greater, then hemostasis and margin exposure often require surgical exposure (crown lengthening) or excision via electrosurgery.

70. Outline the major design criteria for closing space in the anterior dentition.
　1. Most commonly, the maxillary central diastema may be closed by composite bonding and/or porcelain veneers. Careful space analysis with calipers allows the most esthetic result. The width of each central incisor is measured, along with the diastema space. One-half the dimension of the diastema space is normally added to each crown unless the central incisors are unequal. Then adjustment is made to create equal central incisors.
　2. If the central incisors appear too wide esthetically, then one can reduce the distal incisal to narrow the tooth and bond it over to seal any exposed dentin. One then adds to the mesial incisal of the lateral incisor to effect closure of space.
　3. A tooth in the palatal crossbite may even be transformed into a two-cusped tooth by building up the facial to the buccal profile. This bicuspidization is reasonably durable and esthetically pleasing.
　4. Peg laterals and cogenitally absent laterals replaced by cuspids may similarly be transformed by bonding and/or porcelain veneers. Reduction of protrusive contours, followed by addition to mesial and distal incisal areas, establishes esthetic results.

71. Of the following cements—zinc phosphate, zinc polycarboxylate, zinc oxide-eugenol, glass ionomer, and zinc silicophosphate—
　1. **Which are anticariogenic?**
　　Glass ionomer and zinc silicophosphate have fluoride available.
　2. **Which are adhesive to tooth structure?**
　　Zinc polycarboxylate and glass ionomer
　3. **Which need dentin tubules sealed in advance?**
　　Zinc phosphate
　4. **Which require removal of the smear layer?**
　　Zinc polycarboxylate and glass ionomer (sometimes)
　5. **Which are suitable as a base under composites?**
　　All except zinc oxide-eugenol, which inhibits the composite setting reaction
　6. **Which are suitable as a base under amalgams?**
　　All

72. What is the difference between a direct and an indirect restoration?

Direct-bonded composite restorations are constructed chairside, directly on the patient, whereas indirect procelain veneer restorations usually involve impressions and poured casts for laboratory fabrication.

73. List the indications for the porcelain veneer restoration.
1. Stained teeth or teeth in which color changes are desired
2. Enamel defects
3. Malposed teeth
4. Malformed teeth
5. Replacement for multisurfaced composite restoration when adequate tooth structure remains (at least 30%)

Each patient must be evaluated on an individual basis. A general requirement is excellent periodontal health and good hygiene practices. In the case of stained teeth, prior bleaching (either passive home or in-office) helps to ensure better color esthetics.

74. Describe the basic tooth preparation for the porcelain veneer restoration on anterior teeth.
1. **Vital bleaching** (optional)
2. **Preparation:** Enamel reduction of at least 0.5 mm, which may extend to 0.7 mm at the cervical line angles, is necessary to avoid overcontouring. The only exception may be a tooth with a very flat labial contour and slight linguoversion. Chamfer-type labial preparations can be achieved with bullet-type diamonds and the use of self-limiting 0.3-, 0.5-, 0.7-mm diamond burs are essential for consistent depth of preparation.

   The gingival cavosurface margin should be level with the free gingival crest. The mesial and distal proximal margins are immediately labial to the proximal contact area. The contacts are not broken but may be relaxed with fine specialty strips of 10–20-μ thickness. This allows placement of smooth metal matrix strips at the time of placement. The incisal margin is placed at the crest of the incisal ridge. Placing retraction cord into the gingival sulcus prior to preparing the gingival cavosurface margin helps in the atraumatic completion of the preparation.
3. **Impressions:** Standard impression techniques use vinyl polysiloxane materials.
4. **Temporization,** if at all possible, should be limited in use; it may be time-consuming and add to the expense of the procedure. One should use fine discs on the labial enamel surface for polishing the rough surface of the diamond cut preparation to limit the accumulation of stain and debris. If it is necessary to temporize, preconstructed laboratory composite veneers or chairside direct temporization may be used. The techniques are similar. Spot etch two or three internal enamel areas on the labial preparation. Apply unfilled resin and tack-bond the veneer, or place some light-cured composite on the tooth and spread it with a gloved finger dipped in unfilled resin to a smooth finish. The preparation should be light-cured, and one should be able to lift it off relatively easily at the unetched areas and polish down the etched spots.

75. Describe the technique for insertion of porcelain veneers.
1. After isolation, pumicing, and washing, the fragile porcelain veneers are tried on the chamfer-prepared tooth. First, the inside surface of the veneer is wetted with water to increase the adhesion. Margins are then carefully evaluated.
2. Next, try-in pastes are used to determine the correct color-matching. Water-soluble pastes are the easiest to use. The try-in pastes closely match the final resin cements but are not light-activated.
3. The porcelain veneers are prepared for bonding. Apply a 30-second phosphoric acid etchant for cleaning. Wash and dry. Apply a silane coupling agent, and air-dry. Apply the unfilled light-cured bonding resin and cure for 20 seconds.
4. To bond the porcelain veneer to the tooth, first clear interproximal areas with fine strips. Pumice and wash thoroughly. Place strips of dead, soft interproximal matrix, and etch the enamel for 30 seconds. Wash for 60 seconds and dry. Apply the bonding resin. Any known

dentin areas should be primed (with dentin primer materials) before applying the bonding resin. Any opaquers or shade tints may now be applied. The light-cured resin luting cement is now applied to tooth and veneer. The veneer is carefully placed into position, and gross excess composite is removed. Precure at the incisal edge for 10 seconds, and remove any partially polymerized material gingivally and proximally. Light-cure fully for 30–60 seconds. Finish the margins with strips, discs, and finishing burs. Check for protrusive excursions.

5. In general, apply central incisors first, then laterals, then cuspids.

76. What are the technical considerations for posterior cast-porcelain, partial-coverage restorations?

1. Remove all old restorative material, and excavate any caries.

2. Cavosurface margins are butt-jointed at 90°; otherwise a fine porcelain flange is prone to fracture.

3. Hard-setting calcium hydroxide may be placed at the pulpal floor area where dentin thickness is estimated to be 0.5 mm or less.

4. Glass ionomer cement is placed on all exposed dentin, and any undercuts are blocked out accordingly to create an ideal inlay form. The result is a fully bondable surface.

5. Impressions are taken, and temporization is performed with acrylic resin and cemented with *noneugenol* temporary cement.

6. The porcelain inlay received from the laboratory is trial-fitted, but occlusion is not adjusted at this time because of possible fracture.

7. The porcelain and the tooth are prepared in the usual manner for bonding.

8. Cementation with a composite luting cement, preferably with a dual-cured material, allows better polymerization, especially at interproximal areas.

9. Finishing and final occlusal adjustment are done in the usual manner.

77. List advantages of the porcelain inlay.

The restoration is highly esthetic.
The restoration is highly wear-resistant.
As a fully bonded restoration, adjacent tooth structure is strengthened.
Polymerization shrinkage is negligible.
Marginal adaptation is excellent.
Postoperative sensitivities are rare.

78. What is generally considered to be the best technique for cementing a post, either cast or pre-fabricated?

The canal space should be clean and dry with final drying done with a paper point to ensure no puddling at the end of the dowel space. If available the post can be sandblasted to ensure a clean surface and improve the cement bond. A spiral paste filler is used to carry the cement and disperse it into the dowel space. Then lightly coat the post with cement and slowly insert to allow excess cement to escape. After initial set, begin removing excess cement.

79. Describe the technique of enamel microabrasion.

Microabrasion is the controlled removal of discolored enamel using a rubber cup and a mixture of pumice and an acid, usually hydrochloric acid.

80. When is microabrasion indicated?

This technique is effective for treating superficial enamel discolorations, white or brown spots, caused by fluorosis and often seen post orthodontically.

81. Describe methods used to optimize proximal contacts with direct posterior class II composites.

Due to our relative inability to rack and condense composite as we can amalgam and due to the polymerization shrinkage of light-cured composites, proper proximal contacts can be more difficult to obtain. Aggressive wedging, pre-wedging, the use of thin metal matrices, and the use of sectional matrices with tooth separating rings (Bitine ring) have all been advocated to help overcome this problem. If all prove inadequate and the patient demands a tooth-colored restoration, consider an indirect laboratory fabricated composite or porcelain inlay.

82. What are the three dimensions of color as they relate to teeth? Describe them briefly.
1. Hue—the name of the color, such as red or yellow
2. Value—the lightness of a color or its brightness as related to a scale from black to white
3. Chroma—the strength of a color or the degree of color saturation. Chroma is the strength or purity of a given hue and describes the extent to which that hue differs from a gray of the same value.

83. What is the purpose of a vent along the length of a post?
The vent allows excess cement to escape from the dowel space without building up excessive hydraulic pressure. This excessive pressure can cause root fractures, incomplete seating of the post, or extrusion of the cement through the apical seal.

84. What is cracked tooth syndrome?
Cracked tooth syndrome is generally described as an incomplete fracture of a tooth. The patient typically complains of sharp pain with biting hard food. The pain goes away immediately and usually does not hurt otherwise. Occasionally, there is some temperature sensitivity but the inability to bite food on the tooth is the primary complaint.

85. Describe the treatment of cracked tooth syndrome.
Treatment of these teeth can be quite vexing, as the clinician may have difficulty discerning the location and extent of the fracture. Treatment may begin with a relatively simple restorative procedure, but if there is cuspal involvement and the tooth is heavily restored, the tooth should be prepared for a full coverage restoration and temporized. If symptoms are alleviated, proceed to a permanent crown. If not, one should suspect that the fracture has involved pulpal tissue and endodontics should be done. In the worst possible situation, endodontics does not resolve the pain, in which case one assumes the fracture proceeds subgingivally or through the furcation. In this event, extraction must be considered.

86. Dental implants have the highest success rate in which part of the mouth and why?
Implant fixtures, regardless of type, have the highest success rate in the anterior mandible between the mental foramina. In the mandible, fixtures can engage the cortical bone at the inferior border. Also, bone quantity and bone quality tend to be best in this region, the cancellous bone being quite dense and allowing for excellent integration.

87. Why are products like IRM and Temp Bond incompatible with composite resin restorative materials and composite cements?
Both IRM and Temp Bond are zinc oxide-eugenol based products. Eugenol inhibits the setting of composite resin materials.

88. What are the advantages of the full gold crown versus a porcelain fused to gold crown?
This question may be more simply answered by saying that the only real advantage of the porcelain/gold crown is its superior esthetics. The full gold crown requires less tooth reduction, which reduces the risk of endodontic involvement, has margins that are more easily finished, is simpler to fabricate in the laboratory, has much better wear properties against opposing natural teeth, cannot chip or break, and is easily polished after chairside adjustment.

89. Describe the technique for chairside porcelain repair.
Assuming there is not exposed metal, after rubber dam isolation, a chairside sandblaster, if available, is used on the fractured porcelain, and the area is rinsed and treated with a silane

coupling solution for 30 seconds. Bonding resin is then applied followed by a hybrid composite resin. If the sandblaster is not available, an 8% hydrofluoric acid gel is used for 3–4 minutes to etch the porcelain; the restoration is then completed as above.

90. What is the biologic width? Explain its relationship to restorative dentistry.

The biologic width is an area that ideally is approximately 3 mm wide from the crest of bone to the gingival margin. It consists of approximately 1 mm of connective tissue, 1 mm of epithelial attachment, and 1 mm of sulcus. As it relates to restorative dentistry, if a restorative procedure violates this zone, there is a higher likelihood that periodontal inflammation will ensue, causing the attachment apparatus to move apically.

91. When it becomes necessary for restorative reasons to impinge upon the biologic width, what steps can be taken prior to final restoration to create a maintainable periodontal environment prior to final restoration?

Crown lengthening and orthodontic extrusion are the two most common ways to deal with this problem. Crown lengthening exposes more tooth structure surgically and is in effect surgical repositioning of the biologic width. Orthodontic extrusion is done in cases where crown lengthening would unduly compromise the peridontal health of the adjacent teeth or create an unfavorable esthetic situation, as often can occur in the anterior maxilla.

92. What are the indications for light-cured, dual-cured, and auto-cured composite cements?

Light-cured resin cements are generally used for cementation of porcelain veneers. Dual-cured resins may be used for veneers but color stability may change with continued polymerization of the cement. Therefore, dual-cured cements are usually reserved for cementation of porcelain and composite inlays and onlays. In these cases the dentist can light-cure the material at the margins, and the auto-cure feature enables the cement deeper within the restoration, where light is excluded, to set properly. Auto- or self-cure cements are used when the curing light is completely excluded, such as for post and core cementation or the luting of porcelain/gold and full gold crowns.

93. Describe the options for treatment of root surface sensitivity.

Root sensitivity is a very common problem and can be adequately resolved in many instances by modifying the patient's toothbrushing technique and having patients use a desensitizing tooth-paste such as Sensodyne. Other desensitizing agents such as Protect by Butler utilize oxalate precipitates to occlude the dentin tubules. Dentin adhesives such as All Bond 2 work well to reduce sensitivity as well. Others advocate iontophoresis to apply fluoride to the sensitive surface.

94. Describe the criteria for optimal occlusion of natural teeth.

According to Okeson, three criteria satisfy this situation.
　　1. Even, simultaneous contact on posterior teeth in centric relation with forces directed axially along each tooth.
　　2. Adequate tooth-guided contacts on the working side to disclude the nonworking teeth immediately. Canine guidance is the most desireable.
　　3. The anterior teeth should disclude the posterior teeth in protrusion.

95. Describe the proper occlusal scheme for a single unit implant-born crown restoration.

Any single tooth implant restoration should have minimal occlusal contact. Occlusal tables should be kept small in the posterior with very light occlusion in centric. As a rule, lateral and protrusive contacts should be avoided on all implant-supported fixed prostheses supported by less than three fixtures.

96. Describe the technique of internal bleaching.

Teeth that have successful endodontic treatment or have a completely calcified pulp canal and are discolored are candidates for this procedure. The tooth is isolated with a rubber dam and the endodontic access is re-opened. A hard cement base such as zinc phosphate is placed 2–3 mm into the pulp canal to the level of the CEJ. An EDTA solution such as RC Prep is placed in the pulp chamber to remove the smear layer and open the dentinal tubules. Rinse and dry. Mix 35% hydrogen peroxide (Superoxol) with sodium perborate and place into the pulp chamber. Then place a thin cotton pellet over the bleach solution and close the tooth with IRM or similar material to prevent the bleach from leaking out. Caution the patient to avoid eating on the tooth for 24 hours so as not to dislodge the temporary. Repeat as needed.

97. As a general rule, why should you not splint natural teeth and implants in a fixed prosthesis?

Implants have no periodontal ligament and so do not have the same shock-absorbing capability as natural teeth. Under occlusal loading, this difference has been shown to be detrimental to the natural tooth as well as cause bone loss around the implants.

98. What is the theory of "abfraction"?

Abfraction is defined as the pathologic loss of tooth substance caused by biomechanical loading forces. The loss of structure is usually seen as wedge-shaped cervical lesions or cervical erosions. This theory is used as an alternative explanation for areas that have been attributed to toothbrush abrasion.

99. What is the purpose of an altered cast impression in fabricating a mandibular class I or II partial denture?

By definition, a mandibular class I or II partial denture is both tooth and tissue supported. The altered cast technique enables you to accurately record an impression of the edentulous ridge so that functional forces on the denture will be spread more evenly between the abutment teeth and the tissues.

BIBLIOGRAPHY

1. Berry EA: The clinical uses of glass ionomer cements. In Hardin JF (ed): Clark's Clinical Dentistry, vol. 4. Philadelphia, J.B. Lippincott, 1993.
2. Christensen GJ: A look at state of the art tooth colored inlays and onlays. J Am Dent Assoc 123:66–70, 1992.
3. Halpern BG (ed): Restorative Dentistry. Philadelphia, W.B. Saunders, 1993.
4. Hardin JF (ed): Restorative dentistry. In Clark's Clinical Dentistry, vol 4. Philadelphia, J.B. Lippincott, 1993.
5. Heyman H, Baynes S: Current concepts in dentine bonding. J Am Dent Assoc 124(5):27–41, 1993.

9. PROSTHODONTICS

Ralph B. *Sozio,* D.M.D.

FIXED PROSTHODONTICS

1. What is the definition of "fit" for a full-crown restoration? What is the clinical acceptance of the fit of a full-crown restoration?

The fit of a full crown restoration is normally measured in relationship to two reference areas: (1) the occlusal seat and (2) the marginal seal. The two areas are interrelated and affect each other. The ideal fit of a full crown (marginal discrepancy) is related to the film thickness of the cementing medium, normally 10–30 μ. The clinical acceptance of marginal discrepancy is approximately 80 μ.

2. What is the best marginal tooth preparation?

There is no ideal marginal tooth preparation. The selection of the marginal design depends on many factors, including:

1. The material employed in the construction of the full crown:
   All-ceramic restoration—shoulder or deep chamfer
   Metal-ceramic with porcelain extended to marginal edge—shoulder or deep chamfer
   Metal-ceramic with metal collars—shoulder with bevel or chamfer
   Full gold crown—feathered edge, bevel, or chamfer
2. The amount of retention needed: beveled or feathered edge afford the most retention.
3. Seating resistance: shoulder preparation affords the least resistance.
4. Sealing capability: beveled or feathered edge affords the best seal.
5. Pulpal consideration: more tooth reduction is necessary with a shoulder preparation than with a chamfer; and the feathered edge requires the least reduction.

3. How does one determine the number of abutments to be employed?

There is no rigid rule. Determining factors include:

1. The more pontics, the greater the increase in loading forces on the abutments.
2. The position of the pontics affects the loading forces of the abutments: the more posterior the pontics, the greater the loading forces on the abutments.
3. The crown-to-root ratio of the abutments (the bone support): a periodontally compromised mouth increases the abutment-to-pontic ratio.
4. Roots of the abutments that are parallel to each other distribute the loading forces down the long axis of the teeth. When the loading forces do not fall within the long axis of the tooth, then the lateral forces on the abutments are increased. This situation necessitates the use of additional abutments.

4. In periodontally compromised patients, is splinting the entire dental arch with a one-piece, "round-house" fixed bridge the treatment of choice?

Splinting an entire dental arch with a round-house fixed bridge is far from being the treatment of choice, because it is fraught with potential problems:

1. All tooth preparations must be parallel to each other.
2. Impression taking and die construction are extremely difficult.
3. Accuracy of fit and the one-piece unit is extremely difficult.
4. Premature setting of the cement is a major risk, because total seating of the fixed bridge onto the abutments is made extremely difficult by the mobility of the existing teeth.
5. If one of the abutments fails, it may be necessary to replace the entire prosthesis.

It is better to split up the prosthesis in some fashion than to construct a one-piece unit.

5. Is a cantilever fixed bridge sound treatment?

A cantilever fixed bridge is a design that places more torquing forces on terminal abutments than desirable. Certain guidelines should be followed if a cantilever is used:

1. Cantilever pontics are limited to one per fixed bridge.

2. If the cantilever is replacing a molar, the size of the pontic should be the same as for a bicuspid, and at least one more abutment unit should be incorporated than in a conventional bridge. In addition, there should be no lateral occlusal contact on the pontic, and the bridge should be cemented with a rigid medium.

3. If the cantilever pontic is anterior to the abutments, the mesial aspect of the pontic should be designed to allow some interlocking effect.

6. Can a three-quarter crown be used as an abutment for a fixed bridge?

A three-quarter crown can be used successfully as an abutment for a fixed bridge if certain guidelines are followed:

1. Because there is less tooth reduction than with a full crown, retention may be compromised. Internal modifications, such as grooves or pins, must be used to compensate for potential loss of retention.

2. Proper tooth coverage is necessary for a three-quarter crown abutment:
   Anterior: linguoincisal
   Posterior/upper: linguoocclusal
   Posterior/lower: linguoocclusal plus coverage over the buccal cusp tips

3. A three-quarter crown should be made only of metal; therefore, esthetics may be compromised.

7. Must a post and core be constructed for an endodontically treated tooth that is to be used in a fixed bridge?

An endodontically treated tooth is generally a more brittle structure than a vital tooth. Because of the tooth reduction for the full-crown restoration and preparation of the access cavity for the endodontic procedure, the remaining coronal tooth structure is likely to be small. Therefore, a post and core is more likely to be necessary in the anterior and bicuspid region.

If the access cavity is small and sufficient tooth structure remains after tooth preparation in the molor region, a post and core may not be necessary. In this instance, the coronal chamber should be filled, preferably with a bonded material.

8. What is the proper length for the post? Should a post be made for each canal in a multi-rooted tooth?

In general, the length of a post should be such that the fulcrum point, determined from measuring the height of the core to the apex of the tooth, is in bone. This guideline normally places the post approximately two-thirds into the root length. Improper length allows a potential for root fracture.

It is not necessary to construct a post for each canal in a multirooted tooth, provided that the dominant root (i.e., palatal root of maxillary molar) is employed and that proper length has been established. If proper length cannot be obtained, then it is necessary to place posts in at least one of the other remaining roots.

9. Can one use the preformed, single-step post and core in place of the two-step post and core?

A preformed, single-step post and core can be used in fixed prosthodontics, but the potential for failure is greater with many of the single-step systems than with a cast-gold post and core for the following reasons:

1. The canal preparation must be shaped to the configuration of the preformed post. This requirement may lead to overpreparation of the canal and potential root perforation. In contrast, a cast post is made to fit the existing configuration of the canal.

2. A screw-type post has the greatest retentive value, but it also has the greatest stress forces during insertion.

3. The core buildup of the single-step post and core may not be as stable as a cast-gold core.

4. The modulus of elasticity of the single-step post is normally much higher than that of the root. This may lead to root fracture during loading. In contrast, a type-three cast-gold post has a modulus of elasticity similar to that of the root.

10. Where should a crown margin be placed in relationship to the gingiva: supragingivally, equigingivally, or subgingivally?

It is better for gingival health to place a crown margin supragingivally, 1–2 mm above the gingival crest, or equigingivally, at the gingival crest. Such positioning is quite often not possible because of esthetic or caries considerations. Subsequently, the margin must be placed subgingivally. The question then becomes whether the subgingival margin ends slightly below the gingival crest, in the middle of the sulcular depth, or at the base of the sulcus.

When preparing a subgingival margin, the major concern is not to extend the preparation into the attachment apparatus. If the margin of the subsequent crown is extended into the attachment apparatus, a constant gingival irritant has been constructed. Therefore, for clinical simplicity, when a margin is to be placed subgingivally, it is desirable to end the tooth preparation slightly below the gingival crest.

Materials

11. What materials are employed in the construction of a full crown?

Gold alloy	Composite resin
Nongold alloy	Composite resin with a metal alloy
Acrylic resin	Ceramic with a metal alloy
Acrylic resin with a metal alloy	All ceramic

12. Are the same materials used in the construction of a fixed bridge?

In general, a fixed bridge needs a metal support for strength. The veneer coating may be acrylic, composite, or ceramic. Newer ceramic materials, including alumina and zirconium, have increased strength that in some cases may eliminate the metal substructure.

13. What are the major advantages and disadvantages of the metal-ceramic crown?

In general, the metal-ceramic crown combines certain favorable properties of metal in its substructure and of ceramic in its veneer coating. Advantages of this combination include:

1. The metal substructure give high strength that allows the materials to be used in fixed bridgework and for splinting teeth.

2. The fit of a metal casting can also be accomplished with the metal-ceramic crown.

3. Esthetics can be achieved by the proper application of the ceramic veneer.

The disadvantages are:

1. To allow enough space for the metal-ceramic materials, adequate tooth reduction is necessary (1.5 mm or more). The marginal tooth preparation is critical in relation to the design of the metal with the ceramic.

2. The fabrication technique is complex. The longer the span of bridgework, the greater the potential for metal distortion and/or porcelain problems.

14. What tooth preparation is necessary for the metal-ceramic crown?

The amount of tooth reduction necessary for the metal-ceramic crown depends on the metal and ceramic thickness. The necessary thickness of the metal is 0.5 mm, whereas the minimal ceramic thickness is 1.0–1.5 mm. Therefore, the tooth reduction is approximately 1.5–2.0 mm. With this porcelain-metal sandwich, a shoulder preparation is generally necessary for adequate tooth reduction.

15. What happens if tooth preparation or reduction is inadequate in the marginal area?
If the tooth reduction is <1.5 mm at the marginal area, only metal can be present in that area. If porcelain is applied on metal that has been reduced in thickness because of lack of space, marginal metal distortion is likely to occur during the firing cycle. If the porcelain thickness is reduced to compensate for the reduced space, the opaque porcelain layer is likely to be exposed or to dominate, leading to an unesthetic result. If both the porcelain and metal have adequate thickness, then the crown is overcontoured.

16. Can the marginal area of a metal-ceramic crown be constructed in porcelain without metal?
There are many techniques with which to construct a porcelain margin with optimal esthetics, proper fit, and correct contour (emergence profile).

17. If the tooth preparation is sufficient to accept the porcelain edge of the metal without distortion, why is it necessary to construct a margin in porcelain solely for esthetic reasons?
It is possible to cover the metal correctly with porcelain in the marginal area, but most often the esthetic results fall short of expectation in the most critical area. Incident light that transmits through the porcelain and reflects from the metal often creates a shadowing effect. If porcelain is present only at this marginal area, light transmission and reflection occur through the porcelain and the tooth. This creates the proper blend between the marginal aspect of the crown and the tooth.

18. For a successful porcelain marginal construction, how far should the metal extend in relation to the shoulder?
Originally the metal was finished slightly shy of the edge of the shoulder, with porcelain extending to the edge. Another technique finished the metal at the axiocaval line angle of the preparation, creating a porcelain margin that totally covers the horizontal shoulder. With both techniques, however, shadowing was still present. To create a proper light transmission and reflection of the porcelain/tooth interface, the metal should be finished to about 1–2 mm above the axiocaval line angle of the shoulder.

19. What are noble alloys?
Noble alloys in general do not oxidize on casting. This feature is important in a metal substrate so that oxidation at the metal-porcelain interface can be controlled by the addition of trace oxidizing elements. If oxidation cannot be controlled on repeated firings, porcelain color may be contaminated and the bond strength may be weakened. Noble alloys are gold, platinum, and palladium. A silver alloy that oxidizes is considered semiprecious.

20. What is a base metal alloy? Can it be used in the construction of a metal-ceramic crown?
The base metal or nonprecious alloys most often used in the construction of a metal-ceramic crown are nickel and chromium. Because such alloys readily oxidize at elevated temperatures, they create porcelain-to-metal interface problems. The oxidation must be controlled by a metal-coating treatment, which is somewhat unpredictable. Casting and fitting are also difficult. Authorities agree that a noble alloy is preferable.

21. What are the criteria for selecting a specific alloy?
  1. Compatibility of the coefficient of thermal expansion with the selected porcelains
  2. Controllability of oxidation at interface
  3. Ease in casting and fabrication
  4. Fit potential
  5. High yield of strength
  6. High modulus of elasticity (stiffness) to avoid stress in the porcelain

22. How does porcelain bond to the alloy?
Ceramic adheres to metal primarily by chemical bond. A covalent bond is established by sharing O_2 in the elements present in the porcelain and the metal alloy. These elements include

silicon dioxide (SiO_2) in the porcelain and oxidizing elements such as silicon, indium, and iridium in the metal alloy.

23. How is a porcelain selected?
The criteria for selecting a specific porcelain include:
   1. Compatibility with the metal used in regard to their respective coefficients of thermal expansion (of prime importance)
   2. Stability of controlled shrinkage with multiple firings
   3. Color stability with multiple firings
   4. Capability of matching shade selection with various thicknesses of porcelain
   5. Ease of handling (technique-sensitive)
   6. Full range of shades and modifiers

24. How many layers or different porcelains can be applied in the buildup of a metal-ceramic crown?
The different layers or porcelains are as follows:

1. Shoulder	4. Body	7. Modifiers in every layer
2. Opaque	5. Incisal	8. External colorants
3. Opacious dentin	6. Translucent	

25. What is the function of the opaque layer?
The elements in the opaque layer create the chemical bond of the porcelain to the metal substrate. The opaque layer masks the color of the metal and is the core color in determining the final shade of the crown.

26. What is opacious dentin?
Opacious dentin is an intermediary modifying porcelain that affords better light transmission than the opaque layer, in part because of its optical properties. Opacious dentin is less opaque than the opaque layer but less translucent than the body (dentin) porcelain. It is also used for color shifts or effect properties.

27. What differentiates shoulder porcelain from dentin (body) porcelain?
The principal difference between shoulder and body porcelain is the firing temperature. Because the shoulder porcelain is established before the general buildup, its color and dimension must remain stable during subsequent firings. Therefore, the shoulder porcelain matures at a higher temperature than the subsequent body porcelain firings.

28. What is segmental buildup in the construction of the metal-ceramic crown?
Segmental buildup refers to the method of applying the porcelain powders in incremental portions horizontally. Each increment differs from the others in either opacity and translucency or hue, value, or chroma. This technique is used to construct a crown that attempts to mimic the optical properties of a natural tooth.

29. What is coefficient of thermal expansion? What is its importance in prosthodontics?
Coefficient of thermal expansion is the exponential expansion of a material as it is subjected to heat. The coefficient is extremely important during joint firing of two dissimilar materials. For example, the coefficient of thermal expansion should be slightly higher (rather than the same) for the metal substrate than for the porcelain coating. This slight difference results in compression of the fired porcelain coating, which gives it greater strength.

30. What is the proper coping design for the metal-ceramic restoration?
The purpose of the metal coping is to ensure the fit of the crown and to maximize the strength of the porcelain veneer. The metal must have proper thickness so as not to distort during the firing. The coping should be reinforced in load-bearing areas, such as the interproximal space,

and can be strengthened in areas where metal exists alone, such as the lingual collar. To maximize the strength potential of the porcelain, uniform thickness should be attempted in the final restoration. This thickness can be obtained by designing the wax-up of the framework to accommodate the porcelain layer.

31. How does the marginal tooth preparation affect the design of the metal-ceramic crown?

The marginal tooth preparation determines the marginal configuration of the metal-ceramic crown. The three options are:

1. **Beveled or feathered edge:** the preparation is covered only in metal.
2. **Chamfer:** if the depth of the chamfer is at least 1 mm, the porcelain can extend over the metal and a supported porcelain margin can be constructed.
3. **Shoulder:** the preparation must be 1 mm for the porcelain to cover the metal.

32. Is the design of the metal framework of a fixed bridge different from the design of a single unit?

The design of the metal framework must incorporate four basic interrelationships: strength, esthetics, contour, and occlusion. In fixed bridgework, however, strength of the substrate plays the dominant role. Therefore, greater attention must be paid to reinforcement of the framework than of a single unit.

33. How do design problems of the metal framework influence the function of the metal-ceramic restorations?

The function of the metal-ceramic restoration is influenced by the design of the metal framework in the following ways:

1. The color of the porcelain is compromised between abutments and pontics if the thickness of the porcelain varies.
2. If the porcelain veneer is too thick (>2 mm) because of improper framework design, much of the strength of the interface bond is lost.
3. If the porcelain veneer is too thin (≤0.75 mm), the esthetic effect is compromised.
4. The metal framework is designed to resist deformation. If strut-type connector design is not used in the fixed bridgework, the bridge may flex and result in porcelain fracture.

34. What is metamerism? How does it affect the metal-ceramic restoration?

Metamerism is the optical property by which two objects with the same color but different spectral reflectance curves do not match. This property is important in matching the shade of the metal-ceramic restoration to the natural tooth. Even if the colors are the same, different reflectance curves create the "just noticeable difference."

35. What is the importance of fluorescence in porcelain?

Fluorescence is the optical property by which a material reflects ultraviolet radiation. Fluorescence reflects different hues. Natural teeth can fluoresce yellow-white to blue-white hues. Fluorescence in porcelain is important to minimize metamerism of porcelain to natural teeth in varying light conditions.

36. What are hue, value, and chroma? What is their importance in dentistry?

Color consists of three properties:

1. **Hue** refers to color families (e.g., red, green).
2. **Value** refers to lightness or darkness as related to a scale from black to white.
3. **Chroma** refers to the saturation of a color at any given value level.

The properties have a practical use in ordering color.

37. What is opalescence?

Opalescence is the optical property seen in an opal during light transmission and light reflection. During transmission, the opal takes on an orange-white hue, whereas during reflection it takes on a bluish-white hue. This phenomenon also occurs in the natural tooth as a result of light scattering through the crystalline structure of the opal. The structure size is in the submicron range (0.2–0.5 μ). A porcelain restoration can demonstrate the opal effect by incorporating submicron particles of porcelain into the enamel (incisal) layer.

38. How do you select a shade to match the natural teeth?

There is no truly scientific method to analyze the shade of a natural tooth and to apply this information to the selection of porcelain and fabrication of the crown. Attempts to establish such a technique have met with limited success. At present, shade determination is designed to match natural teeth with a man-made replication (shade guide) that results in a range of acceptability rather than an absolute match.

39. Can you change a shade with external stains?

External stains or colorants are frequently used to minimize the differences between natural and ceramic teeth. They should be used rationally rather than empirically. An understanding of the color phenomenon is necessary in all aspects of shade control and is essential if extrinsic colorants are to be used correctly. Extrinsic colorants follow the physical laws of substractive color.

40. What guidelines derived from the color phenomenon apply to the use of external colorants?

The understanding of hue, value, and chroma and their effect on external staining of a crown are essential. The major guidelines are as follow:

Hue: Drastic change of the shade of the ceramic restoration by use of external colorants is quite often impossible. Slight changes in shade may be accomplished (e.g., orange to orange-brown).

Value: External colorants can be used to lower the value of the ceramic. The complementary color of the shade to be altered may have a darkening effect. It is almost impossible to increase the value or shade of the ceramic.

Chroma: Chroma can be successfully increased by external colorants, most frequently in the gingival or interproximal areas.

41. What effects can be created with surface stains?

1. Separation and individualization with interproximal staining
2. Coloration of a cervical area to emulate root surface and to produce the illusion of change of form
3. Coloration of hypocalcified areas
4. Coloration of check lines
5. Coloration of stain lines
6. Neutralization of hue for increase of apparent translucency (usually violet)
7. Highlighting and shadowing
8. Incisal edge modifications—emulated opacities, high chroma areas, stain areas
9. Synthetic restorations
10. Aging

42. Are external colorants stable in the oral cavity?

External colorants are metallic oxides that fuse to the ceramic unit during a predetermined firing cycle. Although quite stable in an air environment, they are susceptible to corrosion when subjected to certain oral environments. Depending on the stain and the pH of the oral fluids, external colorants may be lost from the ceramic unit over a long period of time.

43. What is the most important factor in determining the strength of a ceramic?

The most important factor in the strength of a ceramic material is control of small flaws or microcracks, which often are present both at the surface and internally. In most cases, the strength of the ceramic depends on surface flaws rather than porosity within the normal range.

44. Should porcelain be used on the occlusal surface of a metal-ceramic crown?
In general, the surface hardness of dental porcelains is greater than that of tooth structure, metal alloys, and all other restorative materials. This may lead to excessive wear of the opposing dentition if certain occlusal guidelines are not followed. In the best scenario, the opposing material is porcelain, but results are good if the occlusal loads have good force distribution. Porcelain is contraindicated in patients who indulge in bruxism or parafunctional activities in which occlusal overloading may occur.

45. Can a porcelain fracture of a metal ceramic restoration be repaired?
It is now possible to bond composite or ceramic materials to a fractured restoration. The bond, which may occur on porcelain or on the metal substrate, is sufficiently strong to be resistant in a non- or low–stress-bearing area. However, if the fracture occurs in a stress-bearing area, the probability of a successful repair is low.

46. On what basis do you choose between an all-ceramic or a metal-ceramic crown?
In recent times all-ceramic crowns have been frequently introduced. As with their predecessor, the porcelain jacket crown, which was introduced at the turn of the century, the main reason for their use is superior esthetics. Unlike the metal-ceramic crown, which is hindered by the metal substrate, the all-ceramic crown has the capability to mimic the optical properties of the natural tooth. However, all other factors—including strength, fit, ease of fabrication, and tooth selection and preparation—may inhibit its use.

47. Is tooth preparation the same for an all-ceramic crown as for a metal-ceramic restoration?
The same amount of overall tooth reduction is needed for a metal-ceramic restoration as for an all-ceramic crown (1.0–1.5 mm labially, lingually and interproximally). However, unlike the metal-ceramic restoration, which will accept any marginal design, marginal tooth preparation for the all-ceramic crown must be a shoulder or very deep chamfer (minimum of 1.0 mm tooth reduction).

48. Can the newer all-ceramic materials with high strength values be used in place of metal-ceramic restorations?
Some manufacturers claim that the newer ceramic materials with high theoretical strength values can be used in place of metal-ceramic restorations for any tooth and for small-unit, anterior fixed bridges. However, the guidelines for usage, such as tooth preparation, are more critical and in general more complicated than for metal-ceramic restorations. It is advisable, therefore, to use the all-ceramic crown in the anterior segment, where esthetics is the dominant factor.

49. What are the different types of all-ceramic crowns?
All-ceramic crowns may be categorized by composition and method of fabrication:
  Composition
  1. Feldspathic porcelain, such as a conventional porcelain jacket crown.
  2. Aluminous porcelain: Vitadur, Hyceram, Cerestore, Alceram, Inceram
  3. Mica glass: Dicor, Cerapearl
  4. Crystalline-reinforced glass; Optec, Empress
  Method of Fabrication
  1. Refractory die technique: Optec, Mirage, Hyceram, Inceram
  2. Casting: Dicor
  3. Press technique: Cerestore, Alceram, Empress

50. What is crystalline-reinforced glass?
A crystalline-reinforced glass is a glass in which a crystalline substance such as leucite is dispersed. This composition is employed in the Optec or Empress systems. Strength is derived from the crystalline microstructure within the glass matrix. The higher concentration of leucite crystals in the matrix limits the progress of microcracks within the ceramic.

51. What is the importance of alumina in an all-ceramic restoration?

Alumina (Al_2O_3) is a truly crystalline ceramic—the hardest and probably the strongest oxide known. Alumina is used to reinforce glass (as in Hyceram). The strength is determined by the amount of alumina reinforcement. Alumina is also used in total crystalline compositions (Cerestore, Alceram, Inceram), which may serve as the substructure much like metal coping. With this technique, the ceramic has high strength.

52. Is the cementing of an all-ceramic crown different from the cementing of a metal-ceramic crown?

The major difference is that a trial cement is not recommended for the all-ceramic crown, which obtains much of its strength from the underlying support of the tooth. If the cement washes out, the unsupported crown is susceptible to fracture. In general, all rigid cements can be used, but a bonded resin cement is highly recommended to maximize the underlying support.

53. Can all of the all-ceramic materials be bonded to the tooth preparation?

It is important that the ceramic material be chemically etched for bonding to a tooth. If the ceramic material cannot be properly etched, alumina is used in the substrate.

54. What is the significance of the refractory die?

A refractory die is used in many techniques for the construction of different types of all-ceramic crowns and veneers. Basically it is a secondary die obtained by duplicating the master die. The ceramic material is applied on the refractory die for the firing cycles. Once the cycles have been completed, the refractory die is removed, and the ceramic piece is returned to the master die. Refractory die material must have the following properties:

1. Compatibility with impression materials
2. Dimensional stability for measurements
3. Tolerance of high-heat firing cycles
4. Compatible coefficient of thermal expansion with the ceramic material used
5. Easy removal from the ceramic piece

55. What determines the design of the pontic?

The design of the pontic is dictated by the special boundaries of (1) edentulous ridge, (2) opposing occlusal surface, and (3) musculature of tongue, cheeks, or lips. The task is to design within these boundaries a tooth substitute that favorably compares in form, function, and appearance with the tooth it replaces. The tooth substitute must provide comfort and support to the adjacent musculature, conformity to the food-flow pattern, convenient contours for hygiene, and cosmetic value, if indicated.

56. How should the contact area of the pontic on the edentulous ridge be designed?

Three concepts in pontic design are currently popular:

1. The **sanitary pontic** design leaves space between pontic and ridge.
2. The **saddle pontic** design covers the ridge labiolingually. Total coronal width is usually concave.
3. The **modified ridge** design uses a ridge lap for minimal ridge contact. Labial contact is usually to height of the ridge contour (straight emergence profile).

The selection of the design depends on the following factors:

1. Spatial boundaries
2. Shape of edentulous ridge (normal, blunted, or excessive resorption)
3. Maxillary or mandibular posterior arch (In contrast to the mandibular posterior pontic, the maxillary edentulous ridge is usually broad and blunted and has superior cosmetic effects.)
4. Anterior pontic (The overriding cosmetic requirement is that form and shape reproduce the facial characteristics of the natural tooth.)

57. What is the emergence profile? What is its importance?
The emergence profile is the shape of the marginal aspect of a tooth or a restoration and relates to the angulation of the tooth or restoration as it emerges from the gingiva. This gingival contour is extremely important for tissue health after placement of a crown.

The most obvious error of the emergence profile of a crown is overcontouring, which creates abnormal pressure of the gingival cuff and leads to inflammation in the presence of bacteria. Overcontouring and poor emergence profile are due primarily to (1) inadequate tooth preparation, (2) improper handling of materials and/or (3) inadequate communication between the dentist and the technician.

58. After periodontal therapy, when can the dentist complete the marginal tooth preparation?
A certain period of time is necessary between completion of periodontal therapy and completion of the marginal tooth preparation both to establish and to stabilize the attachment apparatus on the root surface. If this waiting time is not observed, impingement of the restoration into the attachment apparatus quite frequently occurs. The result is an iatrogenic gingival inflammation. The amount of waiting time necessary depends on the aggressiveness of the gingival procedure. A reasonable guideline, however, is to wait at least 6 weeks for tissue resolution.

59. What is a biologically compatible material?
A biologically compatible material elicits no adverse response either in the tissue or systemically. Adverse tissue response may be due to any of the following:
1. Allergic reaction
2. Toxic response
3. Mechanical irritation
4. Promotion of bacterial colonization
In general, highly polished noble alloys and highly glazed porcelains are the most biologically compatible materials.

60. Is any material used to construct crowns suspected of biologic incompatibility?
In general, most materials used in the construction of crowns are biologically compatible. Adverse reactions have occurred to some materials, primarily because of unpolished metal or unglazed porcelain surfaces. However, reports in the literature indicate that nickel-chrome alloys used in castings may be biologically incompatible. An allergic response may occur in 10% of women and 5% of men.

REMOVABLE PARTIAL DENTURES

61. What is the most important factor in determining the success of a bilateral, free-end mandibular removable partial denture (RPD)?
The most important factor in determining success is proper coverage over the residual ridge. Coverage should extend over the retromolar pad to create stability of the RPD and to minimize the torquing forces on the abutment teeth.

62. When clasps are to be used on the abutment teeth, what important factors must be considered?
When clasps are used, it is important to design the prosthesis so that the path of insertion is parallel to the abutment teeth. This is an important factor in eliminating torquing forces on the abutment teeth during insertion and removal of the partial denture. If the planes are not parallel, then the abutment teeth must be adjusted.

The abutment teeth must also be evaluated for placement of the retentive clasps and the reciprocal bracing arm. The abutment teeth are then shaped to accept the clasps.

The proper positioning of occlusal rests on the abutment teeth is extremely important, and the teeth are prepared to optimize positioning.

63. What are the advantages and disadvantages of the cingulam bar as a connector?

Advantages

1. Space problems for bar placement seldom exist unless anterior teeth have been worn down by attrition.

2. No pressure is exerted on the gingival tissues with movement of the RPD.

3. The major connector forms a single unit with the anterior teeth, thus contributing to comfort of the RPD.

4. Indirect retention is provided.

5. Repair of the RPD is simple when natural anterior teeth are lost.

Disadvantages

1. The metal bar situated on the lingual surface of the anterior teeth is relatively bulky, especially where crowding is present.

2. Esthetics are compromised if spacing exists.

3. Marked lingual inclination of the anterior teeth precludes use of the bar.

64. What laboratory requirements should be implemented when a cingulum bar is used?

The laboratory requirements for use of a cingulum bar are as follows:

1. For sufficient rigidity, a minimal height of 4 mm and a thickness of 2.5 mm are necessary. These dimensions should be increased when the cingulum bar traverses more natural teeth.

2. No notches should be made in the metal to stimulate tooth contour because they weaken the bar. In the presence of reduced height, the bar is placed more gingivally and made thicker to provide rigidity.

3. The junction of the bar to the denture base must be sufficiently strong. The bar can cover the lingual surfaces of premolars, if present. The contour of the teeth should be adapted to the path of insertion of the RPD.

65. Are indirect retainers necessary in the construction of an RPD? If so, where should they be placed?

The function of an indirect retainer is to prevent dislodgement of the RPD toward the occlusal plane. In a total tooth-bearing RPD, it is unnecessary to include indirect retainers. However, when the RPD has a free-end saddle portion, it is advisable to include indirect retention to prevent vertical dislodgement.

The ideal positioning of the indirect retainer is at the furthest point from the distal border of the free-end saddle. For example, if the free-end saddle is on the lower right quadrant, the indirect retainer is placed on the lower left canine.

66. Is it advantageous to place stress-breaking attachments adjacent to a free-end saddle in an RPD?

The advantage of constructing a stress-breaking attachment next to a free-end saddle is to relieve torquing forces on abutment teeth that have been periodontally compromised. However, further displacement of the free-end saddle toward the underlying ridge may cause an acceleration of resorbtion of the residual ridge. It is preferable, therefore, to compensate for torquing forces on the abutment teeth by the proper extension of the saddle area.

67. Is it necessary to use clasps around abutment teeth in a RPD?

Clasps may be eliminated around abutment teeth if these teeth are restored with a partial or full crown containing some form of attachment that replaces the functions of the clasps. These functions include:

1. Guide planes for the RPD
2. Prevention of vertical displacement toward the ridge by the occlusal and cingular rest
3. Retentive function from the retentive arm
4. Bracing function from the reciprocal arm

Depending on the type of attachment, all or part of these functions may be replaced. With partial replacement, the remaining functions are incorporated into the RPD.

68. What is the difference between a precision and a semiprecision attachment?
A **precision attachment** is preconstructed with male and female portions that fit together in a precise fashion with little tolerance. Normally, there is no stress, and retention can be adjusted within the attachment. The attachment parts, constructed of a metal that can be placed into the crown and the RPD, normally are joined by solder. In general, no other clasps are necessary.

A **semiprecision attachment** is cast into the crown and the RPD. The female portion is normally made of preformed plastic that is positioned into the wax form and then cast. The male portion is cast with the RPD framework. The female and male parts fit together with much more tolerance than in the precision attachment, resulting in less retention. Secondary retentive clasping is necessary. Less torque is induced on the abutments with a semiprecision than with a precision attachment.

69. Do unlike metals in the male and female portions of the semiprecision attachment pose a problem?
The female portion of the attachment is cast with the crown and is made of the same metal as the crown. The male portion is cast into the RPD. The male portion is made of a harder metal than the female portion, which thus is subjected to greater wear. The wear pattern normally occurs on the vertical walls rather than on the occlusal seat. This creates a loosening of the attachment but no significant vertical displacement of the RPD. The result is the need for an adjustable retentive clasp.

70. What is the difference between an intracoronal and an extracoronal attachment?
An intracoronal attachment is placed within the body of the crown, whereas the extracoronal attachment is attached to the outer portion. The selection of one over the other depends on many factors; if designed properly, both types can be used successfully.

71. What are the advantages and disadvantages of an intracoronal attachment?
   Advantages
   1. Placement of torquing forces near the long access of the tooth, thus minimizing these forces
   2. Elimination of clasps
   3. Parallel guide planes for proper RPD insertion
   4. Capability to establish proper contour at the abutment-RPD interface
   Disadvantages
   1. More tooth reduction
   2. Need for adequate coronal length
   3. Lack of stress-bearing capability
   4. Difficulty in performing repairs

72. What are the advantages and disadvantages of an extracoronal attachment?
   Advantages
   1. Same amount of reduction of the abutment tooth and conventional restoration
   2. Elimination of clasps
   3. Incorporation of stress-breaking into attachment
   4. Ease of replacing parts
   5. Improved esthetics
   Disadvantages
   1. The attachment is positioned away from the long axis of the tooth, creating a potential for torquing forces on the abutment tooth.
   2. Adequate vertical space is necessary for placement of the attachment.
   3. Interproximal contour at the crown-attachment interface is difficult to establish correctly.

73. Is the unilateral RPD an acceptable treatment modality?
In general, a unilateral RPD is not an ideal treatment modality because cross-arch stabilization is necessary for success. A unilateral RPD can be used, however, when a single tooth is replaced and abutment teeth are on either side of the replacement tooth (Nesbitt appliance).

FULL DENTURES

74. What is the best material for taking a full-denture impression?
In taking a full denture impression, it is important to understand that the topography of an edentulous arch includes soft, displaceable tissue with undercut areas. An impression material must not distort the tissues. Therefore, the material must be low in viscosity and elastomeric so that it can rebound in the undercut areas.

75. Is border molding necessary for a full lower denture?
Unlike a full upper denture, a lower denture does not rely on a peripheral seal for retention. Thus one may assume that border molding is an unnecessary procedure during impression taking. This assumption is incorrect because inadvertent overextension can greatly reduce denture stability as well as irritate tissue. Underextension of the peripheral border decreases tissue-bearing surfaces, thereby affecting denture stability.

76. What is the importance of the posterior palatal seal? How is its position determined?
The posterior palatal seal is an important component because it completes the entire peripheral sealing aspect of a maxillary denture. Anatomically, the seal is located at the juncture of the hard and the soft palate and joins the right and left hamular notches. If the seal is positioned more posteriorly, then tissue irritation, gagging reflex, and decreased retention can result. If the seal is positioned more anteriorly, tissue irritation and decreased retention can result. Manual palpation and phonetics (the "ah" sound) are the best ways to determine the anatomic position for the palatal seal.

77. What are the critical areas in the border-molding procedure of taking impressions for a maxillary arch?
The most critical area to capture in an impression is the mucogingival fold above the maxillary tuberosity area. Proper three-dimensional extension of the final prosthesis is extremely important for maximal retention. Other critical areas are the labial frena in the midline and the frena in the bicuspid area. Overextension in these areas often leads to decreased retention and tissue irritation.

78. Should an impression be taken under functional load or passively at one static moment?
The answer to this question has been debated for years. Soft tissue constantly changes, and a static impression captures the tissue at one point in time. On the other hand, a functional impression is taken with abnormal masticatory loads. Therefore, there is no absolute method of taking the impression. Denture stability with occlusal forces and periodic tissue evaluation, however, are critical with both methods.

79. What are the critical areas to capture in an impression of a mandibular arch?
Mandibular dentures do not rely on suction from a peripheral seal for retention but rather on denture stability in covering as much basal bone as possible without impinging on the muscle attachments. Movement of the tongue, lips, and cheeks greatly affects the amount of tissue-bearing area. Therefore, apart from identifying and covering the retromolar areas, the active border molding performed by the lip, cheeks, and tongue determines the peripheral areas of a mandibular arch, thus establishing maximal basal bone coverage.

80. How do you determine the peripheral extent of a denture?
For a peripheral border impression, a moldable material should be used around a well-fitting tray. The material should have moderate or low viscosity so as not to displace tissue and should

set in a brief period of time. The lips, cheeks, and tongue dictate the extent of the peripheral impression. The impression is captured by exaggerated movements of the anatomic structures made by the patient or manipulated by the dentist.

81. If an impression does not capture everything that is intended, can you realign the existing impression?

One must always bear in mind that an edentulous ridge has soft, displaceable tissue. Thus it is important to relieve the pressure before realigning an existing impression. If this is not done, tissue is compressed, and dimensional stability of the final impression is compromised. This inevitability leads to an undersized, ill-fitting denture.

82. How is vertical dimension established in a totally edentulous mouth?

Vertical dimension is established with the aid of bite rims. The most important aspect of vertical dimension is to establish the freeway space. The minimal opening in freeway space, which is determined phonetically (the "s" sound), is normally 1–2 mm.

83. How are overlap and overjet established?

Overlap and overjet are established by the maxillary bite rim, which also establishes the occlusal plane. The bite rim is adjusted by its position relative to the lip and cheek.

84. Is the bite registration taken in the centric relation or centric occlusion position?

This controversy has been argued for years and remains unresolved. However, certain principles are generally accepted:
1. A centric relation position may be duplicated.
2. Centric relation is the same position in various openings of the vertical dimension.
3. Centric relation should be an unstrained position.
4. Centric occlusion may be employed if the bite registration is done without increasing the vertical dimension.

85. Is it necessary to take multiple bite registrations?

It is not necessary to take multiple bite registrations to capture a maxillary/mandibular relationship. However, because tissue displacement makes it difficult to obtain a stable bite with wax rims, a single accurate bite registration is unlikely. It is advisable, therefore, to take multiple bite registrations throughout the fabrication procedure and even after insertion of the final dentures.

86. What does the tooth try-in appointment accomplish?

The most obvious reason for the try-in appointment is to visualize the esthetics of the final teeth in regard to lip line, overbite and overjet, shape, and arrangement. The try-in appointment can also determine the fullness of the labial flanges in relationship to the cheeks and lips. Occlusal relationship can be checked and verified, and a new bit registration can be performed. Above all, the try-in appointment affords both the dentist and the patient a preview of the final completed denture.

87. How is posterior occlusion selected with regard to tooth morphology?

Posterior occlusion can range from monoplane (flat plane) to steep anatomic occlusal cusps. In general, the more anatomic the occlusion, the more efficient its function. However, it is more difficult to establish "balanced" occlusion with a steep anatomic denture, and lack of balance leads to denture instability. It is, therefore, easier to establish occlusal harmony with monoplane teeth. Overbite and overjet of the anterior teeth also affect selection of the posterior teeth.

88. How do overbite and overjet affect the selection of cuspid inclines of the posterior teeth?

Overbite and overjet of the anterior teeth affect selection of the cuspid inclines of the posterior teeth when balanced occlusion is to be achieved in lateral and protrusive movements:

Steep overbite . . . . steep cuspal incline
Small overbite . . . . monoplane
Wide overjet . . . . monoplane
Narrow overjet . . . . steep cuspal incline

89. Of what materials are denture teeth composed? How are they selected?

Denture teeth are made from basically three materials: porcelain, acrylic, and composite-filled resin. All three materials afford excellent esthetic capabilities.

Porcelain teeth afford the greatest degree of hardness and best withstand wear. However, they are brittle and difficult to change or adjust; they also have a low mechanical bond strength to the resin base.

Acrylic teeth, on the other hand, are the softest of the materials and therefore the least resistant to wear. They are, however, easy to use, they can be easily changed or adjusted, and they have the best bond strength to the denture base.

Composite-filled resin teeth have hardness and strength values between porcelain and acrylic; they bond well to denture base and can be adjusted easily.

90. What procedure should be followed for insertion of a full upper and full lower denture?

During the processing of the denture base, the probability of dimensional change is high. Dimensional change affects the adaptation of the base to the tissue-bearing area and also affects the occlusion. It is advisable, therefore, to verify the adaptation of the dentures to the tissue-bearing areas. This procedure can be accomplished by placing some type of pressure-indicating material inside the denture. The extension of the peripheral borders, especially in the frenum area, should be evaluated. Once the individual bases are adjusted, the occlusal balance should be carefully checked and adjusted. A remount procedure is recommended for this equilibration.

91. When the treatment plan calls for an immediate (transitional) denture, what are the expectations?

If the anterior teeth are to be extracted at the time of denture insertion, the patient should be informed that the denture teeth can be placed in the same position as the existing teeth. However, facial appearance will change because of the presence of the labial flange, which affects the fullness of the lip. The patient also should be made aware of the necessary process of adaptation to the palate and of the increase in salivary flow that over time will become normal. Finally, the patient should be told that most people adapt well to such oral changes.

92. Is the impression procedure the same for a transitional denture as for a conventional denture?

The impression procedure is approximately the same for establishing the peripheral border. The major concern in taking an impression around existing teeth and exaggerated undercut area is to select a material that has the lowest viscosity and is nonrigid after setting. These properties are important to avoid damage of existing teeth during the removal of the impression.

93. How is vertical dimension established in the construction of a transitional denture?

It is important to use the existing teeth to establish the centric occlusal position, regardless of the amount and position of the teeth. At the bite registration phase, a bite rim is constructed in the edentulous space adjacent to the existing teeth, and the teeth with the wax rim are used to capture the occlusal relationship.

94. If the master casts are altered in a transitional denture procedure (e.g., elimination of gross tissue undercuts), how is the surgical procedure altered?

It is necessary during the surgical procedure to know exactly how the master cast has been altered. This knowledge is critical for successful insertion of the transitional denture. It is advisable to construct a second denture base that is transparent. This surgical stent is placed over the ridge after the teeth are extracted. Pressure points and undercuts are readily visible, and surgical ridge correction can be performed.

95. When a transitional denture is inserted, what procedures should be followed?

It is always beneficial to have a surgical stent available to ascertain the fit of the denture base. Because many soft-tissue undercut areas may be present, it is critical to establish a single path of insertion of the denture. Gross removal of areas inside the dentures may lead to poor adaptation of the denture base and instability. In this situation an immediate soft-lining material is indicated.

96. During the healing phase, what procedures should be followed?

The patient should be instructed not to remove the denture and to return after 24 hours. At that time, tissue irritation and occlusion are checked, and the denture is adjusted. Then the patient is instructed about insertion and removal of the denture and told that as the ridges heal, resorption will occur. Each case varies, but in general resorption leads to a loosening of the denture. Therefore, transitional soft-lining procedures should be performed throughout the healing phase, on approximately a monthly basis. The final healing may take from 3–6 months, at which time a permanent lining in the existing denture or a new denture is constructed.

97. Is a face-bow transfer necessary in jaw registration in the full-denture construction?

It is advisable to take a face-bow transfer in the construction of a full denture. The purpose of the registration is to relate the maxillary bite rims to the temperomandibular joint and facial planes. This registration aids in determining not only esthetic factors but also the type of occlusal plane.

98. Is it necessary to take eccentric bite registrations in the construction of full dentures?

Although eccentric bite registrations are not essential, they aid in establishing a balanced occlusion. A stable occlusion is important for the retention and stability of dentures as well as for functional efficiency.

99. What is the neutral zone? How does it relate to the alveolar ridge?

The neutral zone is defined as the potential space between the lips and cheeks on one side and the tongue on the other. Natural or artificial teeth in this zone are subject to equal and opposite forces from the surrounding musculature. The alveolar ridge, which normally dictates the position of the denture teeth, may conflict with the neutral zone. Therefore, the neutral position zone also should be considered when denture teeth are positioned.

100. Are there any advantages to retaining roots under a denture apart from retention properties?

Retention is a critical aspect in root-retained dentures. Of equal importance, however, retained roots help to prevent resorbtion of the residual ridges. Retained roots also afford the patient some proprioceptive sense of "naturalness" in function of dentures.

101. What is the ideal type of attachment in a root-retained denture?

The ideal type of attachment affords maximal retentive forces for the denture with minimal torquing forces to the roots. Because these ideal properties cannot be totally obtained, a compromise is necessary. Many factors determine how much retention a tooth can withstand without subjection to harmful forces, including:

1. The amount of supportive bone around the retained roots
2. The number of existing roots
3. The type and amount of occlusal forces
4. The type of attachment (i.e., intra- or extraradicular, rigid or stress-bearing attachments)
5. Splinting or nonsplinting of roots

102. In a root-retained denture, which is better—intraradicular or extraradicular attachment?

Both attachments can be equally retentive, but the intraradicular attachment places the fulcrum forces more deeply into the bone than an extraradicular attachment and thus helps to withstand deleterious torquing forces. The intraradicular attachments, however, are more difficult to implement because of (1) length of existing root, (2) width of existing root, (3) paralleling to other roots, (4) inability to splint, and (5) difficulty in hygiene.

103. Is splinting a preferred treatment in a root-retained denture?

The main purpose of splinting roots in a tooth-borne denture is to dissipate the forces, thus minimizing the torque on the existing roots. Splinting does not necessarily result in increased denture retention, but it creates a more difficult construction procedure. Splinting should be attempted after certain aspects are evaluated, such as (1) paralleling, (2) amount of freeway space, (3) placement of bar to ridge, and (4) type of bar.

104. What is the difference between a rigid and a stress-breaking attachment?

In **rigid attachment** the male and female components join in a precise fashion, allowing almost no movement between the two parts. This creates a rigid, nonflexible attachment that affords the greatest amount of retention but also produces the greatest amount of torque on the retained roots. A rigid attachment is not recommended on periodontically compromised teeth.

A **stress-bearing attachment** affords movement between the male and female components, thereby relieving torque. In most cases, a stress-bearing attachment is recommended.

105. How many roots must be retained to construct a root-retained denture?

There is no fixed rule. A root-retained denture can be constructed with only one root. The fewer the roots, the less the retentive force that should be applied to them. The ideal distribution of retained roots would be both cuspid regions and bilateral molar regions.

106. Is it necessary to place attachments or to cover the roots of a root-retained denture?

It is not always necessary to cover a root beneath an overdenture. Retention is not the only goal of this treatment modality. Equally important is preservation of the residual ridge by retaining the roots. However, if a root is not covered, the exposed surfaces are highly susceptible to decay. Oral hygiene must be stringently maintained.

107. Are the principles the same for a maxillary as for a mandibular overdenture?

Many of the principles for root-retained dentures are the same for the maxillary arch as for the mandible, including (1) selection of roots to be retained with regard to position and stability, (2) types of attachments, (3) paralleling, and (4) splinting. One aspect that may differ is related to morphologic differences of the residual ridges. The maxillary arch has a greater probability of undercut areas in the anterior region above the roots. This difference is quite apparent in the canine area. It is necessary to design the path of insertion to take the undercuts into consideration. Therefore, attachment selection may have to be altered, and the peripheral border of the denture may have to be reduced or eliminated.

108. Can the palate be eliminated in a root-retained maxillary denture?

If retention is adequate from the retained roots with their attachments, it is possible to eliminate the palate. It must be remembered that the palatal area affords the denture the greatest bearing area and also creates cross-arch stabilization.

109. What are the causes of denture stomatitis? How can it be treated?

Denture stomatitis is caused by trauma from poorly fitting dentures, by poor oral and denture hygiene, and by the oral fungus *Candida albicans.*

Denture stomatitis can be treated by using resilient denture liners that stabilize ill-fitting dentures, thereby treating the inflamed tissue. Some liners may also inhibit fungal growth.

BIBLIOGRAPHY

1. Chiche GJ, Pinault A: Esthetics of Anterior Fixed Prosthodontics. Chicago, Quintessence, 1993.
2. Lucia VO: Treatment of the Edentulous Patient. Chicago, Quintessence, 1986.
3. McLean JW: The Science and Art of Dental Ceramics, Vol. I. Chicago, Quintessence, 1979.
4. McLean JW: The Science and Art of Dental Ceramics, Vol. II. Chicago, Quintessence, 1980.
5. Morrow RM, Rudd KD, Rhoads JE: Dental Laboratory Procedures: Complete Dentures, Vol. 1, 2nd ed. St. Louis, Mosby, 1986.
6. Phillips R: Skinner's Science of Dental Materials, 9th ed. Philadelphia, W.B. Saunders, 1991.
7. Shillingburg HT Jr, et al: Fundamentals of Fixed Prosthodontics, 2nd ed. Chicago, Quintessence, 1981.
8. Rudd KD, Morrow RM, Rhoads JE: Dental Laboratory Procedures: Removable Partial Dentures, Vol. 3. St. Louis, Mosby, 1986.
9. Yamamoto M: Metal Ceramics: Principles and Methods of Makoto Yamamoto. Tokyo, Quintessence, 1990.

10. ORAL SURGERY

Stephen T. Sonis, D.M.D., D.M.Sc., and Willie L. Stephens, D.D.S.

GENERAL QUESTIONS

1. What are the elements of a SOAP note used for patient assessment?
S = Symptoms
O = Objective findings
A = Assessment
P = Plan

2. Why should a patient be hospitalized for routine oral surgical procedures?
The most common reason for hospitalizing a patient for routine oral surgical procedures is behavioral management. Patients who are severely handicapped, for example, may not be able to tolerate care in an office setting. Patients who are at high medical risk are often best treated in the controlled environment of the operating room where constant monitoring and quick treatment of a problem can be more easily managed. The final reason for treating a patient in the operating room is an inability to tolerate or obtain local anesthesia.

3. What are the basic technical considerations in performing an incision?
- Use a sharp blade of appropriate size.
- A firm, continuous stroke is preferable to short, soft, repeated strokes.
- Avoid vital structures; incising the lingual artery can ruin your morning.
- Use incisions that are perpendicular to epithelial surfaces.
- Consider the anatomy of the site in placement of the incision.

4. What factors influence the placement of incisions in the mouth?
- Anatomy and location of vital structures
- Convenience and access

5. For making an incision in an epithelial surface, how should the scalpel blade be oriented?
To avoid bias, the incision should be made perpendicular to the epithelial surface.

6. What are the principles of flap design?
- Flap design should ensure adequate blood supply; the base of the flap should be larger than the apex.
- Reflection of the flap should adequately expose the operative field.
- Flap design should permit atraumatic closure of the wound.

7. What are the most frequent causes of the tearing of mucogingival flaps?
(1) Flaps are too small to provide adequate exposure, or (2) too much force is used to elevate the flaps.

8. What are the means of promoting hemostasis?

Pressure	Ligation with sutures
Thermal coagulation	Use of vasoconstrictive substances

9. Describe and discuss the function of Allis forceps in oral surgery.
Allis forceps have a locking handle similar to a needle holder and small beaks at the working end of the instruments. These beaks are useful in grasping tissue for removal.

10. What are the indications for tooth transplantation? Which teeth are most often transplanted?
Severe caries of the first molar is the most common indication for tooth transplantation. The first molar is atraumatically removed, and the third molar is placed into the socket. Success of the transplant is most predictable when the apices of the roots of the tooth to be transplanted are one-third to one-half formed with open apices and the bordering bony plates are intact.

11. What is genioplasty?
Genioplasty is a procedure by which the position of the chin is surgically altered. The most common techniques for genioplasty are osteotomy or augmentation with natural or synthetic materials.

12. How are facial and palatal clefts classified?

Class I	Cleft lip only
Class II	Cleft lip and cleft palate
Class III	Cleft palate only
Class IV	Facial cleft

13. What is the role of the general dentist in managing oral cancer?
The general dentist has three major roles in managing oral cancer:
   1. Perhaps the most important is detection. As the primary provider of oral health care, the dentist is in the position to detect the presence of early lesions. A high degree of suspicion should lead to aggressive evaluation of any abnormality of the oral soft tissues. Biopsy of most areas of the mouth is within the realm of the generalist.
   2. Once a diagnosis of oral cancer has been established, the dentist has the responsibility of ensuring that there are no areas of latent oral infection that may predispose to the development of osteoradionecrosis or other complications of therapy.
   3. Because xerostomia and subsequent caries are common among patients receiving radiation therapy to the head and neck, the generalist should educate the patient about factors and behavior that increase the risk and should provide the patient with trays for the self-application of fluoride gels. An aggressive recall schedule should be established.

14. What are the major oral side effects of radiation to the head and neck?

Xerostomia	Caries
Mucositis	Osteoradionecrosis

SUTURES: TECHNIQUES AND TYPES

15. What is the most common suture method? What are its advantages?
The interrupted suture is the most common method. Because each suture is independent, this procedure offers strength and flexibility in placement. Even if one suture is lost or loosens, the integrity of the remaining sutures is not compromised. The major disadvantage is the time required for placement.

16. What are the advantages of a continuous suture?
   • Ease and speed of placement
   • Distribution of tension over the whole suture line
   • A more watertight closure than interrupted sutures

17. What are the factors that determine the type of suture to be used?

Tissue type	Healing process
Wound condition	Expected postoperative course

18. How are sutures sized?
Size refers to the diameter of the suture material. The smallest size that provides the desired wound tension should be used. The higher the number, the smaller the suture. For example, 3-0 sutures are thicker than 4-0 sutures. The larger the diameter, the stronger the suture. In general, sutures for intraoral wound closure are 3-0 or 4-0.

19. What are the types of resorbable sutures? Nonresorbable sutures?

Resorbable	Nonresorbable
Plain gut	Silk
Chromic gut	Synthetic
Synthetic	Nylon
Vicryl	Mersilene
Dexon	Prolene

20. What is the difference between monofilament and polyfilament sutures?
Monofilament sutures consist of material made from a single strand. They resist infection by not harboring organisms. Plain and chromic gut are examples. Polyfilament sutures are made of multiple fibers that are either braided or twisted. They generally have good handling properties. The most common examples used in oral surgery are silk, Dexon, and Vicryl.

21. What are the principles of suturing technique?
- The suture should be grasped with the needle holder three-fourths of the distance from the tip.
- The needle should be perpendicular when it enters the tissue.
- The needle should be passed through the tissue to coincide with the shape of the needle.
- Sutures should be placed at an equal distance from the wound margin (2–3 mm) and at equal depths.
- Sutures should be placed from mobile tissue to fixed tissue.
- Sutures should be placed from thin tissue to thick tissue.
- Sutures should not be overtightened.
- Tissues should not be closed under tension.
- Sutures should be 2–3 mm apart.
- The suture knot should be on the side of the wound.

22. When should intraoral sutures be removed?
In uncomplicated cases, sutures generally may be removed 5–7 days after placement.

TOOTH EXTRACTION

23. What are the components of extraction forceps?
Handle
Hinge
Beaks

24. What forceps are typically used for the removal of maxillary teeth?
Single-rooted teeth are usually removed with a maxillary universal forceps (150) or a No. 1 forceps. Premolars can be extracted with the maxillary universal forceps. To extract maxillary molars, 150 forceps usually can be used. Alternatively, the upper molar cowhorn can be used for fractured or carious teeth if care is applied.

25. What forceps are typically used for the removal of mandibular teeth?
Ashe forceps are generally the most effective for the removal of mandibular incisors, canines, and premolars. A lower universal forceps (151) is an alternative. The 151 also can

be used for most molars, although a mandibular cowhorn forceps (No. 23) or No. 17 forceps are alternatives.

26. Name the indications for tooth extraction.

- Severe caries resulting in a nonrestorable tooth
- Pulpal necrosis that is not treatable with endodontic therapy
- Advanced periodontal disease resulting in severe, irreversible mobility
- Malpositioned, nonfunctional teeth
- Cracked or fractured teeth that are not amenable to conservative therapy
- Prosthetic considerations
- Impacted teeth when indicated (Not all impacted teeth require extraction.)
- Supernumerary teeth
- Teeth associated with a pathologic lesion, such as a tumor, that cannot be eliminated completely without sacrificing the tooth
- Before severe myelosuppressive cancer therapy or radiation therapy, any tooth that has a questionable prognosis or may be a potential source of infection should be extracted.
- Teeth involved in jaw fractures

27. What are the major contraindications for tooth extraction?

Contraindications may be either systemic or local. Systemic contraindications are related to the patient's overall health and may include the presence of a coagulopathy, uncontrolled diabetes mellitus, hematologic malignancy such as leukemia, uncontrolled cardiac disease, and certain drug therapy. Elective extractions in pregnant patients is contraindicated. Local factors include radiation therapy to the area, active infection, and nonlocalized infection. The presence of a localized, dentoalveolar abscess is not an arbitrary contraindication for extraction.

28. What factors affect the difficulty associated with tooth extraction?

- Position of the tooth in the arch. In general, anterior teeth are more easily extracted than posterior teeth. Maxillary teeth are less difficult than mandibular teeth.
- Condition of the crown. Carious teeth may be easily fractured, thus complicating the extraction.
- Mobility of the tooth. Teeth that are mobile as a consequence of periodontal disease are more easily extracted. Ankylosis or hypercementosis increases the difficulty of tooth removal. In assessing mobility, the operator needs to ensure that the crown is not fractured; fracture may produce a false sense of overall tooth mobility.
- Root shape and length
- Proximity of associated vital structure
- Patient attitude and general health

29. What conditions may influence the difficulty of extraction of an erupted tooth?

Root form
Caries
Hypercementosis
Prior endodontic therapy
Internal or external root resorption

30. How are cases classified according to their difficulty?

Type 1: Easy patient, easy case
Type 2: Easy patient, difficult case
Type 3: Difficult patient, easy case
Type 4: Difficult patient, difficult case

31. What are the major forces used for tooth extraction?

Rotation and luxation are the major forces used for tooth extraction.

32. For multiple extractions, what is the appropriate order of tooth removal?
In general, maxillary teeth are removed before mandibular teeth and posterior teeth before anterior teeth.

33. What principles guide the use of elevators in tooth extraction?
- Elevators may be used to assess the level of anesthesia and to release the periodontal ligament.
- The bone, not adjacent teeth, should be used as the fulcrum for elevator assistance in tooth extraction.
- Elevators are most useful in multiple extractions.
- Elevators may assist in the removal of root tips by using a wedge technique.

34. What are the steps in postoperative management of an extraction site?
1. Irrigate the site with sterile saline.
2. Remove tissue tags and granulation tissue from the soft tissue of the site.
3. Aggressive curettage of the socket is contraindicated. Pathologic tissue should be removed by gentle scraping of the socket.
4. Compress the alveolar bone with finger pressure.
5. Suture if necessary at the papillae bordering the extraction site and across the middle of the site.
6. Review postoperative instructions with the patient.

35. What are the indications for third-molar extraction?
Pericoronitis
Nonrestorable caries
Advanced periodontal disease
Position that prohibits adequate home care of the third molar or compromises
    maintenance of the second molar
Cyst formation
Malposition
Chronic pain
Association with a neoplasm
Resorption of adjacent tooth

36. Should all impacted third molars be extracted?
No. Fully impacted third molars that do not communicate with the oral cavity need not be extracted. The teeth should be followed regularly, however, to ensure that no pathologic process develops. No data support the suggestion that impacted third molars contribute to crowding of anterior teeth.

37. What are the major complications of tooth extraction?
Fracture of the root or alveolar plate
Displacement of a root tip
Bleeding
Dry socket (localized osteitis)
Fracture of the tuberosity
Infection
Perforation of the maxillary sinus
Paresthesia
Soft-tissue injury

38. What is the most common complication of tooth extraction? How can it be prevented?
The most common complication of tooth extraction is root fracture. The best method of prevention is to expose the tooth surgically and to remove bone before extraction.

39. Which tooth root is most likely to be displaced into an unfavorable anatomic site during extraction?

The palatal root of the maxillary first molar is most likely to be displaced into the maxillary sinus during extraction.

40. Describe the prevention and treatment of postoperative bleeding.

A thorough preoperative medical history helps to identify most patients at systemic risk for postoperative bleeding. On leaving the office, patients should receive both verbal and written instructions for postoperative wound care. Of particular relevance regarding bleeding is the avoidance of rinsing, spitting, and smoking during the first postoperative day. The patient should be specifically instructed to avoid aspirin. Patients should be instructed to bite on a gauze sponge for 30 minutes after the extraction.

A patient with postoperative bleeding should return to the office. The wound should be cleared of residual clot or debris, and the source of the bleeding identified. Local anesthesia should be administered, and existing sutures removed. The wound should be irrigated copiously with saline. Residual granulation tissue should be removed. A hemostatic agent, such as gelatin sponge, oxidized cellulose, or oxidized regenerated cellulose, may be placed into the extraction site. The wound margins should be reapproximated and carefully sutured.

41. What is a dry socket?

Dry socket is a localized osteitis of the extraction site that typically develops between the third and fourth postoperative day. The term applies to the clinical appearance of the socket, which is devoid of a typical clot or granulating wound. Consequently, patients develop moderate-to-severe throbbing pain. The frequency of dry socket after routine tooth extractions is around 2%. However, the condition may occur in as many as 20% of cases after extraction of impacted mandibular third molars.

42. How can dry socket be prevented?

Prevention of dry socket is somewhat controversial. It is generally agreed that careful technique with minimal trauma is helpful in minimizing the frequency of this complication. The literature contains mixed data relative to the efficacy of topical and systemic antibiotic postoperative regimens.

43. How is dry socket treated?

Curettage of the extraction site is contraindicated. The extraction site should be gently irrigated with warm saline. A medicated dressing is then placed into the socket. The medication used for this purpose has been the topic of much discussion. One alternative consists of eugenol, benzocaine, and balsam of Peru. Alternatively, a dressing composed of equal amounts of zinc oxide, eugenol, tetracycline and benzocaine impregnated on gauze can be used.

44. Describe pain control after extraction.

For the majority of patients, adequate control of postoperative pain is obtained with the use of nonsteroidal antiinflammatory drugs (NSAIDs). A large number of compounds are available. Data indicate that postoperative pain can be minimized if the first dose of NSAIDs is administered immediately after the procedure. No evidence supports that preoperative administration of NSAIDs favorably alters the postoperative course. For patients unable to take NSAIDs because of allergies, ulcer disease, or other contraindications, various narcotic analgesics are available. Patients taking such medications must be cautioned about drowsiness and concurrent use of alcohol or other medication. In no instance is persistent postoperative pain (> 2 days) to be expected, and patients should be instructed to call if they have prolonged discomfort, which may indicate infection or another complication.

45. Which teeth are most commonly impacted?

The most commonly impacted teeth are the third molars and the maxillary canines.

INFECTIONS AND ABSCESSES

46. What are the major origins of odontogenic infections?
The two major sources of odontogenic infection are periapical disease, which occurs as a consequence of pulpal necrosis, and periodontal disease.

47. What are the three clinical stages of odontogenic infection?
1. Periapical osteitis occurs when the infection is localized within the alveolar bone. Although the tooth is sensitive to percussion and often slightly extruded, there is no soft tissue swelling.
2. Cellulitis develops as the infection spreads from the bone to the adjacent soft tissue. Subsequently, inflammation and edema occur, and the patient develops a poorly localized swelling. On palpation the area is often sensitive, but the sensitivity is not discrete.
3. Suppuration then occurs and the infection localizes into a discrete, fluctuant abscess.

48. What are the significant complications of untreated odontogenic infection?
Tooth loss
Spread to the cavernous sinus and brain
Spread to the neck with large vein complications
Spread to potential fascial spaces with compromise of the airway
Septic shock

49. What are the principles of therapy for odontogenic infections as defined by Peterson?
1. Determine the severity of the infection.
2. Evaluate the state of the host defense mechanisms.
3. Determine whether the patient should be treated by a general dentist or a specialist.
4. Treat the infection surgically.
5. Support the patient medically.
6. Choose and prescribe the appropriate antibiotic.
7. Administer the antibiotic properly.
8. Evaluate the patient frequently.

50. What is the treatment of choice for an odontogenic abscess?
The treatment of choice for an odontogenic abscess is incision and drainage, which may be accomplished in one of three ways: (1) exposure of the pulp chamber with extirpation of the pulp, (2) extraction of the tooth, or (3) incision into the soft-tissue surface of the abscess. Antibiotic therapy is indicated in the presence of fever or lymphadenopathy.

51. How is incision and drainage of soft tissue best performed?
Local anesthesia should be obtained first. Care must be taken not to inject through the infected area and thus spread the infection to noninvolved sites. Once adequate anesthesia has been obtained, an incision should be placed at the most dependent part of the swelling. The incision should be wide enough to facilitate drainage. Blunt dissection is often helpful. After irrigation, a drain of either iodoform gauze or rubber should be placed to maintain the patency of the wound. Postoperative instructions should include frequent rinses with warm saline, appropriate pain medication, and, when indicated, antibiotic therapy. The patient should be instructed to return for follow-up evaluation in 24 hours.

52. When infection erodes through the cortical plate, it does so in a predictable manner. What factors determine the location of infection from a specific tooth?
- Thickness of bone overlying the tooth apex; the thinner the bone, the more likely it is to be perforated by spreading infection.
- The relationship of the site of bony perforation to muscle attachments to the maxilla or mandible.

53. State the usual site of bone perforation, the relationship to muscle attachment, the determining muscle, and the site of localization for each tooth for odontogenic infections.

INVOLVED TEETH	USUAL SITE OF PERFORATION OF BONE	RELATION OF PERFORATION TO MUSCLE ATTACHMENT	DETERMINING MUSCLE	SITE OF LOCALIZATION
Maxilla				
Central incisor	Labial	Below	Orbicularis oris	Labial vestibule
Lateral incisor	Labial	Below	Orbicularis oris	Labial vestibule
	(palatal)*	—	—	(palatal)
Canine	Labial	Below	Levator anguli oris	Oral vestibule
	Labial	(above)	Levator anguli oris	(canine space)
Premolars	Buccal	Below	Buccinator	Buccal vestibule
Molars	Buccal	Below	Buccinator	Buccal vestibule
	Buccal	Above	Buccinator	Buccal space
	(palatal)	—	—	(palatal)
Mandible				
Incisors	Labial	Above	Mentalis	Labial vestibule
Canine	Labial	Above	Depressor anguli oris	Labial vestibule
Premolars	Buccal	Above	Buccinator	Buccal vestibule
First molar	Buccal	Above	Buccinator	Buccal vestibule
	Buccal	Below	Buccinator	Buccal space
	Lingual	Above	Mylohyoid	Sublingual space
Second molar	Buccal	Above	Buccinator	Buccal vestibule
	Buccal	Below	Buccinator	Buccal space
	Lingual	Above	Mylohyoid	Sublingual space
	Lingual	Below	Mylohyoid	Submandibular space
Third molar	Lingual	Below	Mylohyoid	Submandibular space

* Parentheses indicate rare occurences.
Modified from Laskin DM: Anatomic considerations in diagnosis and treatment of odontogenic infections. J Am Dent Assoc 69:308, 1964, with permission.

54. What is osteoradionecrosis?

Osteoradionecrosis is a chronic infection of bone that occurs after radiation therapy. It is most commonly noted in the mandible of patients who receive treatment for head and neck cancer and have preexisting dental infection. Thus, the frequency is higher in dentulous patients compared with edentulous patients. Prevention of osteoradionecrosis involves the elimination of infected teeth before initiation of radiation therapy. The patient who receives radiation to the head and neck remains at risk for osteoradionecrosis.

55. What are the indications for hospitalization of patients with infection?

Fever > 101°F

Dehydration

Trismus

Marked pain

Significant and/or spreading swelling

Elevation of the tongue

Bilateral submandibular swelling

Neurologic changes

Difficulty breathing or swallowing

Leukocytosis (WBC > 10,000)

Shift of WBC to the left (increased immature neutrophils)

Systemic disease known to modify the patient's ability to fight infection

Need for parenteral antibiotics

Inability of patient to comply with traditional treatment

Need for extraoral drainage

56. What are the indications for antibiotic therapy in orofacial infection?
- Evidence of systemic involvement, such as fever, leukocytosis, malaise, fatigue, weakness, lymphadenopathy, or increased pulse
- Infection that is not localized but extending or progressing
- No response to standard surgical intervention
- Increased risk for endocarditis or systemic infection because of cardiac status, immune status, or systemic disease

57. What are fascial space infections?
Fascial spaces potentially exist between fascial layers and may become filled with purulent material from spreading orofacial infections. Spaces that become directly involved are termed spaces of primary involvement. Infections may spread to additional spaces, which are termed secondary.

58. What are the primary maxillary fascial spaces?
Canine
Buccal
Infratemporal

59. What are the primary mandibular fascial spaces?
Submental   Submandibular
Buccal   Sublingual

60. What are the secondary fascial spaces?
Masseteric   Lateral pharyngeal
Pterygomandibular   Retropharyngeal
Superficial and deep temporal Prevertebral

61. What is Ludwig's angina?
Ludwig's angina is bilateral cellulitis affecting the submandibular and sublingual spaces. Patients develop marked brawny edema with elevation of the floor of the mouth and tongue that results in airway compromise.

62. What is cavernous sinus thrombosis?
Cavernous sinus thrombosis may occur as a consequence of the hematogenous spread of maxillary odontogenic infection via the venous drainage of the maxilla. The lack of valves in the facial veins permits organisms to flow to and contaminate the cavernous sinus, thus resulting in thrombosis. Patients present with proptosis, orbital swelling, neurologic signs, and fever. The infection is life-threatening and requires prompt and aggressive treatment, consisting of elimination of the source of infection, drainage, parenteral antibiotic therapy, and neurosurgical consultation.

63. What is the antibiotic of choice for odontogenic infection?
Penicillin is the drug of choice; 95% of bacteria causing odontogenic infections respond to penicillin. For most infections, a dose of penicillin VK, 500 mg every 6 hours for 7–10 days, is adequate; 5–7% of the population, however, is allergic to penicillin.

64. What are alternative antibiotics for patients who are allergic to penicillin?
Erythromycin
Clindamycin
Tetracycline

65. Despite the advent of numerous new antibiotics, penicillin remains the drug of choice for odontogenic infections. Why?
- It is bactericidal with a narrow spectrum of activity that includes the most common pathogens associated with odontogenic infection.

- It is safe; the toxicity associated with penicillin is low.
- It is cheap. A 10-day supply of penicillin cost under $5, compared, for example, with Augmentin, which costs the patient approximately $70.

66. What is the major side effect associated with erythromycin?
Stomach upset and cramping are common after ingestion of erythromycin. Such side effects may be minimized by prescribing an enteric-coated formulation, by having the patient eat with the medication, or by prescribing a form of erythromycin that is absorbed from the intestine rather than the stomach.

67. What factors govern the selection of a particular antibiotic?

Specificity	Cost
Toxicity	Ease of administration

68. When should cultures be used for odontogenic infection?
- Infection in patients with immunocompromise due, for example, to cancer chemotherapy, diabetes mellitus, or immunosuppressive drugs
- Before changing antibiotics in a patient who has failed to respond to empirical therapy
- Before initiating antibiotic therapy in a patient who demonstrates signs of systemic infection

69. Why may antibiotic therapy fail?
Lack of patient compliance
Failure to treat the infection locally
Inadequate dose or length of therapy
Selection of wrong antibiotic
Presence of resistant organisms
Nonbacterial infection
Failure of antibiotic to reach infected site
Inadequate absorption of antibiotic, as when tetracycline is taken with milk products

70. Why is phenoxymethyl penicillin (penicillin V) more desirable than benzyl penicillin (penicillin G) for the treatment of odontogenic infections?
Penicillin V has the same spectrum of activity as penicillin G but is not broken down by gastric acid. It is absorbed well orally.

71. Does the initiation of antibiotic therapy obviate the need for surgical intervention in a patient with an infection?
No. Failure to eliminate the source of infection through surgical intervention ultimately results in the failure of other forms of therapy.

DENTAL TRAUMA

72. What are the most important questions to ask in evaluating a patient with acute trauma?
1. How did the injury occur?
2. Where did the injury occur?
3. When did the injury occur?
4. Was the patient unconscious or have nausea, vomiting, or headache?
5. Was there prior injury to the teeth?
6. Is there any change in the occlusion?
7. Is there any thermal sensitivity of the teeth?
8. Review of the medical history

Andreasen JO, Andreasen FM: Essentials of Traumatic Injuries to the Teeth. Copenhagen, Munksgaard, 1990.

73. Discuss the primary assessment and management of the patient with trauma.

The initial assessment and management of the patient with trauma are centered on identification of life-threatening problems. The three most significant aspects are (1) establishing and maintaining an airway, (2) evaluation and support of the cardiopulmonary system, and (3) control of external hemorrhage. The patient should be assessed and treated for shock.

74. What are the diagnostic methods of choice for evaluation of the pediatric patient with trauma?

History and physical examination are the mainstays in evaluating the pediatric patient with trauma. The clinician should determine the cause of the trauma, the type of injury and the direction from which it occurred. In the case of a younger child, it is helpful if an adult witnessed the traumatic event. Physical examination should determine the child's mental state, facial asymmetry, trismus, occlusion, and vision. The radiographic evaluation of choice is computerized tomography.

Kaban L: Diagnosis and treatment of fractures of facial bones in children. J Oral Maxillofac Surg 51:722–729, 1993.

75. What are the four best ways for a patient to preserve a recently avulsed tooth until he or she is seen by a dentist?

The four best ways for a patient to preserve a recently avulsed tooth are (1) to replace it immediately into the socket from which it was avulsed; (2) to place it in the mouth, under the tongue; (3) to place the tooth in milk; or (4) to place the tooth in saline (1 teaspoon of salt in a glass of water).

76. How should an avulsed tooth be managed?

1. Whenever possible, avulsed teeth should be replaced into the socket within 30 minutes of avulsion. After 2 hours, associated complications such as root resorption increase significantly.

2. The tooth should not be scraped or extensively cleaned or sterilized because such procedures will damage the periodontal tissues and cementum. The tooth should be gently rinsed with saliva only.

3. The tooth should be placed in the socket with a semirigid splint for 7–14 days.

77. What should be included in the clinical evaluation of the traumatized dentition?

Mobility testing   Electric pulp testing
Percussion sensitivity   Soft-tissue evaluation

Andreasen JO, Andreasen FM: Essentials of Traumatic Injuries to the Teeth. Copenhagen, Munksgaard, 1990.

78. Describe the injuries involving the supporting structures of the dentition.

Concussion: Injury to the tooth that may result in hemorrhage and edema of the periodontal ligament, but the tooth remains firm in its socket. Treatment: occlusal adjustment and soft diet.

Subluxation: Loosening of the involved tooth without displacement. Treatment: same as for concussion.

Intrusion: Tooth is displaced apically into the alveolar process. Treatment: if root formation is incomplete, allow the tooth to reerupt over several months; if root formation is complete, then the tooth should be repositioned orthodontically. Pulpal status must be monitored, because pulpal necrosis is frequent in the tooth with an incomplete root and close to 100% in the tooth with complete root formation.

Extrusion: Tooth is partially displaced out of the socket. Treatment: manually reposition tooth into socket, and splint in position for 2–3 weeks. A radiographic examination should be performed after 2–3 weeks to rule out marginal breakdown or initiation of root resorption.

Lateral luxation: Tooth is displaced horizontally, therefore resulting in fracture of the alveolar bone. Treatment: gentle repositioning of tooth into socket followed by splinting for 3 weeks. A radiographic examination should be performed after 2–3 weeks to rule out marginal breakdown or initiation of root resorption.

Avulsion: Total displacement of the tooth out of the socket. Treatment: rapid reimplantation is the ideal. The tooth should be held by the clinical crown and not by the root. Rinse the tooth in saline, and flush the socket with saline. Replant the tooth, and splint in place with semirigid splint for 1 week. Place the patient on antibiotic therapy (e.g., penicillin VK, 1 gram loading dose followed by 500 mg qid for 4 days). Assess the patient's tetanus prophylaxis status and treat appropriately. If the apex is closed, a calcium hydroxide pulpectomy should be initiated at the time the splint is removed. If the tooth cannot be replanted immediately, placing it in Hank's medium, milk, or saliva aids in maintaining the vitality of the periodontal and pulpal tissues. Follow-up radiographic examinations should be performed at 3 and 6 weeks and at 3 and 6 months.

79. What are the types and characteristics of the resorption phenomenon that may follow a traumatic injury?

Inflammatory external and internal resorption occurs when necrotic pulp has become infected, leading to resorption of the external surface of the root or the pulp chamber and/or canal. Immediate treatment with a calcium pulpectomy is indicated to arrest the process.

Replacement resorption occurs after damage to the periodontal ligament results in contact of cementum with bone. As the root cementum is resorbed, it is replaced by bone, resulting in ankylosis of the involved tooth.

80. When can the above forms of resorption be detected radiographically?

It is possible to detect periapical radiolucencies that indicate internal and external resorption after 3 weeks. Replacement resorption may be detected after 6 weeks.

81. Why should radiographs of the soft tissue be included in evaluation of a patient with dental trauma?

It is not uncommon for fragments of fractured teeth to puncture and imbed themselves into the oral soft tissue. Clinical examination is often inadequate to detect these foreign bodies.

82. When a lip laceration is encountered, what part of the lip is the most important landmark and the first area to be reapproximated?

The vermilion border, the area of transition of mucosal tissue to skin, is evaluated and approximated first. An irregular vermilion margin is unesthetic and difficult to correct secondarily.

83. How should a small avulsion of the lip be managed?

Avulsions can be treated with primary closure if no more than one-fourth of the lip is lost. The tissue margins should be excised so that the wound has smooth, regular margins.

84. How should a full-thickness, mucosa-to-skin laceration of the lip be closed? Which layers should be sutured?

A layer closure ensures an optimal cosmetic and functional results. First a 5-0 nylon suture is placed at the vermilion border. The muscle layer, the subcutaneous layer, and the mucosa layer are closed with 4-0 resorbable sutures; then the skin layer is closed with a 5-0 or 6-0 nylon suture.

85. How should a facial laceration that extends into dermis or fat be closed?

Wounds that extend into dermis or fat should be closed in layers. The dermis should be closed with 4-0 absorbable sutures, the skin with 5-0 or 6-0 nonabsorbable sutures.

86. Why is a layered closure important?
A layered wound closure reestablishes anatomic alignment and avoids dead space, thus reducing the risk of infection and scar formation. Closure of the muscle and subcutaneous tissue layers minimizes tension in the skin layer and thus allows eversion of the skin edges, which results in the most esthetic scar.

87. What structures are at risk when a facial laceration occurs posterior to the anterior margin of the masseter muscle and inferior to the level of the zygomatic arch?
The buccal branch of the facial nerve and the parotid gland duct are at risk with lacerations in this position. When such a laceration is encountered, facial nerve function must be tested, along with salivary flow from the parotid duct.

88. What is a dentoalveolar fracture? How is it treated?
A dentoalveolar fracture is a fracture of a segment of the alveolus and the tooth within that segment. This fracture usually occurs in anterior regions.

Treatment consists of reduction of the segment to its original position or best position relative to the opposing dentition, because it may not be possible to determine the exact position before injury. The segment is then stabilized with a rigid splint for 4–6 weeks.

89. What is the modified Le Fort classification of fractures?

Le Fort I	Low maxillary fracture
Ia	Low maxillary fracture/multiple segments
Le Fort II	Pyramidal fracture
IIa	Pyramidal and nasal fracture
IIb	Pyramidal and nasoorbitoethmoidal (NOE) fracture
Le Fort III	Craniofacial dysjunction
IIIa	Craniofacial dysjunction and nasal fracture
IIIb	Craniofacial dysjunction and NOE
Le Fort IV	Le Fort II or III fracture and cranial base fracture
IVa	Supraorbital rim fracture
IVb	Anterior cranial fossa and supraorbital rim fracture
IVc	Anterior cranial fossa and orbital wall fracture

90. Describe the Ellis classification of dental fractures.

Class I	Enamel only	Class III	Dentin, enamel, and pulp
Class II	Dentin and enamel	Class IV	Whole crown

91. Describe the management of each of the above fractures.

Class I	Enameloplasty and/or bonding
Class II	Dentin coverage with calcium hydroxide and bonded restoration or reattachment of fractured segment
Class III	Pulp therapy via pulp capping or partial pulpotomy
Class IV	If the fracture is supragingival, remove the coronal segment and perform appropriate pulp therapy, then restore. If the fracture is subgingival, remove the coronal segment and perform appropriate pulp therapy, then reposition the remaining tooth structure coronally either orthodontically or surgically. The surgical approach results in loss of pulpal vitality and therefore requires a pulpectomy.

92. What are the most likely signs and symptoms of a mandibular body or angle fracture?

Alteration in occlusion	Mobility at the fracture site
A step or change in the mandibular occlusal plane	Pain at the fracture site
Lower lip numbness	Bleeding at the fracture site or submucosal hemorrhage

93. How is a displaced fracture of the mandibular body or angle treated?
A displaced mandibular fracture is treated by open reduction and internal fixation in combination with several weeks of intermaxillary fixation. This procedure involves exposing the mandible through an incision, reducing the fracture, and fixing the fracture segments with interosseous wires. Arch bars are placed on the teeth and used with either intermaxillary wires or elastics to maintain intermaxillary fixation for several weeks.

In many cases, rigid internal fixation can be used to avoid intermaxillary fixation. These cases are treated by exposing the fracture area and applying a compression plate that provides absolute interosseous stability for the fracture. Intermaxillary fixation usually is not required.

94. What are the two causes of displacement of mandibular fractures?
Mandible fractures are displaced by the force that causes the fractures and by the muscles of mastication. Depending on the orientation of the fracture line, the attached muscles may cause significant displacement of fractures.

95. Are most fractures of the mandibular condyle treated by closed or open reduction?
Most fractures of the mandibular condyle are treated by closed reduction. Treatment usually consists of 1–4 weeks of intermaxillary fixation followed by mobilization and close follow-up.

96. What radiographs are used to diagnose mandibular fractures?
Panoramic radiograph
Occlusal radiography
Periapical radiography
Mandibular series
   Lateral oblique views
   Posteroanterior view
   Towne's view
Plain tomography
CT scan

97. What are the likely signs and symptoms of a zygomatic fracture?

Pain over zygomatic region	Submucosal hemorrhage or ecchymosis
Numbness in the infraorbital nerve distribution	Subconjunctival hemorrhage or ecchymosis
	Submucosal or subconjunctival air emphysema
Swelling in the zygomatic region	Palpable step at the infraorbital rim
Depression or flatness of the zygomatic prominence	Exophthalmos
	Diplopia
Nasal bleeding	Unequal pupil level

98. Which radiographs are used to evaluate and diagnose zygomatic fractures?
1. Plain film
   Waters' (posteroanterior obliques)
   Submental vertex
   Tomograms
2. CT scan

99. Which bones articulate with the zygoma?

Frontal bone	Maxillary bone
Sphenoid bone	Temporal bone

100. How may mandibular function be affected by a fracture of the zygoma or zygomatic arch?
A depressed zygomatic or zygomatic arch fracture can impinge on the coronoid process or temporalis muscle, causing various degrees of trismus.

LOCAL ANESTHESIA

101. What are the major classifications of local anesthetics used in dentistry?
Classification of local anesthetics is based on the molecular linkage between hydrophilic and lipophilic groups of the molecule. The amides, such as xylocaine and mepivacaine, are the most commonly used class of local anesthetics and for the most part have replaced esters, such as procaine.

102. What is the role of pH in determining the effectiveness of a local anesthetic?
Anesthetic solutions are acid salts of weak bases and have a pH in the range of 3.3–5.5. For the molecule to be active, the uncharged base must be available. If the tissue into which the solution is placed has a pH lower than the anesthetic solution, dissociation does not occur, and the amount of active base available is not adequate for a substantial anesthetic effect. A clinical example of this phenomenon is the injection of local anesthesia into an area of inflammation.

103. What are the advantages of including epinephrine in a local anesthetic solution?
There are two major advantages of including epinephrine in local anesthesia: (1) because epinephrine is a vasoconstrictor, it helps to maintain an optimal level of local anesthesia at the site of injection and thus reduces permeation of the drug into adjacent tissue, and (2) the vasoconstrictive properties of epinephrine also result in reduced intraoperative bleeding.

104. How significant is the concentration of epinephrine in local anesthetic solutions in affecting their hemostatic properties?
No difference in the degree or duration of hemostasis has been noted when solutions containing epinephrine of 1:100,000, 1:400,000 or 1:800,000 were compared. Five minutes should be allowed for epinephrine to achieve its maximal effect.

105. Which nerves are anesthetized using the Gow-Gates technique?
  1. Inferior alveolar nerve
  2. Lingual nerve
  3. Mylohyoid nerve
  4. Auriculotemporal nerve
  5. Buccal nerve

106. Describe the best type of injections of local anesthesia for extractions of the following teeth.

Maxillary lateral incisor	Infiltration at apex
	Infiltration of buccal soft tissue
	Nasopalatine block
Maxillary first molar	Infiltration at apex
	Infiltration over mesial root and over apex of maxillary second molar
	Anterior palatine block
Mandibular canine	Inferior alveolar block
	Lingual nerve block
Mandibular second molar	Inferior alveolar block
	Lingual nerve block

Peterson LJ, Ellis E, Hupp JR, Tucker MR: Contemporary Oral and Maxillofacial Surgery. St. Louis, C.V. Mosby, 1988.

107. What are the symptoms and treatment for inadvertent injection of the facial nerve during the administration of local anesthesia?
The patient develops symptoms of Bell's palsy. The muscles of facial expression are paralyzed. The condition is temporary and self-limiting. However, the patient's eye should be protected, because closure of the eye on blinking may be limited.

108. How does a hematoma form after the administration of a local anesthetic? How is it treated?

Hematoma may occur when the needle passes through a blood vessel and results in bleeding into the surrounding tissue. Posterosuperior alveolar nerve blocks are most often associated with hematoma formation, although injection into any area, particularly a foramen, may have a similar result. Treatment of hematoma includes direct pressure and immediate application of cold. The patient should be informed of the hematoma and reassured. In healthy patients, the area should resolve in about 2 weeks. In patients at risk for infection, hematomas may act as a focus of bacterial growth. Consequently, such patients should be placed on an appropriate antibiotic. Penicillin, 500 mg orally every 6 hours for 1 week, is a reasonable choice.

109. What are the reasons for postinjection pain following the administration of a local anesthetic?

The most common causes of postinjection pain are related to injury of the periosteum, which results either from tearing of the tissue or from deposition of solution beneath the tissue.

110. What causes blanching of the skin after the injection of local anesthesia?

Arterial spasms caused by needle trauma to the vessel may result in sudden blanching of the overlying skin. No treatment is required.

111. What is the toxic dose of most local anesthetics used in dentistry? What is the maximal volume of a 2% solution of local anesthetic that can be administered?

The toxic dose for most local anesthetics used in dentistry is 300–500 mg. The standard carpule of local anesthetic contains 1.8 cc of solution. Thus, a 2% solution of lidocaine contains 36 mg of drug (2% solution = 20 mg/ml × 1.8 ml = 36 mg). Ten carpules or more are in the toxic range.

112. What is the most common adverse reaction to local anesthesia? How is it treated?

Syncope is the most common adverse reaction associated with administration of local anesthesia. Almost half of the medical emergencies that occur in dental practice fall into this category. Syncope typically is the consequence of a vasovagal reaction. Treatment is based on early recognition of a problem; the patient often feels uneasy, queasy, sweaty, or lightheaded. The patient should be reassured and positioned so that the feet are higher than the head (Trendelenburg position); oxygen is administered. Tight clothing should be loosened and a cold compress placed on the forehead. Vital signs should be monitored and recorded. Ammonia inhalants are helpful in stimulating the patient.

POSTOPERATIVE MANAGEMENT AND WOUND HEALING

113. What are the principal components of postoperative orders?
- Diagnosis and surgical procedure
- Patient's condition
- Allergies
- Instructions for monitoring of vital signs
- Instructions for activity and positioning
- Diet
- Medications
- Intravenous fluids
- Wound care
- Parameters for notification of dentist
- Special instructions

Peterson LJ, Ellis E, Hupp JR, Tucker MR: Contemporary Oral and Maxillofacial Surgery. St. Louis, C.V. Mosby, 1988.

114. What is "dead space"?

Dead space is the area in a wound that is free of tissue after closure. An example is a cyst cavity after enucleation of the cyst. Because dead space often fills with blood and fibrin, it has the potential to become a site of infection.

115. What are the four ways that dead space can be eliminated?

1. Loosely suture the tissue planes together so that the formation of a postoperative void is minimized.
2. Place pressure on the wound to obliterate the space.
3. Place packing into the void until bleeding has stopped.
4. Place a drain into the space.

116. What is postoperative ecchymosis? How does it occur? How is it managed?

Ecchymosis is a black and blue area that develops as blood seeps submucosally after surgical manipulation. It is a self-limiting condition that looks more dramatic than it actually is. Patients should be warned that it may occur. Although no specific treatment is indicated, moist heat often speeds resolution.

117. What are the causes of postoperative swelling after an oral surgical procedure?

The most common cause of swelling is edema. Swelling due to edema usually reaches its maximum 48–72 hours after the procedure and then resolves spontaneously. It can be minimized by application of cold to the surgical site for 20-minute intervals on the day of surgery. Beginning on the third postoperative day, moist heat may be applied to swollen areas. Patients should be informed of the possibility of swelling. Swelling after the third postoperative day, especially if it is new, may be a sign of infection, for which patients need appropriate assessment and management.

118. What is primary hemorrhage? How should it be treated?

Primary hemorrhage is postoperative bleeding that occurs immediately after an extraction. In essence, the wound does not stop bleeding. To permit clear visualization and localization of the site of bleeding, the mouth should be irrigated thoroughly with saline. The patient's overall condition should be assessed. Once the general site of bleeding is identified, pressure should be applied for 20–30 minutes. Extraneous granulation tissue or tissue fragments should be carefully debrided. If the source of the bleeding is soft tissue (e.g., gingiva), sutures should be applied. If the source is bone, the bone may be burnished. Bee's wax can be applied. Placement of a hemostatic agent, such as a surgical gel, in the socket may be followed by the placement of interrupted sutures. The patient then should be instructed to bite on gauze for 30 minutes. At the end of that time, coagulation should be confirmed before the patient is dismissed.

A clot may fail to form because of a quantitative or functional platelet deficiency. The former is most readily assessed by obtaining a platelet count. The normal platelet count is 200,000–500,000 cells/mm^3. Prolonged bleeding may occur if platelets fall below 100,000 cells/mm^3. Treatment of severe thrombocytopenia may require platelet transfusion. Qualitative platelet dysfunction most often results from aspirin ingestion and is most commonly measured by determining the bleeding time. Prolonged bleeding time requires consultation with a hematologist.

119. What is secondary hemorrhage? How is it treated?

Secondary hemorrhage occurs several days after extraction and may be due to clot breakdown, infection, or irritation to the wound. The mouth first should be thoroughly irrigated and the source of the bleeding identified. The wound should be debrided. Sources of local irritation should be eliminated. The placement of sutures or a hemostatic agent may be necessary. Patients with infection should be placed on an antibiotic. If local measures fail to stem the bleeding, additional studies, especially relative to fibrin formation, are indicated.

120. Describe the stages of wound healing.
The **inflammatory stage** begins immediately after tissue injury and consists of a vascular phase and a cellular phase. In the vascular phase initial vasoconstriction is followed by vasodilatation, which is mediated by histamine and prostaglandins. The cellular phase is initiated by the complement system, which acts to attract neutrophils to the wound site. Lymphocytic infiltration follows. Epithelial migration begins at the wound margins.

During the **fibroplastic stage,** wound repair is mediated by fibroblasts. New blood vessels form, and collagen is produced in excessive amounts. Foreign and necrotic material is removed. Epithelial migration continues.

In the **remodeling stage,** the final stage of wound healing, collagen fibers are arranged in an orderly fashion to increase tissue strength. Epithelial healing is completed.

121. What is the difference between healing by primary and secondary intention?
In healing by primary intention, the edges of the wound are approximated as they were before injury, with no tissue loss. An example is the healing of a surgical incision. In contrast, wounds that heal by secondary intention involve tissue loss, such as an extraction site.

122. What are the five phases of healing of extraction wounds?
1. Hemorrhage and clot formation
2. Organization of the clot by granulation tissue
3. Replacement of granulation tissue by connective tissue and epithelialization of the wound
4. Replacement of the connective tissue by fibrillar bone
5. Recontouring of the alveolar bone and bone maturation

IMPLANTOLOGY

123. What are dental implants?
Dental implants are devices that are placed into bone to act as abutments or supports for prostheses.

124. Describe the differences in the bone–implant interface between osseointegrated implants and blade implants.
Osseointegrated (osteointegrated) implants interface directly with the bone, resulting in a relationship that mimics ankylosis of a tooth to bone. Osseointegrated implants are typically cylinders made of titanium. In contrast, blade implants are usually fabricated of surgical stainless steel. The interface between the implant and bone is filled with connective tissue fibers similar to the periodontal ligament.

125. What type of implants are currently favored?
Osseointegrated implants.

126. What are the requirements for successful implant placement?
• Biocompatibility
• Mucosal seal
• Adequate transfer of force

127. The surgical placement of most osseointegrated implants usually requires two steps. What are they? How long between them?
The first step is the actual placement of the implant. Most implants are covered with soft tissue during the time that they integrate with bone. This process takes between 3–6 months. After this period, a second surgical procedure is performed, during which the implant is exposed. Some brands of implants are not "buried" during the period of osseointegration, and therefore do not require a second surgical procedure.

128. Describe some of the indications for the consideration of implants as a treatment alternative.

- Resorption of alveolar ridge or other anatomic consideration does not allow for adequate retention of conventional removable prostheses.
- Patient is psychologically unable to deal with removable prostheses.
- Medical condition for which removable prostheses may create a risk, i.e., seizure disorder.
- Patient has a pronounced gag reflex that does not permit the placement of a removable prothesis.
- Loss of posterior teeth, particularly unilaterally

129. What are some contraindications for the placement of implants?

- Presence of pathology within the bone
- Presence of limiting anatomic structures such as the inferior alveolar nerve or maxillary sinus
- Unrealistic outcome expectations from patient
- Poor oral health and hygiene
- Patient inability to tolerate implant procedures because of a medical or psychological condition

130. What is the prognosis of osseointegrated implants placed in an edentulous mandible? Maxilla?

According to studies done with implants developed by Branemark, the stability of implant-supported continuous bridges in the mandible for a 5- to 12-year period was 100%, and of the maxilla, 90%.

131. What are the steps in the assessment of patients prior to implant placement?

Medical and dental history
Clinical examination
Radiographic examination

132. Which radiographic studies are used for patient assessment prior to implant placement?

For many implant cases, panoramic and periapical radiographs provide adequate information relative to bone volume and the location of limiting anatomic structures. In some instances, CT may be especially useful in providing information relative to multiplanar jaw configuration.

133. During preparation of the implant recipient site, what is the maximum temperature that should develop at the drill-bone interface?

To prevent necrosis of bone, a maximum temperature of 40° C has been recommended. This is achieved through the use of copious external or internal saline irrigation and low-speed, high-torque drills. In the final step of implant site preparation, the drill rotates at a speed of only 10–15 rpm.

134. What is the best way to ensure proper implant placement and orientation?

Careful pretreatment evaluation and preparation by *both* the surgeon and the restoring dentist are critical. A surgical stent fabricated to the specifications of the restoring dentist is an extremely helpful technique. Lack of pretreatment communication and planning may result in implants that are successfully integrated but impossible to restore.

135. Do any data suggest that osseointegration of implants may occur when implants are placed into an extraction site?

Some data suggest that placement of an implant into an extraction site may be successful, especially if the implant extends apically beyond the depth of the extraction site. Conventional treatment, however, consists of a period of 3 months from extraction to implant placement.

136. What anatomic feature of the anterior maxilla must be evaluated prior to the placement of an implant in the central incisor region?
The incisor foramen must be carefully evaluated radiographically and clinically. Variations in size, shape, and position determine the position of maxillary anterior implants. Fixtures should not be placed directly into the foramen.

137. Which anatomic site is the most likely to yield failed implants?
Implants placed in the maxillary anterior region are the most likely to fail. Because short implants are more likely to fail than longer implants, the longest implant that is compatible with the supporting bone and adjacent anatomy should be used.

138. Are there definitive data to support the contention that implanted supported teeth should not be splinted to natural teeth?
This is controversial. There are data to refute the claim that bridges that have both implant and natural tooth abutments do more poorly than bridges that are supported by only implants.

Gunne J, Astrand P, Ahlen K, et al: Implants in partially edentulous patients: A longitudinal study of bridges supported by both implants and natural teeth. Clin Oral Implant Res 3:49–56, 1992.

139. Is there any reason to avoid the use of fluorides in implant recipients?
Yes. Acidulated fluoride preparations may corrode the surface of titanium implants.

140. Do implants need periodic maintenance once they are placed?
Like natural teeth, poorly maintained implants may demonstrate progressive loss of supporting bone, which may result in implant failure. Aggressive home care is necessary to ensure implant success. Plastic-tipped instruments are available for professional cleaning.

141. What is the most common sign that an implant is failing?
Mobility of the implant is regarded as an unequivocal sign of implant failure.

PAIN SYNDROMES AND TEMPOROMANDIBULAR JOINT (TMJ) DISORDERS

142. What is trigeminal neuralgia?
Trigeminal neuralgia, or tic douloureux, results in severe, lancinating pain in a predictable anatomic location innervated by the fifth cranial nerve. The pain typically is of short duration but extremely intense. Stimulation of a trigger point initiates the onset of pain. Possible etiologies include multiple sclerosis, vascular compression of the trigeminal nerve roots as they emerge from the brain, demyelination of the gasserian ganglia, trauma, and infection.

143. Discuss the treatment of trigeminal neuralgia.
Drug therapy is the primary treatment for most forms of trigeminal neuralgia. Carbamazepine and antiepileptic drugs are used most often. If drug therapy fails, surgical intervention may be necessary. Surgical options include rhizotomy and nerve compression.

144. What symptoms are associated with TMJ disorders?
TMJ disorders are characterized by the presence of one or more of the following:
- Preauricular pain and tenderness
- Limitation of mandibular motion
- Noise in the joint during condylar movement
- Pain and spasm of the muscles of mastication

145. What are the two most common joint sounds associated with TMJ disorders? How do they differ?
Clicking and crepitus are the two most common joint sounds associated with TMJ disorders. Whereas clicking is a distinct popping or snapping sound, crepitus is a scraping, continous sound. Sounds are best distinguished by use of a stethoscope.

146. What are the components of evaluation of the patient with TMJ symptoms?
Evaluation of the patient with TMJ symptoms should include a detailed history of the problem, a thorough physical examination, and appropriate radiographic and imaging studies.

147. What should be included in the physical examination of the patient with TMJ symptoms?
- Gross observation of the face to determine asymmetry
- Palpation of the muscles of mastication
- Observation of mandibular motion
- Palpation of the joint
- Auscultation of the joint
- Intraoral examination of the dentition and occlusion

148. What are parameters for normal mandibular motion?
The normal vertical motion of the mandible results in 50 mm of intraincisor distance. Lateral and protrusive movement should range to approximately 10 mm.

149. What radiographic and imaging studies are of value in evaluating the TMJ?
No single radiographic study can be applied universally to provide definitive evaluation of the TMJ. Instead, a combination of lateral and anteroposterior views may be appropriate to diagnose intraarticular bony pathology. Lateral techniques include transcranial, panoramic, and tomographic studies. Anteroposterior views include transorbital, modified Towne, and tomographic examinations. Computerized tomographic studies may provide the most definitive information for the assessment of bony disease of the joint and surrounding structures. Magnetic resonance imaging (MRI) is the technique of choice to evaluate soft-tissue changes within the joint.

150. What is the likelihood that a patient with TMJ symptoms will demonstrate identifiable pathology of the joint?
Only 5–7% of patients presenting with TMJ symptoms have identifiable pathology of the joint. Based on this frequency, it clearly makes sense to proceed initially with conservative, reversible treatment.

151. What is the most common disorder associated with the TMJ?
Myofascial pain dysfunction (MPD) is the most common clinical problem associated with the TMJ.

152. What is the etiology of MPD?
The etiology of MPD is multifactorial. Functional, occlusal, and psychological factors have been associated with its onset. Fortunately, most cases are self-limiting.

153. What occlusal factors may contribute to MPD?
Clenching and bruxing may be associated with MPD, because each may result in muscle spasm or soreness. Lack of posterior occlusion, which results in changes in the relationship of the jaws, also is a potential cause. The placement of restorations or prostheses that alter the occlusion may cause MPD directly or indirectly through the patient's attempt to accommodate changes in vertical dimension.

154. What patient group is at highest risk for MPD?
Of patients with MPD, 70–90% are women between the ages of 20 and 40 years.

155. What are the diagnostic criteria for myofascial pain syndrome?
1. Tender areas in the firm bands of the muscles, tendons, or ligaments that elicit pain on palpation
2. Regional pain referred from the point of pain initiation
3. Slightly diminished range of motion

Sturdivant J, Fricton JR: Physical therapy for temporomandibular disorders and orofacial pain. Curr Opin Dent 1:485–496, 1991.

156. What signs and symptoms are associated with MPD?

Patients with MPD may have some or all of the following:
- Pain on palpation of the muscles of mastication
- Pain of the joint on palpation
- Pain on movement of the joint
- Altered TMJ function, including trismus, reduced opening, and mandibular deviation on opening
- Joint popping, clicking or crepitus
- Stiffness of the jaws
- Facial pain
- Pain on opening

157. What radiographc findings are associated with MPD?

None. Radiographic studies of the joint of patients with MPD fail to demonstrate the presence of pathology.

158. Describe the treatment approach to MPD.

Because most cases of MPD are self-limiting, a conservative, reversible approach to intervention is recommended. Patients should be informed of the condition and its frequency in the overall population (patients always feel better knowing that they have something that is "going around" rather than some rare, exotic disease), then reassured. Mobility of the joint should be minimized. A soft diet, limited talking, and elimination of gum chewing should be recommended. Moist heat, applied to the face, is often helpful in relieving muscle spasms. Diazepam has two pharmacologic actions that make it an especially good medication in the treatment of MPD: it is a major muscle relaxant, and it is anxiolytic. A typical dose might be 5 mg 1 hour before sleep and then 2 mg 2–3 times during the day. Patients should be cautioned that the drug may cause drowsiness. In general, diazepam rarely needs to be continued for more than 1 week to 10 days. Pain symptoms generally respond to nonsteroidal antiinflammatory agents. For patients with evidence of occlusal trauma or abnormal function, fabrication of an occlusal appliance may be helpful.

159. What are the indications for superficial heat in the treatment of facial muscle and TMJ pain?

1. To reduce muscle spasm and myofascial pain
2. To stimulate removal of inflammatory byproducts
3. To induce relaxation and sedation
4. To increase cutaneous blood flow

Sturdivant J, Fricton JR: Physical therapy for temporomandibular disorders and orofacial pain. Curr Opin Dent 1:485–496, 1991.

160. What are the contraindications for using superficial heat to treat facial pain?

1. Acute infection
2. Impaired sensation or circulation
3. Noninflammatory edema
4. Multiple sclerosis

Sturdivant J, Fricton JR: Physical therapy for temporomandibular disorders and orofacial pain. Curr Opin Dent 1:485–496, 1991.

161. What is the function of ultrasound in the therapy of myofascial pain?

Ultrasound provides deep heat to musculoskeletal tissues through the use of sound waves. It is indicated for treatment of muscle spasm or contracture, inflammation of the TMJ, and increased sensitivity of the joint ligament or capsule, and as a technique to push antiinflammatory drugs, such as steroid ointments, into the tissue. It is contraindicated in areas of acute inflammation, infection, cancer, impaired sensation, or noninflammatory edema. Ultrasound is typically administered by a physical therapist.

162. What is internal derangement of the TMJ?
Although internal derangement refers to disturbances among the articulating components within the TMJ, it is generally applied to denote changes in the relationship of the disc and the condyle.

163. What are the main categories of internal derangement?
- Anterior displacement of the disc with reduction, in which the meniscus is displaced anteriorly when the patient is in a closed-mouth position but reduces to its normal position on opening. Patients experience a click on both opening and closing.
- Anterior displacement of the disc without reduction (also called a closed lock)
- Disc displacement with perforation

164. What are the common symptoms of internal derangement?
- Pain, usually in the preauricular area and usually constant, increasing with function
- Earache
- Tinnitus
- Headache
- Joint noise
- Deviation of the mandible on opening

165. What imaging techniques are useful in the diagnosis of internal derangement?
MRI and arthrography are the imaging techniques of choice for evaluating soft-tissue changes of the joint. Because of its lack of invasiveness, MRI is preferred.

166. What is the treatment of internal derangement?
Initial treatment should be similar to MPD and is successful in a reasonable number of cases, particularly in patients with anterior disc displacement with reduction. Surgical intervention may be required in patients who do not respond to conservative therapy.

167. What are the most common causes of ankylosis of the TMJ?
Infection and trauma are the most common causes of ankylosis caused by pathologic changes of joint structures. Severe limitation of TMJ function also may be caused by non-TMJ factors, such as contracture of the masticatory muscles, tetanus, psychogenic factors, bone disease, tumor, or surgery.

168. Are tumors of the TMJ common?
No. Tumors of the joint itself are rare. However, benign connective tumors are common, including osteomas, chondromas, and osteochondromas. Both benign and malignant tumors also may affect structures adjacent to the joint and thereby affect TMJ function.

169. What is the effect of radiation therapy on the TMJ?
Patients receiving radiation therapy for the treatment of head and neck cancer may experience fibrotic changes of the joint. Consequently, they have difficulty with opening. Exercise may help to minimize such functional changes.

170. What is the effect of orthodontic therapy on the development of temporomandibular dysfunction?
The results of many well-controlled scientific studies have revealed no causal relationship between orthodontics and temporomandibular dysfunction.

171. What about extraction therapy?
Again, the results of several well-controlled studies offer no support to the contention that extraction therapy may precipitate TMJ disorders.

172. What degenerative diseases can affect the TMJ?

Osteoarthritis, osteoarthrosis, and rheumatoid arthritis may affect the TMJ. Over time, radiographs may demonstrate degenerative changes of joint structures. Often patients have a history of one of these conditions elsewhere in the body.

BIBLIOGRAPHY

1. Andreasen JO, Andreasen FM: Essentials of Traumatic Injuries to the Teeth. Copenhagen, Munksgaard, 1990.
2. Branemark P, Zarb G, Alberktsson T (eds): Tissue-integrated Prostheses. Chicago, Quintessence Books, 1985.
3. Donoff RB (ed): Manual of Oral and Maxillofacial Surgery. St. Louis, C.V. Mosby, 1987.
4. Kwon PH, Kaskin DM (eds): Clinician's Manual of Oral and Maxillofacial Surgery. Chicago, Quintessence Publishing, 1991.
5. Laskin DM (ed): Oral and Maxillofacial Surgery. St. Louis, C.V. Mosby, 1980.
6. Peterson LJ, Ellis E, Hupp JR, Tucker MR: Contemporary Oral and Maxillofacial Surgery. St. Louis, C.V. Mosby, 1988.
7. Smith RA; New developments and advances in dental implantology. Curr Opin Dent 2:42, 1992.
8. Tarnow DP: Dental implants in periodontal care. Curr Opin Periodontol 157, 1993.

THE FAR SIDE

By GARY LARSON

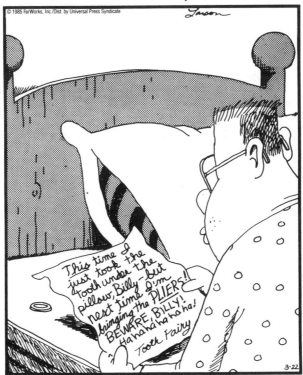

11. PEDIATRIC DENTISTRY AND ORTHODONTICS

Andrew L. Sonis, D.M.D.

1. What is the current schedule of systemic fluoride supplementation?

Fluoride Supplementation

	FLUORIDE CONCENTRATION IN LOCAL WATER SUPPLY (ppm)		
AGE	<0.3	0.3–0.6	>0.6
6 months to 3 yr	0.25 mg/day	0	0
3–6 yrs	0.50 mg/day	0.25 mg/day	0
6–16 yrs	1.00 mg/day	0.50 mg/day	0

2. What is the earliest macroscopic evidence of dental caries on a smooth enamel surface?
A white-spot lesion results from acid dissolution of the enamel surface, giving it a chalky white appearance. Optimal exposure to topical fluorides may result in remineralization of such lesions.

3. Which teeth are often spared in nursing caries?
The mandibular incisors often remain caries-free as a result of protection by the tongue.

4. What is the first step in treating a child who has ingested an amount of fluoride greater than the safely tolerated dose?
In acute toxicity, the goal is to minimize the amount of fluoride absorbed. Therefore, syrup of ipecac is administered to induce vomiting. Calcium-binding products, such as milk or milk of magnesia, decrease the acidity of the stomach, forming insoluble complexes with the fluoride and thereby decrease its absorption.

5. What is the appropriate amount of toothpaste to apply to the toothbrush of a preschool aged child?
Because children this age tend to ingest all the toothpaste on the toothbrush, no more than a pea-sized drop should be applied. Although the ingestion of even greater amounts of toothpaste does not represent a health risk, it may result in clinically evident fluorosis of the permanent dentition.

6. What are the indications for an indirect pulp cap in the primary dentition?
Because of the low success rate, most pediatric dentists feel indirect pulp caps are contraindicated in the primary dentition.

7. Which branchial arch gives rise to the maxilla and mandible?
The first branchial or mandibular arch gives rise to the maxilla, mandible, Meckel's cartilage, incus, malleus, muscles of mastication, and the anterior belly of the digastric.

8. How does the palate form?
The paired palatal shelves arise from the intraoral maxillary processes. These shelves, originally in a vertical position, reorient to a horizontal position as the tongue assumes a more inferior position. The shelves then fuse anteriorly with the primary palate, which arises from the median nasal process posteriorly and with one another. Failure of this fusion results in a cleft palate.

9. When do the primary teeth develop?
At approximately 28 days in utero, a continuous plate of epithelium arises in the maxilla and mandible. By 37 days in utero, a well-defined, thickened layer of epithelium overlying the cell-derived mesenchyme of the neural crest delineates the dental lamina. Ten areas in each jaw become identifiable at the location of each of the primary teeth.

10. After the eruption of a tooth, when is root development completed?
In the primary dentition, root development is complete approximately 18 months after eruption; in the permanent dentition, the period of development is approximately 3 years.

11. How should dosages of local anesthetic be calculated for a pediatric patient?
Because children's weights vary dramatically for their chronologic age, dosages of local anesthetic should be calculated according to a child's weight. A dosage of 4 mg/kg of lidocaine should *not* be exceeded in the pediatric patient.

12. What is the treatment for a traumatically intruded primary incisor?
In general, the treatment of choice is to allow the primary tooth to reerupt. This usually occurs in 2–4 months. If the primary tooth is displaced into the follicle of the developing permanent incisor, the primary tooth should be extracted.

13. What are the potential sequelae of trauma to a primary tooth?
1. **Pulpal necrosis** usually manifests as a gray or gray-black color change in the crown of the involved primary tooth at any time after the injury (weeks, months, years). No treatment is indicated unless other pathologic changes occur (e.g., periapical radiolucency, fistulation, swelling, or pain).

2. **Damage to the succedaneous permanent tooth,** including hypoplastic defects, dilaceration of the root, or arrest of tooth development, has also been reported.

14. What are the common signs of acute fluoride toxicity?
Acute fluoride toxicity can result in nausea, vomiting, hypersalivation, abdominal pain, and diarrhea.

15. Does the administration of prenatal fluoride result in any anticaries effect in the primary dentition?
Although there is little question that fluoride passes through the placental barrier, few data support the use of prenatal fluorides.

16. What are the advantages of fixed versus removable orthodontic appliances?
Fixed orthodontic appliances offer controlled tooth movement in all planes of space. Removable appliances are generally restricted to tipping teeth.

17. What is the straightwire appliance?
The straightwire appliance is a version of the edgewise appliance with several features that allow placement of an ideal rectangular archwire without bends (a so-called straightwire). These features include (1) variations in bracket thickness to compensate for differences in the labiolingual position and thickness of individual teeth; (2) variations in angulation of the bracket slot relative to the long axis of the tooth to allow for mesiodistal differences in root angulation of individual teeth; and (3) variations in torque of the bracket slot to compensate for buccal-lingual differences in root angulation of individual teeth.

18. What are so-called functional appliances? Do they work?
Functional appliances are a group of both fixed and removable appliances generally used to promote mandibular growth in patients with class II malocclusions. Although these appliances have been shown to be effective in correcting class II malocclusions, most studies indicate that their effects are mainly dental, with little if any effect on the growth of the mandible.

19. Is thumbsucking abnormal? Does it adversely affect the permanent dentition?

Almost all children engage in some form of nonnutritive sucking, whether it is a thumb, other digit, or pacifier. If such habits stop before the eruption of the permanent teeth, they have no lasting effects. If the habits persist, openbites, posterior crossbites, flared maxillary incisors, and class II malocclusions may result.

20. What are the indications for a lingual frenectomy?

Tongue-tie, or ankyloglossia, is relatively rare and usually requires no treatment. Occasionally, however, a short lingual frenum may result in lingual stripping of the periodontium from the lower incisors, which is an indication for frenectomy. A second indication is speech problems secondary to tongue position as diagnosed by a speech pathologist. Nursing problems have been reported in infants who were "cured" after frenectomy.

21. When should orthodontic therapy be initiated?

There is no one optimal time to initiate treatment for every orthodontic problem. For example, a patient in the primary dentition with a bilateral posterior crossbite may benefit from palatal expansion at age 4 years. Conversely, the same-aged patient with a severe class III malocclusion due to mandibular prognathism may be best treated by waiting until all craniofacial growth is completed.

22. What is the difference between a skeletal and dental malocclusion?

Skeletal malocclusion refers to a disharmony between the jaws in a transverse, sagittal, or vertical dimension or in any combination of these. Examples of skeletal malocclusions include retrognathism, prognathism, openbites, and bilateral posterior crossbites. **Dental malocclusion** refers to malpositioned teeth, generally the result of a discrepancy between tooth size and arch length. This discrepancy often results in crowding, rotations, or spacing of the teeth. Most malocclusions are neither purely skeletal nor purely dental but rather a combination of the two.

23. If a child reports a numb lip, can you be certain that the child has a profoundly anesthetized mandibular nerve?

Children, especially young ones, often do not understand what it means to be numb. The mandibular nerve is the only source of sensory innervation to the labial-attached gingiva between the lateral incisor and canine. If probing of this tissue with an explorer evokes no reaction from the patient, a profound mandibular block is assured. No other sign can be used to diagnose profound anesthesia of the mandibular nerve.

24. Does slight contact with a healthy approximal surface while preparing a class II cavity have any significant consequences?

Even slight nicking of the mesial or distal surface of a tooth greatly increases the possibility for future caries. Placement of an interproximal wedge before preparation significantly decreases the likelihood of tooth damage and future pathosis.

25. Why bother with restoring posterior primary teeth?

Caries is an infectious disease. As at any location in the body, treatment consists of controlling and eliminating the infection. With teeth, caries infection can be eliminated by removing the caries and restoring or extracting the tooth. However, extraction of primary molars in children may result in loss of space needed for permanent teeth. To ensure arch integrity, decayed primary teeth should be treated with well-placed restorations.

26. How should a primary tooth be extracted if it is next to a newly placed class II amalgam?

Two steps can be taken to eliminate the possibility of fracturing the newly placed amalgam: (1) The primary tooth to be extracted can be disked to remove bulk from the proximal surface. Care still must be taken to avoid contacting the new restoration. (2) Placing a matrix band (tee-band) around the newly restored tooth offers additional protection.

27. Can composites be used to restore primary teeth?
If good technique is followed, composite material is not contraindicated. Interproximally, however, it may be quite difficult to get the kind of isolation required for optimal bonding. There is no scientific advantage to using composite instead of amalgam for these restorations, and one has to evaluate whether esthetic effects justify the additional time required for the composite technique in primary teeth.

28. Which syndromes or conditions are associated with supernumerary teeth?

Apert's syndrome

Cleidocranial dysplasia

Cleft lip and palate

Crouzon's syndrome

Down syndrome

Gardner's syndrome

Hallermann-Streiff syndrome

Oral-facial-digital syndrome type 1

Sturge-Weber syndrome

29. Which syndromes or conditions are associated with congenitally missing teeth?

Achondroplasia

Cleft lip and palate

Crouzon's syndrome

Chondroectodermal dysplasia

Down syndrome

Ectodermal dysplasia

Hallermann-Streiff syndrome

Incontinentia pigmenti

Oral-facial-digital syndrome type 1

Rieger's syndrome

30. What is the difference between fusion, gemination, and concrescence?
Fusion is the union of two teeth, resulting in a double tooth, usually with two separate pulp chambers. Fusion is observed most commonly in the primary dentition.

Gemination is the attempt of a single tooth bud to give rise to two teeth. The condition usually presents as a bifid crown with a single pulp chamber in the primary dentition.

Concrescence is the cemental union of two teeth, usually the result of trauma.

31. What is the incidence of natal/neonatal teeth?
1/2,000–3,500.

32. What is the incidence of inclusion cysts in the infant?
Approximately 75%.

33. What are the three most common types of inclusion cysts and their etiology?
Epstein's pearls are due to entrapped epithelium along the palatal raphe.

Bohn's nodules are ectopic mucous glands on the labial and lingual surfaces of the alveolus.

Dental lamina cysts are remnants of the dental lamina along the crest of the alveolus.

34. What are the most common systemic causes of delayed exfoliation of the primary teeth and delayed eruption of the permanent dentition?

Cleidocranial dysplasia	Gardner's syndrome	Vitamin D–resistant rickets
Chondroectodermal dysplasia	Down syndrome	Hypothyroidism
Achondroplasia	DeLange syndrome	Hypopituitarism
Osteogenesis imperfecta	Apert's syndrome	Ichthyosis

35. What are some systemic causes of premature exfoliation of the primary dentition?

Fibrous dysplasia	Cyclic neutropenia	Acatalasia
Vitamin D–resistant rickets	Histiocytosis	Gaucher's disease
Prepubertal periodontitis	Juvenile diabetes	Dentin dysplasia
Papillon-Lefevre syndrome	Scurvy	Odontodysplasia
Hypophosphatasia	Chediak-Higashi disease	

Murphy's Laws of Dentistry

1. The easier a tooth looks on radiograph for extraction, the more likely you are to fracture a root tip.
2. The shorter a denture patient, the more adjustments he or she will require.
3. The closer it is to 5:00 PM on Friday, the more likely someone will call with a dental emergency.
4. The cuter the child, the more difficult the dental patient.
5. Parents who type their child's medical histories are trouble.
6. The more you need specialists, the less likely they are to be in their office.
7. When a patient localizes pain to one of two teeth, you will open the wrong one.
8. The less a patient needs a procedure for dental health, the more the patient will want it (e.g., anterior veneer vs. posterior crown).

36. What are the appropriate splinting times for an avulsed tooth, a root fracture, and an alveolar fracture?

Avulsed tooth: 7 days
Root fracture: 3 months
Alveolar fracture: 3–4 weeks

37. What can be done to prevent impaction of permanent maxillary canines?
Within 1 year after the total eruption of the maxillary lateral incisors, either a panoramic radiograph or intraoral radiographs should be taken to determine the axial inclination of the developing permanent canine. If mesial angulation is noted, extraction of the maxillary primary canine and maxillary first primary molars may often eliminate the impaction of the maxillary canine.

38. What is the most important technique of behavioral management in the pediatric dental patient?
Tell the child what is going to happen, show the child what is going to happen, and then perform the actual procedure intraorally. The major fear in the pediatric dental patient is the unknown. The tell, show, and do technique eliminates fear and enhances the patient's behavioral capabilities.

39. What pharmacologic agents are indicated for behavioral control of the pediatric dental patient in an office setting?
There are no absolutely predictable pharmacologic agents for controlling the behavior of the pediatric dental patient. Unless the operator has received specific training in sedation techniques for children, patients with behavioral problems are best referred to a specialist in pediatric dentistry.

40. If a primary first molar is lost, is a space maintainer necessary?
Before eruption of the six-year molar and its establishment of intercuspation, mesial migration of the second primary molar will occur, and a space maintainer is indicated to prevent space loss.

41. When should crossbites be corrected?
Whenever a crossbite is noted and the patient is amenable to intraoral therapy, correction is indicated. Although a crossbite can be corrected at a later date, optimal time for correction is as soon as possible after diagnosis.

42. What technique may be used if a pediatric patient refuses to cooperate for conventional bitewing radiographs?
A buccal bitewing is taken. The tab of the film is placed on the occlusal surfaces of the molar teeth, and the film itself is positioned between the buccal surfaces of the teeth and cheek. The

cone is directed from 1 inch behind and below the mandible upward to the area of the second primary molar on the contralateral side. The setting is three times that which is normally used for a conventional bitewing exposure.

43. What are the morphologic differences between primary and secondary teeth? How does each difference affect amalgam preparation?

1. Occlusal anatomy of primary teeth is generally not as defined as that of secondary teeth, and supplemental grooves are less common. The amalgam preparation therefore can be more conservative.

2. Enamel in primary teeth is thinner than in secondary teeth (usually 1 mm thick); therefore, the amalgam preparation is more shallow in primary teeth.

3. Pulp horns in primary teeth extend higher into the crown of the tooth than pulp horns in secondary teeth; therefore, the amalgam preparation must be conservative to avoid a pulp exposure.

4. Primary molar teeth have an exaggerated cervical bulge that makes matrix adaptation more difficult.

5. The generally broad interproximal contacts in primary molar teeth require wider proximal amalgam preparation than those in secondary teeth.

6. Enamel rods in the gingival third of the primary teeth extend occlusally from the dentinoenamel junction, eliminating the need in class II preparations for the gingival bevel that is required in secondary teeth.

44. What is the purpose of the pulpotomy procedure in primary teeth?

The pulpotomy procedure preserves the radicular vital pulp tissue when the *entire* coronal pulp is amputated. The remaining radicular pulp tissue is treated with a medicament such as formocresol.

45. What is the advantage of the pulpotomy procedure on primary teeth?

The pulpotomy procedure allows resorption and exfoliation of the primary tooth but preserves its role as a natural space maintainer.

46. What are the indications for the pulpotomy procedure in primary teeth?

1. Primary tooth that is restorable with carious or iatrogenic pulp exposure
2. Deep carious lesions without spontaneous pulpal pain
3. Absence of pathologic internal or external resorption but intact lamina dura
4. No radiographic evidence of furcal or periapical pathology
5. Clinical signs of a normal pulp during treatment (e.g., controlled hemorrhage after coronal amputation)

47. What are the contraindications for pulpotomy in primary teeth?

1. Interradicular (molar) or periapical (caries and incisor) radiolucency
2. Internal or external resorption
3. Advanced root resorption, indicating imminent exfoliation
4. Uncontrolled hemorrhage after coronal pulp extirpation
5. Necrotic dry pulp tissue or purulent exudate in pulp canals
6. Fistulous tracks or abscess formation
7. Contraindication to pulpotomy procedure

48. How does rubber-dam isolation of the tooth improve management of pediatric patients?

1. The rubber dam seems to calm the child as it acts as both physical and psychological barrier, separating the child from the procedure being performed.
2. Gagging from the water spray or suction is alleviated.
3. Access is improved because of tongue, lip, and cheek retraction.
4. The rubber dam reminds the child to open.

5. The rubber dam ensures a dry field that otherwise would be impossible in many children.

49. When do the primary and permanent teeth begin to develop?

The primary dentition begins to develop during the sixth week in utero; formation of hard tissue begins during the fourteenth week in utero. Permanent teeth begin to develop during the twelfth week in utero. Formation of hard tissue begins about the time of birth for the permanent first molars and during the first year of life for the permanent incisors.

50. What is the sequence and approximate age of eruption for primary teeth?

The primary teeth erupt in the following order: central incisor, lateral incisor, first molar, canine, and second molar.

In the mandible, the primary central incisor erupts at about 7–8 months of age, the lateral incisor at about 13 months, the first molar at 16 months, the canine at 20–22 months, and the second molar at about 27–30 months.

In the maxilla, the primary central incisor erupts at about 9–10 months of age, the lateral incisor at about 11 months, the first molar at 16 months, the canine at 19–20 months, and the second molar at 29–30 months.

51. What is the sequence and approximate age of eruption for permanent teeth?

In the mandible, the permanent teeth erupt as follows: first molar and central incisor (age 6–7 years), lateral incisor (age 7–8 years), canine (age 9–10 years), and first premolars (age 11–13 years).

In the maxilla, the sequence and approximate ages for eruption of permanent teeth is as follows: first molar (age 6–7 years), central incisor (7–8 years), lateral incisor (8–9 years), first premolar (10–11 years), second premolar (10–12 years), canine (11–12 years), and second molar (12–13 years).

52. What is leeway space?

Leeway space is the difference in the total of the mesiodistal widths between the primary canine, first molar, and second molar and the permanent canine, first premolar, and second premolar. In the mandible, leeway space averages 1.7 mm (unilaterally); it is usually about 0.9–1.1 mm (unilaterally) in the maxilla.

53. What changes occur in the size of the dental arch during growth?

From birth until about 2 years of age, the incisor region widens and growth occurs in the posterior region of both arches. During the period of the full primary dentition, arch length and width remain constant. Arch length does not increase once the second primary molars have erupted; any growth in length occurs distal to the second primary molars and not in the alveolar portion of the maxilla or mandible. There is a slight decrease in arch length with the eruption of the first permanent molars, but a slight increase in intercanine width (and some forward extension of the anterior segment of the maxilla) with the eruption of the incisors. A further decrease in arch length may occur with molar adjustments and the loss of leeway space when the second primary molar exfoliates.

54. What is ectopic eruption? How is it treated?

Ectopic eruption occurs when the erupting first permanent molar begins to resorb the distal root of the second primary molar. Its occurrence is much more common in the maxilla, and it is often associated with a developing skeletal class II pattern. It is seen in about 2–6% of the population and spontaneously corrects itself in about 60% of cases. If the path of eruption of the first permanent molar does not self-correct, a brass wire or an orthodontic separating elastic can be placed between the first permanent molar and the second primary molar, if possible. In severe cases, the second primary molar may exfoliate or require extraction, necessitating the need for space maintenance or space regaining.

55. When is the proper time to consider diastema treatment?

A thick maxillary frenum with a high attachment (sometimes extending to the palate) is common in the primary dentition and does not require treatment. However, a large midline diastema in the primary dentition may indicate the presence of an unerupted midline supernumerary tooth (mesiodens) and often warrants an appropriate radiograph.

The permanent maxillary central incisors erupt labial to the primary incisors and often exhibit a slight distal inclination that results in a midline diastema. This midline space is normal and decreases with the eruption of the lateral incisors. Complete closure of the midline diastema, however, does not occur until the permanent canines erupt. Treatment of residual midline space is addressed orthodontically at this time.

56. What is the effect of early extraction of a primary tooth on the eruption of the succedaneous tooth?

If a primary tooth must be extracted prematurely and 50% of the root of the permanent successor has developed, eruption of the permanent tooth is usually delayed. If >50% of the root of the permanent tooth has formed at the time of extraction of the primary tooth, eruption is accelerated.

57. Where are the primate spaces located?

In the maxilla, primate spaces are located distal to the primary lateral incisors.
In the mandible, primate spacing is found distal to the primary canines.

58. What is the normal molar relationship in the primary dentition?

Historically both the flush terminal plane and mesial step have been considered normal. More recent studies demonstrate that this may not be the case, because about 45% of children with a flush terminal plane go on to develop a class II molar relationship in the permanent dentition.

59. What is meant by the term "pseudo class III"?

This term refers to the condition in which the maxillary incisors are in crossbite with the mandibular incisors. Although the patient appears to have a prognathic mandible, it is due not to a skeletal disharmony but rather to the anterior positioning of the jaw as a result of occlusion. The ability of the patient to retrude the mandible to the edge-to-edge incisal relationship is often considered diagnostic.

60. What is the space maintainer of choice for a 7-year-old child who has lost a lower primary second molar to caries?

The lower lingual arch (LLA) is the maintainer of choice. The 6-year-old molars are banded. The connecting wire lies lingual to the permanent lower incisors in the gingival third and prevents mesial migration of the banded molars. Unlike the band and loop space maintainer, the LLA is independent of eruption sequence. (The band and loop serve no purpose after the primary first molar exfoliates.)

61. What is the space maintainer of choice for a 5-year-old child who has lost an upper primary second molar to caries?

The distal shoe is the appliance of choice. This appliance extends backward from a crown on the primary first molar and subgingivally to the mesial line of the unerupted first permanent molar, thus preventing mesial migration.

62. A 4-year-old child with generalized spacing loses three primary upper incisors to trauma. What space maintainer is needed?

No space maintainer is necessary.

63. What is the best space maintainer for any pulpally involved primary tooth?

Restoring the tooth with pulpal therapy is the best way to preserve arch length and integrity.

64. If a primary tooth is lost to caries but has no successor, is it necessary to maintain space?
Sometimes it is necessary to maintain the space, sometimes it is not. The decision is based on the patient's skeletal and dental development. Either way orthodontic evaluation is of utmost importance to formulate the future plan for this space.

65. When do you remove a space maintainer once it is inserted?
The space maintainer can be removed as soon as the succedaneous tooth begins to erupt through the gingiva. Space maintainers that are left in place too long make it more difficult for patients to clean. Furthermore, it may be necessary to replace a distal shoe with another form of space maintainer once the 6-year molar has erupted to prevent rotation of the molar around the bar arm.

66. What are the various types of headgear and their indications?
There are four basic types of headgear. Each type of headgear has two major components: intraoral and extraoral. The extraoral component is what generally categorizes the type of headgear.
    1. **Cervical-pull headgear.** The intraoral component of this type of headgear is composed of a heavy bow that engages the maxillary molars through some variation on a male-female connector. The anterior part of the bow is welded to an extraoral portion that is connected to an elasticized neck strap, which provides the force system for the appliance. The force application is in a down and backward direction. This headgear is generally used in Class II, division 1 malocclusions where distalization of the maxillary molars and/or restriction of maxillary growth, as well as anterior bite opening, are desired.
    2. **Straight-pull headgear.** The intraoral component is similar to the cervical-pull headgear. However, the force application is in a straight backward direction from the maxillary molar, parallel to the occlusal plane. Like cervical-pull headgear, this appliance is also used for the Class II, division 1 malocclusions. Due to the direction of force application, this appliance may be chosen when excessive bite opening is undesirable.
    3. **High-pull headgear.** The intraoral components of this headgear are similar to those described above. However, the force application is in a back and upward direction. Consequently, it is usually chosen for the Class II, division 1 malocclusions where bite opening is contraindicated, i.e., Class II malocclusion with an open bite.
    4. **Reverse-pull headgear.** Unlike the other headgears mentioned, the extraoral component of this headgear is supported by the chin, cheeks, forehead, or a combination of these structures. The intraoral component of this headgear usually attaches to a fixed appliance in the maxillary appliance via elastics. This type of headgear is most often used for Class III malocclusions, where protraction of the maxilla is desirable.

67. What is the basic sequence of orthodontic treatment?
    1. **Level and align.** This phase establishes preliminary bracket alignment generally with a light round wire, braided archwire, or a nickel-titanium archwire.
    2. **Working archwires.** This phase corrects vertical discrepancies (i.e., bite opening) and sagittal position of the teeth. A heavy round or rectangular archwire is usually employed.
    3. **Finishing archwires.** This phase idealizes the position of the teeth. Generally, light round archwires are used.
    4. **Retention.** Retention of teeth in their final position may be accomplished with either fixed or removable retainers.

68. What is a tooth positioner?
A tooth positioner is a removable appliance composed of rubber, silicone, or a polyvinyl material. Its appearance is not unlike that of a heavy mouthguard, except it engages both the maxillary and mandibular dentition. It is generally used to idealize final tooth position at or near the completion of orthodontic therapy. The appliance is usually custom fabricated by taking models of the teeth and then repositioning them to their ideal position. The positioner

is then fabricated to this ideal setup. The elasticity of the appliance provides for minor positional changes of the patient's teeth. Following completion of treatment, the positioner may then be used as a retainer.

BIBLIOGRAPHY

1. Andreasen JO, Andreasen FM: Essentials of Traumatic Injuries to the Teeth. Copenhagen, Munksgaard, 1990.
2. Enlow DH: Facial Growth, 3rd ed. Philadelphia, W.B. Saunders, 1990.
3. Gorlin RJ, Cohen MM Jr, Levin LS: Syndromes of the Head and Neck. New York, Oxford University Press, 1990.
4. Kaban LB: Pediatric Oral and Maxillofacial Surgery. Philadelphia, W.B. Saunders, 1990.
5. McDonald RE, Avery DR: Dentistry for the Child and Adolescent. St. Louis, Mosby, 1994.
6. Moyers R: Handbook of Orthodontics. Chicago, Year Book, 1986.
7. Pinkham JR, Casamassimo PS, Fields HW, et al: Pediatric Dentistry: Infancy through Adolescence, 2nd ed. Philadelphia, W.B. Saunders, 1994.
8. Proffit W, Fields HW: Contemporary Orthodontics. St. Louis, Mosby, 1993.
9. Scully C, Welbury R: Color Atlas of Oral Diseases in Children and Adolescents. London, Mosby-Year Book Europe Limited, 1994.

12. INFECTION AND HAZARD CONTROL

Helene Bednarsh, R.D.H., B.S., M.P.H.,
Kathy J. Eklund, R.D.H., B.S., M.H.P., and
John A. Molinari, PhD

EXPOSURE CONTROL

1. What is the difference between infection control and exposure control?
Infection control encompasses all policies and procedures to prevent the spread of infection, i.e., the transmission of disease. A newer term, exposure control, is the practice of preventing the exposure to begin with.

2. What is required to be contained in a written exposure control plan?
The following three elements must be included:
1. The employer's "exposure determination" identifying at-risk employees.
2. An implementation schedule and discussion of specific methods of implementing requirements of the standard.
3. The method for evaluating and documenting exposure incidents.

3. How often must a written exposure control plan be reviewed?
The Occupational Safety and Health Administration (OSHA) Bloodborne Pathogens Standard requires an annual review of a written exposure control plan. The plan must also be reviewed and updated if necessary should there be any change in knowledge, practice, or personnel that can affect occupational exposure.

4. What is an exposure incident?
As OSHA defines it, an exposure incident is any reasonably anticipated eye, skin, mucous membrane, or parenteral contact with blood or other potentially infectious fluids during the course of one's duties. In more general terms, an exposure incident is an occurrence that puts one at risk of a biomedical or chemical contact/injury while on the job.

5. What should be included in the procedure for evaluating an exposure incident?
1. What engineering controls and work practices were in place at the time of the incident?
2. What personal protective equipment was in use at the time of the incident?
3. What policies were in place at the time of the incident?

6. What is the OSHA definition of a "source individual" with respect to an exposure incident?
The standard defines "source individual" as "any individual, living or dead, whose blood or other potentially infectious materials may be a source of occupational exposure to the employee."

7. Are students covered by OSHA Standards?
In accordance with the Occupational Safety and Health Act of 1970, OSHA jurisdiction extends only to employees and does not cover students if they are not considered to be employees. Regardless of employee status, however, most aspects of the OSHA Bloodborne Pathogens Standard are considered to be standards of practice for exposure/infection control.

8. How do you determine who is at risk for an exposure?
Risk assessment begins by evaluating the tasks that are always done, sometimes done, and never done at all by an employee. If any one task carries with it a chance for exposure to blood

or other potentially infectious fluid or if a person may, even once, be asked to do a task that carries an exposure risk, then that employee is an at-risk employee who must learn to lessen, control, or eliminate the risk.

9. Can the receptionist help out in the clinic?
Only if that person has been trained to work in a manner that reduces his or her chance of an exposure incident and understands the risks.

10. What is an engineering control?
A technologically derived device that isolates or removes a hazard from the environment and thereby reduces a person's risk of an exposure incident is an engineering control.

11. Can you give some examples?
A needle recapping device is an engineering control, as is a sharps container which isolates sharps, wires, and glass. A rubber dam for certain dental procedures reduces the amount of aerosolization of fluids and, in so doing, reduces the amount of infectious fluids to which one is exposed.

12. Where should sharps containers be located?
Close to where they are used. To be most effective in reducing the hazard associated with nonreusable sharps, the container should be placed in a site near where the sharps are used and not in an area apart that would require transport or additional handling.

13. What needle recapping devices are acceptable?
If recapping must be done, it must be through the use of a mechanical device or a one-handed technique ("scoop technique") so as to ensure that needles are never in direct contact with a hand.

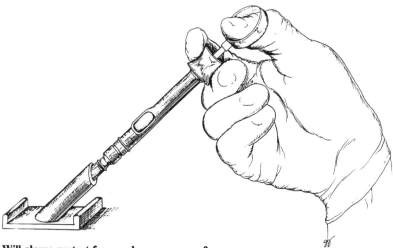

14. Will gloves protect from a sharps exposure?
To a limited degree only. The mechanical action of passing through the glove may reduce some of the microbial load. However, a glove will not stop something sharp from penetrating it.

15. If I cut myself while working on a patient, can I call that patient's personal physician to ask about the medical history?
In almost all states, you cannot. Calling without a written informed consent from the patient may violate medical confidentiality. You may discuss the situation with the patient, but no matter what, you should be evaluated by an appropriate health care provider or physician as soon as feasible.

16. What is aerosolization and how can it be reduced?
Aerosolization is the process whereby an artificially generated collection of particles is suspended in air and is capable of causing airborne infection. The particle size of a true aerosol is less than 50 μ in diameter. As a broad definition in infection control, aerosols are biologic contaminants that occur in solid or liquid form that may remain suspended in air for long periods of time.

Wilkins EM: Clinical Practice of the Dental Hygienist, 6th ed. Philadelphia, Lea & Febiger, 1989.

17. What is a work practice control? How does it differ from an engineering control?
Work practice controls are determined by behavior instead of technology, as are engineering controls. Quite simply, a work practice control is the manner in which a task is performed and the means of changing that manner to reduce the likelihood of an exposure. An example is how you recap a needle, how you use a device, or whether or not you use one at all. Also, something as simple as how you wash your hands so that it is protective is a work practice control.

18. What is the best work practice control for instrument precleaning?
Probably the best technique for precleaning instruments, which also reduces the potential of injury from sharps instruments, is to use an ultrasonic cleaner. If one is not available, then the work practice control would be to select one or two instruments at a time, hold them low in the sink under running water, and scrub them with a long-handled brush.

19. What should a proper handwashing agent be expected to accomplish?
At a minimum, it should:

   1. have the capacity to kill most bacteria and viruses;
   2. continue to kill bacteria and viruses, i.e., it should have a residual antimicrobial effect; and
   3. be dispensed without the risk of cross-contamination.

20. What is the purpose of flushing water lines?
Water lines should be flushed for at least 60 seconds between patients and for at least 3 minutes at the beginning of a clinic day. This process does not remove all contamination. To enhance the removal of contamination would require a specific filtration system in the water line, a sterile water source, or a chemical disinfection process in the lines. Flushing lines mechanically reduces the microbial contamination from resident biofilms. Biofilms are microbial masses that form a matrix on the inner walls of the water lines. As water flows through the matrix, some microorganisms may be released into the patient's mouth. Examples are *Actinomyces*, *Staphyloccocus*, *Legionella*, *Pseudomonas*, *Streptococcus*, and others.

21. What are some measures that will reduce the risk of cross-contaminating dental charts?
Cross-contamination risks can be minimized if charts are not taken into the operatory. If, however, they must be accessible during treatment, then they should not be handled with gloved hands. Overgloves, though, may be used atop clinic gloves to handle records (be sure not to contaminate the outside), or the record itself can be protected with a barrier.

PERSONAL PROTECTIVE EQUIPMENT

22. What type of personal protective equipment (PPE) should a dental health care worker use?
The selection of PPE should be based upon the type of exposure anticipated and the quantity of blood or other potentially infectious materials that reasonably may be anticipated to be encountered in the performance of one's duties. The material should be such that, with normal use, fluids cannot pass through to skin, undergarments, eyes, mouth, or mucous membranes.

23. Does clinic attire, a lab coat, protect me from disease?

The intent of clinic attire is to prevent infectious fluids from reaching the skin, especially nonintact skin, that can serve as a portal of entry for pathogenic organisms. Putting an effective barrier, such as a lab coat, between your body and these fluids reduces the risk of infection.

24. How do you determine if eyewear is protective?

The best evaluation is to look to the same experts OSHA did, the ANSI (American National Standards Institute) standards. These standards describe protective eyewear as being impact resistant, having coverage above the eyebrows down to the cheek, and having solid side-shields to provide peripheral protection. The eyewear should protect not just from fluids but also from flying debris that may be generated during a dental procedure.

25. Is a mask needed under a faceshield?

Yes, unless the faceshield has full peripheral protection at the sides and under the chin. Without comprehensive protection, aerosols can enter under and around the faceshield and may even become trapped in it.

26. What is the recommended bacterial filtration effectiveness for a face mask?

The recommendation is for 95 to 99% filtration of 1–3-μm particles, except in the case of *Mycobacterium tuberculosis*, for which 0.5–1-μm filtration is recommended.

27. How long can a mask be worn?

The Centers for Disease Control and Prevention (CDC) suggest a new mask for each patient. However, if the procedure lasts for more than 20 minutes, if excess aerosols are generated, or if the mask becomes wet from your breath, then the mask may have to be changed more often.

28. What is the purpose of wearing puncture-resistant gloves?

Puncture-resistant gloves, such as those made of nitrile rubber, should be worn whenever contaminated sharps are handled. These gloves are worn during instrument reprocessing for safe pick-up, transport, cleaning, and packaging of contaminated instruments. They should also be used for housekeeping procedures such as surface cleaning and disinfection. Routine cleaning and disinfection are necessary because the gloves become contaminated. They should not be worn when handling or contacting clean surfaces or items.

How to Select Task-Appropriate Gloves

FOR THIS TASK:	USE THIS GLOVE:
Contact with sterile body cavities	Sterile latex gloves
Routine intraoral procedures, routine contact with mucous membranes	Latex exam gloves
Routine contact with mucous membranes, cases of latex allergy	Vinyl exam gloves
Nonclinical care or treatment procedures, such as processing radiographs, writing in a patient record, etc.	Copolymer gloves or over-glove
Contact with chemical agents, contaminated sharps, and other potential exposure incidents not related to patient treatment	Nitrile rubber gloves

29. Name some causes of dermatitis associated with glove use.

Perspiration, a reaction to the powder in a glove, and a true latex allergy are some examples.

30. If my hands break out while wearing latex gloves, what should I do?
First, determine if it is the glove or perhaps a powder used in it. Also, look at your handcare: are your nails short, have you removed all jewelry? Do you use an antimicrobial handwash, and if so, are you allergic to the handwash? What lotion do you use and when? If the problem persists, you should consult a dermatologist to determine if this is a true latex allergy.

31. A patient notes a latex allergy on her medical record and says that if a glove touches her, she will break out. What type of glove should be used?
New and better nonlatex gloves are now on the market that have good fit and eliminate an allergic response. For patients with true latex allergies, a clinical vinyl glove should be worn.

32. Which are more permeable, medical-grade vinyl gloves or unsterile latex gloves?
Medical-grade vinyl gloves are more permeable.

33. Why are lanolin handcreams contraindicated with glove use?
The fatty acids in lanolin break down the latex and cause a build-up of film on the hands.

34. What personal protective equipment is needed when handling chemical agents?
At a minimum, protective eyewear, a mask, and the appropriate type of gloves such as heavy-duty utility or nitrile gloves should be worn when handling chemical agents.

BLOODBORNE INFECTIONS AND VACCINATION

35. What are universal precautions?
Universal precautions is the term for a concept of infection control that requires that all blood and certain other body fluids be considered infectious for human immunodeficiency virus (HIV), hepatitis B virus (HBV), and other bloodborne pathogens.

36. What is the "chain of infection"?
The "chain of infection" consists of three prerequisites for infection to occur by either direct or indirect contact:
1. a susceptible host;
2. a pathogen with sufficient infectivity and numbers to cause infection; and
3. a portal of entry to the host.

37. Why is hepatitis B vaccination so important?
Hepatitis B has been a long-standing occupational threat in dentistry. Transmission from providers to patients and vice versa has been documented. HBV is a hardy virus, and it takes a low concentration to transmit the virus and infect someone. In 1982, a vaccine became available to protect from HBV, and its safety and efficacy are well established.

38. If I am an employee in a dental practice, do I pay for the hepatitis B vaccine?
No. If an employee is potentially exposed to blood or other infectious fluids in the course of work, then it is the responsibility of the employer to make this vaccine available, including paying for the series of shots.

39. What if I refuse the vaccination?
You have a right, in most states, to refuse the vaccination. You should realize, however, that without immunization you will always be at some risk of acquiring the HBV infection. OSHA requires that any employee sign a special statement if he or she refuses the employer's offer.

40. What is the risk of acquiring HBV infection from a single injury with a needle contaminated by an HBV carrier?
The risk of acquiring HBV infection as shown by serologic markers is between 10 and 30%; the risk that this will result in clinically significant hepatitis is 10–20%.

Management Protocol for Accidental Exposures

1. *Most Importantly*, give appropriate first aid to contain or stop bleeding, then clean the wound:

Parenteral	Bleed the wound, and cleanse it
Mucous membrane	Flush the exposed area with copious amounts of water
Nonintact skin	Cleanse area with antimicrobial agent

2. Report incident to employer or other designated personnel to initiate written documentation of incident.

3. Determine source patient if possible. Employer or other designated personnel must discuss incident with source individual and offer to test his or her blood for the presence of HIV or HBV, with written informed consent.

4. If source patient, with written informed consent, releases information regarding HIV or HBV status, this information may be conveyed to exposed worker. Employees should be aware of laws protecting confidentiality of medical history and prohibiting disclosure of HIV status.

5. Contact designated health care professional for immediate medical evaluation of incident, for HIV counseling, and HIV/HBV testing.

6. If baseline HIV test is not desired, counsel or recommend drawing a blood sample for storage at test site. Within 90 days, employee may have blood sample tested for HIV.

7. If zidovudine will be taken as prophylactic measure, this must be started immediately and not longer than 2–4 hours after incident.

8. Follow OSHA steps for reporting, including the use of OSHA form 101 (or equivalent if practice employs less than 11 persons).

9. Ensure health care professional treating the incident has been provided all information required by OSHA, including but not limited to:
   Injury report form
   Description of exposed employee's tasks
   Source individual's information, with written consent to release this
   Copy of OSHA Bloodborne Standard
   Information on exposed employee's vaccination status

10. Health care professional must, within 15 days of the medical evaluation, report to the employer. The report only contains information regarding vaccination status and whether HBV vaccination was provided. All other information is confidential to the exposed employee.

11. Ensure appropriate follow-up occurs.

---

41. How should a health care worker who has sustained a needlestick from a hepatitis-B-positive patient be treated?

The health care worker's own hepatitis B titer should be checked. Hepatitis B immune globulin (HBIG) should be administered as soon as possible, and hepatitis B active immunization should be initiated. Consider the possibility of HIV exposure in the same setting.

42. When must a needlestick be reported to OSHA?

All occupational injuries, including needlesticks, must be recorded on an incident report form if they:

1. were worked related;
2. resulted in medical treatment; or
3. resulted in seroconversion.

43. Can a dental health care worker who is a carrier of hepatitis B resume work involving patient contact?
Yes, in most states, with use of appropriate infection control precautions.

44. What is the risk of HIV transmission via a needlestick?
The average risk of transmission in a large group of health care workers having percutaneous exposure was 1 in 250 exposures, or 0.4%. However, there is tremendous variation in the degree of exposure, and the likelihood of seroconversion will depend on the significance of the exposure.

45. What is the difference between a documented occupational transmission and a possible occupational transmission of HIV?
A documented occupational transmission requires that the exposed health care worker be tested for HIV at the time of the incident and that the baseline test be negative. If, after a designated time, HIV seroconversion occurs, then it is considered to be the result of the exposure incident.

46. How accurate is the HIV antibody test?
At 6 months after an exposure incident, the ability of the test to detect the presence of HIV antibody is 99.9% accurate. After 1 year, it is 99.9999% accurate.

47. What would you recommend to a health care worker who has been potentially infected with HIV?
The first recommendation is to seek voluntary, anonymous testing and counseling. This step allows the health care worker to access early medical intervention to treat and contain the situation.

48. When were the last reports of HBV transmission from dentists to patients?
Since 1987 there have been no reports of HBV transmission from a dentist to a patient. From 1970 through 1987, nine clusters were reported in which HBV infection was associated with dental treatment by an infected dental health care worker. Some of the reasons may include:
1. Routine glove use
2. Use of HBV vaccine
3. Universal precautions
4. Incomplete reporting

INSTRUMENT REPROCESSING AND STERILIZATION

49. What is the difference between sterilization and disinfection?
Sterilization is the act or process of killing all forms of microorganisms on an instrument or surface; disinfection is the process of destroying pathogenic organisms but not necessarily all organisms.

50. Describe the types of sterilization procedures available.
1. Steam-under-pressure, or autoclaving, is the most widely used method.
2. Dry-heat sterilization involves placing instruments in an FDA-approved dry heat sterilizer for a specified period of heating at a required temperature.

51. What is the underlying doctrine of sterilization?
Do not disinfect what you can sterilize.

52. According to the "Spaulding Classification," what are critical, semicritical and noncritical items?

CDC/Spaulding Classification of Surfaces

	DESCRIPTION	EXAMPLES	DISEASE TRANSMISSION RISK	REPROCESSING TECHNIQUE
Critical	Pointed/sharp Penetrates tissue Blood present	Needles Cutting instruments Implants	High	Sterile, disposable Heat sterilization
Semicritical	Mucous membrane contact No tissue penetration No blood or other secretions present	Medical "scopes" Nonsurgical dental instruments Specula Catheters	Intermediate	Heat sterilization High-level disinfection
Noncritical	Unbroken skin contact	Face masks Clothing Blood pressure cuffs Diag electrodes	Low	Sanitize (no blood) Intermediate-level disinfection (blood present)
Environmental Surfaces	Usually no direct patient contact			Sanitize (no blood) Intermediate-level disinfection
Medical equipment		Knobs, handles of x-ray machine Dental units	Minimal	
Housekeeping		Floors, walls Countertops	Least	

Table courtesy of James A. Cottone, DMD, MS, April 1993.

53. How are critical and semicritical items treated after use?
All critical and semicritical instruments that are heat stable should be sterilized. Semicritical items require either heat or chemical-vapor sterilization, immersion chemical sterilization, or high-level disinfection.

54. What does the term "cold sterilization" refer to in dentistry?
Cold sterilization refers to the use of immersion disinfectants for semicritical instruments and items used in the delivery of dental services.

55. What is the appropriate use of a 2% glutaraldehyde solution?
Immersion disinfection.

56. What disadvantages are associated with 2% glutaraldehydes?
The 2% glutaraldehydes have been associated with allergenic properties, corrosiveness to instruments, and tissue irritations.

57. What is the purpose of an antiretraction valve?
To prevent aspiration of patient material into water lines and thereby reduce the risk of transmission of infectious fluids to another patient.

58. What is the best way to reprocess a handpiece?
The only acceptable method of reprocessing between patients is to heat-treat the unit. Manufacturers' instructions for precleaning and lubrication should be followed and the appropriate heat-treatment method used.

59. What is the function of a glass bead sterilizer?
The glass bead sterilizer is used during endodontic procedures for one patient for the safe storage of files and not for sterilization of files between patients.

60. Can a disposable saliva ejector be reused?
No. It cannot be adequately sterilized between patients and is a single-use item only.

61. How must a reusable air-water syringe tip be sterilized?
The most acceptable methods are steam heat-under-pressure, dry heat, or unsaturated chemical vapor.

62. What is the minimum required temperature for an autoclave for proper sterilization?
121° Celsius.

63. Name a disadvantage of an autoclave.
One disadvantage is that instrument cutting surfaces and burs may become dulled. Another is that carbide/carbon steel items may corrode.

64. What can be done to retard bur corrosion during autoclaving?
Burs should be dipped into a 1% sodium nitrite emulsion preparation to minimize corrosion.

65. In a dry-heat oven preheated to 160°C, how long will it take to sterilize instruments?
Sterilization will be achieved in 2 hours in a properly working unit. However, additional time is required for "cool down" before metal items can be used.

66. What is a disadvantage of dry-heat oven sterilizers?
One disadvantage is that the cycle time is long. In addition, many plastics and material items are not compatible with dry heat.

67. Can a dental handpiece withstand dry-heat sterilization?
Currently, it cannot, and manufacturers do not recommend dry-heat sterilization. However, it can safely and appropriately be sterilized by saturated steam-under-pressure or unsaturated chemical-vapor sterilization.

68. Which agency is responsible for regulating handpieces and making recommendations for sterilization procedures for them?
The Food and Drug Administration (FDA) under the Medical Devices Branch and Safe Medical Devices Act. The FDA also approves all medical devices, including sterilizers, for market.

69. What packaging material is suitable for steam-under-pressure sterilization (autoclave)?
The most suitable material for autoclaving is one which the steam can penetrate. Such materials include paper, plastic, or surgical muslin.

70. What packaging material cannot be used in dry-heat sterilizers?
Plastic cannot be used for packaging items or instruments for dry-heat sterilization. It melts.

71. What packaging material is compatible with unsaturated chemical-vapor sterilizers?
Perforated metal trays and paper are suitable, since the vapor must be able to penetrate the material.

72. What is an easy method to demonstrate that sterilization "conditions" have been reached in a cycle?
Process indicators demonstrate that the conditions to achieve sterilization were reached, but they do not imply that actual sterilization—killing of spore-forming organisms and other lifeforms—occurred.

73. What are some common reasons for sterilization failure?
1. Improper maintenance of equipment
2. Damaged gasket or seal on the chamber door
3. Improper cycle time
4. Improper loading
5. Inappropriate packaging material
6. Interruption of a cycle to add or remove items

74. What is the difference between process indicators and biological monitors?
Biological monitors measure spore growth and death, whereas process indicators measure heat and pressure.

75. In biologically monitoring sterilization equipment, which nonpathogenic organisms are used for each type of unit?
For autoclaves and chemical-vapor sterilizers, *Bacillus stearothermophilus* is used. For dry-heat and ethylene oxide units, *Bacillus subtilis* is used.

76. How often should biological monitoring of sterilization units be performed?
At a minimum, it should be done on a weekly basis.

Indications for More Frequent Biological Monitoring of Sterilization Units

1. If the equipment is new and being used for the first time
2. During the first operating cycle after a repair
3. If there is a change in packaging material used
4. If new employees are using the unit or being trained in use of equipment or procedure for monitoring
5. After an electrical or power source failure
6. If door seals or gaskets are changed
7. If cycle time and/or temperature are changed
8. For all cycles treating implantable items or materials
9. For all cycles to render infectious waste as noninfectious
10. If the method of biological monitoring is changed

77. When should a holding solution be used and why?
A holding solution is indicated when it is not possible to clean instruments or items immediately after patient use. The solution is used only to keep debris moist until cleaning and preparation for sterilization are feasible. Holding solutions are not disinfectants. The bioburden on the instruments decreases the potential effectiveness of chemical disinfectants, rendering the process an ineffective, unnecessary step if used as disinfection.

78. Do instruments need to be precleaned before sterilization?
Instruments should be thoroughly cleaned prior to sterilization. Two methods of instrument cleaning are ultrasonic cleaning and handscrubbing. Ultrasonic cleaning is recognized as the method of choice since it minimizes hand contact with contaminated instruments. If an ultrasonic unit is not available, handscrubbing in a safe manner so as to avoid injury from instruments can be best accomplished by cleaning only one or two items at a time. These should be held low in the sink, under running water, and scrubbed with a long-handled brush. No matter which cleaning method is used, puncture-resistant gloves should be worn until the items are securely packaged.

79. How do you ensure that an ultrasonic cleaning unit is in proper working order?
A function test should be performed according to the manufacturers' instructions on ultrasonic units on a routine basis. In general, a function test requires that fresh solution be activated in the unit, that a specified size piece of aluminum foil be cut and placed vertically into the

activated solution for exactly 20 seconds, and then the foil be removed and examined under a light source. A functional unit will cause holes and/or pitting in the foil; if no holes are present, the unit is not working properly and should be repaired.

DISINFECTANTS

80. When is high-level disinfection appropriate?
Instruments that do not penetrate sterile areas of the body (noncritical instruments) can be treated with high-level disinfectants. Any item that penetrates sterile areas (critical items) requires sterilization.

81. What does the efficiency of a disinfectant depend upon?
1. The concentration of microorganisms, or bioburden, left on surfaces and/or items
2. An accurate dilution of the disinfectant
3. The length of exposure time between the agent and the surfaces or items
4. Shelf life of agent.

82. What are two properties of an ideal chemical disinfectant?
1. A residual biocidal effect on treated surfaces
2. An ability to penetrate bioburden

83. What are Spaulding's classifications of biocidal activity?
1. **High level:** sterilants which kill vegetative bacteria, tubercle bacillus, bacterial spores, and lipid and nonlipid viruses.
2. **Intermediate level:** disinfectants that kill vegetative bacteria, tubercle bacillus, and lipid and nonlipid viruses
3. **Low level:** agents which kill only vegetative bacteria and lipid viruses, but not *Mycobacterium tuberculosis.*

84. Which agency(ies) regulates germicidal chemicals?
Initial regulation is by the Environmental Protection Agency (EPA), and if the germicide is marketed and labeled for medical use, then there is dual regulation with the FDA under the 1976 Device Amendment to the Food, Drug, and Cosmetic Act.

85. Does the term "contaminated" refer to wet or dry materials or both?
Contaminated refers to both wet and dry materials since the hepatitis B virus can remain viable in dried materials for up to 7 days.

86. Is household bleach acceptable for surface decontamination?
In the OSHA Instruction CPL 2-2.44C, "Enforcement Procedures for The Occupational Exposure to Bloodborne Pathogens Standard," it is stated that disinfectant products registered by the US Department of Environmental Protection as tuberculocidal are considered "appropriate" for the cleanup of contaminated surfaces. Although *generic* sodium hypochlorite solutions are not registered as such, they are generally recommended by the US Public Health Service, Centers for Disease Control and Prevention, for disinfection of environmental surfaces. A dilution of 1:10 to 1:100 with water is acceptable following initial cleanup of the surface.

87. When and how should laboratory items and materials be cleaned and disinfected?
These items should be cleaned and disinfected after handling in the laboratory and before placement in a patient's mouth. Prior to disinfecting, consult manufacturer's directions for specific materials. In general, an intermediate-level or high-level disinfectant is suitable (i.e., a tuberculocidal hospital disinfectant approved by the EPA).

88. What microbiologic lifeforms do EPA-registered hospital disinfectants generally claim to kill?
Under EPA registration, the kill claim is for *Mycobacterium tuberculosis, Salmonella, Staphylococcus,* and *Pseudomonas* organisms.

89. What are the categories under which a manufacturer may apply for registration of a hospital disinfectant?
Under the disinfectant heading, a manufacturer can apply for four separate categories for registration: microbiological, virucidal, pseudomicidal, and tuberculocidal activity.

90. When choosing a chemical disinfectant, what is the more important kill claim, *Mycobacterium tuberculosis* or HIV?
The more important claim is that *M. tuberculosis* is killed, since this is the more virulent organism and therefore is more difficult to kill. HIV is a fragile virus and easier to kill than the mycobacterium.

91. What is the designation for the highest level of disinfectant activity that the EPA registers?
"High-level" disinfectant is the highest designation, although some manufacturers use either hospital-level or hospital-grade to describe this level of disinfectant activity. It is important to read and understand the product label to be sure of what you are buying.

92. Do EPA tests on germicidal chemicals indicate efficacy?
No. The EPA tests potency, not efficacy. The EPA tests are standardized lab tests for comparing the potency of one germicide to another and are based on descending order of general microbial resistance to germicides. All results are inference.

93. How do you determine use and reuse life for a surface disinfectant?
The EPA requires that use and reuse life information be obvious on a label. Special attention should be given to whether or not the stated use and reuse life is for all organisms or if it differs between organisms.

94. Are manufacturers' data on chemical agents checked for accuracy?
No, monitoring is not done. There have been no regulations for truth in advertising since 1982, when the EPA testing lab was shut down.

95. For a disinfectant product to be appropriate for use in a dental setting, what would its minimum label requirements be?
A disinfectant would require registration as an EPA hospital disinfectant with additional registration of tuberculocidal activity and, under Spaulding, be classified as an intermediate-level disinfectant.

96. When would low-level disinfectants be used in dentistry?
There are no uses for low-level surface disinfectants in dentistry, except perhaps in a nonclinical area such as a restroom. Chemical agents used to achieve disinfection must be at least intermediate level.

97. What items require high-level disinfectants?
High-level disinfectants may be used to decontaminate semicritical items that cannot withstand heat or ethylene oxide sterilization. These agents must be used according to the manufacturer's directions for a chemical sterilant, including appropriate time and temperature, in order to kill spore-forming organisms.

98. What happens when synthetic phenols are used as surface disinfectants?
A synergistic antimicrobial effect occurs when synthetic phenols are used as surface disinfectants.

99. What is substantivity?
Substantivity is the ability to develop a residual antimicrobial effect with repeated usage.

100. What is an antiseptic?
An antiseptic is a chemical agent that can be applied to living tissue and can destroy or inhibit microorganisms on that tissue (for example, antimicrobial handwash or antimicrobial mouth rinse).

101. How does an antiseptic differ from chemical sterilants and disinfectants?
Chemical sterilants and disinfectants cannot be applied to living tissue, whereas antiseptics can.

102. Should a disinfectant be used in a holding tank?
No. It is not necessary. The purpose of a holding solution and tank is to keep debris on hand instruments moist until they can be appropriately heat-treated; it is not to disinfect or sterilize them. Indeed, a presoak in a disinfectant only adds an unnecessary step and a chemical; the instruments still need heat-treatment for sterilization.

103. What is the preferred holding solution?
It is soapy water, using a detergent that is noncorrosive or low in corrosives.

HAZARD MANAGEMENT

104. What is the best source for safety information on a hazardous product?
The Material Safety Data Sheet (MSDS) provides the most comprehensive product information and is the best source for safety information as well as precautions, emergency procedures, and personal protective equipment requirements. These must be provided by the manufacturer or distributor of the product if it is covered under the Hazard Communication Standard. The product label is also a good source of information, but it is not as complete as an MSDS.

105. If I transfer a chemical agent from its primary container to a secondary container, must I label that container?
No, not if it is for your immediate use during that workday. If, however, it is intended for use by other employees, then it must be appropriately labeled.

106. What ventilation requirements are followed when using high-level disinfectants?
All chemical agents should be used in well-ventilated areas. Additional ventilation is not indicated with appropriate use unless required by the manufacturer.

107. Are there special ventilation requirements for surface disinfectants?
Again, all chemical agents should be used in a well-ventilated area. The EPA label or MSDS will provide any additional precautions or requirements for personal protective equipment.

108. Who regulates dental waste?
OSHA regulates how the waste is handled in a dental or medical facility. Federal, state, and local laws govern the disposal itself.

109. What is the intent of the Resource Conservation and Recovery Act (RCRA) of EPA?
The intent of the RCRA is that the generator of a hazardous waste be held responsible for its ultimate disposal or treatment and for any clean-up costs associated with improper disposal. For individual dentists, it means that each is responsible for ensuring proper disposal of his or her own waste, and any improper disposal by an unscrupulous disposal company is ultimately the responsibility of the dentist.

110. What is infectious waste?
Infectious waste is waste that contains strong enough pathogens in sufficient quantity to cause disease.

111. Is all contaminated waste infectious waste?
No, but all infectious waste is contaminated. Some contaminated waste, although it contains pathogens, may not have them in a quantity or type strong enough to cause disease.

112. What is toxic waste?
Toxic waste is waste that is capable of causing a poisonous effect.

113. What is hazardous waste?
Hazardous waste is waste that causes a peril to the environment.

114. Is all hazardous waste toxic?
No. It may not have the poisonous capability.

115. If infectious waste is autoclaved to render it noninfectious, how can you guarantee the sterility of the waste?
If using sterilization equipment to render waste noninfectious, you must biologically monitor each waste load to ensure that the waste is actually noninfectious when the cycle is complete. Each waste load must be labeled with a date and batch number so that if a sterilization failure occurs, that load can be retrieved and resterilized.

116. How should blood-soaked gauze be disposed of? Extracted teeth? Used masks? Gloves?
Blood-soaked gauze, extracted teeth, and any other material that is contaminated by patient fluids, saliva or blood, should be considered infectious waste and disposed of accordingly. Masks, provided they are not blood stained, can be disposed of with ordinary office trash. Used gloves should be thrown away with infectious waste.

117. What is the proper method for disposal of used needles and sharps? Should needles be bent before disposal?
Needles may be recapped (not by hand) after use and inserted, along with other sharps instruments, into an appropriate sharps container for disposal as infectious waste. Needles should not be bent before disposal, because doing so increases one's risk of injury.

BIBLIOGRAPHY

1. Bell DM, Shapiro CN, et al: Risk of hepatitis B and human immunodeficiency virus transmission to a patient from an infected surgeon due to percutaneous injury during an invasive procedure: Estimates based on a model. Infect Agents Dis 1:263–269, 1992.
2. Centers for Disease Control and Prevention: Recommended infection control practices for dentistry. MMWR 41:(RR-8):1–12, 1993.
3. Centers for Disease Control and Prevention: Recommended infection control practices for dentistry. MMWR 42:(RR-8), 1993.
4. Cottone JA, Teerezhalmy GT, Molinari J: Practical Infection Control in Dentistry. Philadelphia, Lea & Febiger, 1990, pp 98–104, 105–118.
5. Councils on Dental Materials, Instruments and Equipment, Dental Practice, Dental Therapeutics: Infection control recommendations for the dental office and dental laboratory. J Am Dent Assoc 116:1988.
6. Food and Drug Administration (FDA): Heat sterilization on dental handpieces. FDA Bulletin, March 1993.
7. Lo B, Steinbrook R: Health care workers infected with the human immunodeficiency virus. JAMA 267:1992.
8. Martin MV: Infection Control in the Dental Environment. London, Martin Dunitz, Ltd., 1991, pp 27–32.

9. Mayo JA, Oertling KM, Andrieu SC: Bacterial biofilm: A source of contamination in dental air-water syringes. Clin Prevent Dent 12:13–20, 1990.

10. Miller C: Cleaning, sterilization, and disinfection: Basics of microbial killing for infection control. J Am Dent Assoc 124:1993.

11. Miller C: Sterilization and disinfection: What every dentist needs to know. J Am Dent Assoc 123:1992.

12. Miller C: Update on heat sterilization and sterilization monitoring. Compendium XIV (No. 2), March 1993.

13. Miller C, Palenik CJ: Sterilization, disinfection and asepsis in dentistry. In Bloc SS (ed): Sterilization, Disinfection and Preservation. Philadelphia, Lea & Febiger, 1991, pp 676–694.

14. Molinari JA, et al: Cleaning and disinfectant properties of dental surface disinfectants. J Am Dent Assoc 117:1988.

15. Molinari JA, et al: Comparison of dental surface disinfectants. Gen Dent, May-June, 1987.

16. Molinari JA, et al: Tuberculosis in the 1990's: Current implications for dentistry. Compendium XIV (No. 3), March 1993.

17. Occupational Safety and Health Administration: Regulations for protection against occupational exposure to bloodborne pathogens. 29 CFR 1919.1030: December 6, 1991.

18. Young JM: Dental air-powered handpieces: Selection, use, and sterilization. Compendium XIV (No. 3), March 1993.

13. DENTAL PUBLIC HEALTH

Edward S. Peters, D.M.D.

PUBLIC HEALTH PROMOTION

1. What are the three tenets of public health?
1. A problem exists.
2. Solutions to the problem exist.
3. The solutions to the problem are applied.

2. What constitutes a public health problem?
A public health problem fulfills two criteria of the public, government, or public health authorities. It is
- a condition or situation that is a widespread actual or potential cause of morbidity or mortality, and
- a perception exists that the condition is a public health problem.

3. Describe the current infection control recommendations.
Recommendations for infection control undergo frequent revision, and the reader is urged to refer to the most up-to-date source.

The principles behind infection control involve *exposure control*, which refers to personal protective barriers such as gloves, masks, and eye protection. In addition, *heat sterilization* of all dental equipment, including handpieces, is required. Finally, the *handling and disposal* of all potentially infectious material must be properly performed.

4. What are primary, secondary, and tertiary prevention?
Primary prevention involves health services that provide health promotion and protection with the goal of preventing the development of disease. An example is community-based fluoridation for caries prevention.

Secondary prevention includes services that are provided once the disease is present to prevent further progression. Such services include dental restorations.

Tertiary prevention services are provided when disease has advanced to the point where loss of function or life may occur. Extractions of diseased teeth to eliminate infection would be an example.

5. What is health promotion?
Health promotion is a set of educational, economic, and environmental incentives to support behavioral changes that lead to better health.

6. How has health promotion been achieved in dentistry?
Examples of health-promoting activities include community fluoridation and sealant programs. On the individual level, health promotion is encouraged through oral hygiene procedures.

7. Of dental public health programs employed in community-based settings, give examples of those geared toward school children.
School-based fluoride delivery, dental screening, hygiene instruction.

8. Prior to the implementation of any community-based program, the process of planning and evaluation is necessary. What are the basic steps involved in planning for a program?
Planning involves making choices to achieve specific objectives. Thus, a planner should review a list of alternative programs, assess the effectiveness of the program under consideration,

examine the community and determine if the program is needed, and initiate the process to implement the program.

9. What skills must an individual possess prior to managing dental public health programs?
The implementation of a public health program requires such skills as planning, marketing, communications, human resources management, financial management, and quality assurance.

10. Differentiate between need and demand for oral health services.
Need can be defined as the quantity of dental treatment that expert opinion deems necessary for people to achieve the status of being dentally healthy. **Demand** for dental care is an expression by patients to receive dental treatment. **Utilization** is expressed as the proportion of the population who visits a dentist.

11. What factors influence the need and demand for oral health services in the U.S.?
Demographic and other variables influence the use of dental services—most notably, gender, age, socioeconomic status, race, ethnicity, geographic location, medical health, and the presence of insurance. Women utilize more dental services than men, although the reasons are unclear. Dental visits are most frequent for patients in their late teenage years and early adulthood, with a gradual tapering of visits with increasing age. Socioeconomic status is directly related to the use of dental services. There are fewer dental visits in patients of lower socioeconomic status and in nonwhite or Hispanic populations.

12. The utilization of health care has been explained through behavioral models. One model demonstrates how variables influence the utilization of health care from the individual's perspective. What factors play a role in explaining a person's health care utilization?
These factors can be broken down into three groups: **Predisposing factors** influence the person to use services and include (1) demographic variables, such as sex and age; (2) societal variables, such as education and job; and (3) health beliefs, such as how susceptible to disease the person believes he or she is and how serious he or she believes the consequences of the disease are. **Enabling factors** allow the services to be used and include such items as personal income, community resources, and accessibility to health care. **Need factors** determine how the services should be used; this factor is simply the presence of disease.

13. What are the risks associated with smokeless tobacco?
Smokeless tobacco increases an individual's risk of developing oral cancer. The use of smokeless tobacco leads to the development of leukoplakia in areas where the tobacco is placed. There is about a 5% chance of leukoplakia becoming cancerous. Leukoplakia may resolve with early cessation of smokeless tobacco use.

14. What is meant by the term "acidogenic"?
Particular foods have the ability to reduce the pH of plaque when consumed and are considered to be acidogenic. The reduction in pH is considered a necessary condition for the development of caries.

15. Describe how the benefits of fluoride were first discovered.
In the early 1900s Dr. Frederick McKay, having recently graduated from dental school, moved to Colorado where he observed an unusual blotching of tooth enamel in many of his patients. This pattern was localized to communities with artesian wells that provided the drinking water. He also observed that this blotching was associated with decreased caries activity. Eventually fluoride was identified as the agent in drinking water responsible for this pattern. This finding led to fluoridation trials that demonstrated that artificial fluoride prevents dental caries.

16. Health economists have concluded that water fluoridation is one of the few public health measures that saves more money than it costs to implement. Why is water fluoridation so cost-effective?

Fluoridation is a low-cost and low-technology procedure that benefits an entire community. It requires no patient compliance and is therefore easy to administer. The major costs are those associated with the initial equipment purchase; afterwards, costs are for maintenance and fluoride supplies. For each dollar invested in fluoridation, $80 in costs for dental treatment are avoided.

17. What are the major mechanisms of action for fluoride in caries inhibition?

1. The topical effect of constant infusion of a low concentration of fluoride into the oral cavity is thought to increase remineralization of enamel.

2. Fluoride inhibits glycolysis in which sugar is converted to acid by bacteria.

3. During tooth development, fluoride is incorporated into the developing enamel hydroxyapatite crystal, which reduces enamel solubility.

18. What percentage of the U.S. population has access to fluoridated water?

Approximately 54% of the total U.S. population has a fluoridated water supply.

19. What is the recommended level of fluoride in the water supply?

The U.S. Public Health Service sets the optimal F level at 1.0 to 1.2 ppm. This has recently been revised to 0.7 ppm.

20. At what policy level is the decision to fluoridate the water supply made?

Local governments make the decision. However, seven states have laws requiring water fluoridation.

21. A parent of a 6-year-old child asks about fluoride supplementation. The child weighs 20 kg and lives in a fluoride-deficient area with less than 0.3 ppm of fluoride ion in drinking water. What do you recommend?

You should prescribe sodium fluoride, 1-mg tablets, to be chewed and swallowed at bedtime.

22. What are the recommended fluoride supplementation dosages for children?

Tablets are available in doses of 1.0 mg and 0.5 mg for children and toddlers. For infants, supplemental fluoride is available as 0.125-mg drops.

Supplemental Fluoride Dosage Schedule

Age (years)	CONCENTRATION OF FLUORIDE ION IN DRINKING WATER		
	Less than 0.3	0.3 to 0.6	Greater than 0.6 ppm
6 months to 3	0.25 mg	0	0
3–6	0.50 mg	0.25 mg	0
6–16	1 mg	0.50 mg	0

23. What are alternatives to systemic fluoride supplementation (i.e., tablets)?

• Topically applied gels of 2.0% NaF, 0.4% SnF, 1.23% acidulated phosphate fluoride (APF).

• Mouth rinses of 0.2% NaF weekly, 0.05% NaF daily, 0.1% SnF daily.

• Daily dentrifice.

24. When prescribing fluoride supplementation, what tradeoffs must be considered?

The benefit of caries reduction must be considered against the risk of fluorosis. Fluorosis occurs with the presence of excessive fluoride during tooth development and causes a discoloration of tooth enamel. Affected teeth appear chalky white on eruption and later turn brown. This risk is especially important during the development of the incisors in the second to third years. To avoid this, it is crucial that you assess the fluoride content of the drinking water prior to dispensing fluoride supplementation. The fluoride in water along with any supplemental fluoride must not exced 1 ppm. If 1 ppm is exceeded, the probability that fluorosis may develop increases as the fluoride concentration increases.

25. Where is ingested fluoride absorbed?
Eighty percent of the absorption of ingested fluoride occurs in the upper gastrointestinal tract.

26. What are the manifestations of fluoride toxicity?
The ingestion of 5 g of fluoride or greater in an adult results in death within 2 hours if the person does not receive medical attention. In a child, the ingestion of a single dose greater than 400 mg will result in death due to poisoning in about 3 hours. Doses of 100 to 300 mg in children result in nausea and diarrhea.

27. How much fluoride is contained in an average 4.6-ounce tube of toothpaste?
Either sodium monoflurophosphate or sodium fluoride toothpaste contains approximately 1.0 mg of fluoride per gram of paste. Therefore, a 4.6-oz tube of toothpaste contains 130 mg of fluoride. A level of 435 mg of fluoride consumed in a 3-hour period is considered fatal for a 3-year-old child. Therefore, only a little over 3 tubes of toothpaste need to be consumed to reach a fatal level.

28. What is the rationale behind the use of pit and fissure sealants in caries prevention?
Occlusal surfaces, particularly fissures, have not experienced as rapid a decline in the caries incidence as have proximal surfaces. This is because fluoride's protective effect is confined to smooth surfaces only. It has been observed that sealing the fissures from the oral environment prevents the development of occlusal caries. Sealants should be part of an early preventive program.

29. Do dentists have an obligation to report child abuse?
Yes. Dentists are morally, ethically, and legally obligated to report a suspected case of child abuse. Reports should be made to the local department of social services, although this may vary from state to state.

30. Where is the dentist's code of ethics found?
The American Dental Association (ADA) established a code of ethics that describes dentistry's responsibility to society. The code is published in the *Journal of the American Dental Association, JADA*. The code deals with issues of patient care, fees, practice guidelines, advertising, and referrals.

31. What does the ADA code of ethics state about the removal of dental amalgam to prevent mercury toxicity?
"The removal of amalgam restorations from the non-allergic patient for the alleged purpose of removing toxic substances from the body, when such treatment is performed solely at the recommendation or suggestion of the dentist, is improper and unethical."

32. How does the Americans with Disabilities Act affect dentists?
- Dentists cannot deny anyone care due to a disability.
- Offices must undergo architectural changes to allow access for the disabled.
- Employees are protected against dismissal due to a disability.
- Offices must accommodate disabled workers to perform jobs.

EPIDEMIOLOGY AND BIOSTATISTICS

33. Define epidemiology.
It is the study of the distribution and frequency of disease or injury in human populations and those factors making groups susceptible to disease or injury.

34. Differentiate between incidence and prevalence.

Incidence is the number of *new* cases of disease occurring within a population during a given time period. It is expressed as a rate (cases)/(population)/(time).

Prevalence is the proportion of a population affected with a disease at a given point in time, i.e., (cases)/(population).

Example:

A dentist counts the number of patients presenting to the office with newly diagnosed periodontal disease in a 6-month period. Ten of the 100 people who came to the office had periodontal disease. The incidence rate is calculated as 10/100 in 6 months, or 0.2 per year. The range for incidence rates is from zero to infinity. The prevalence of periodontal disease may be obtained by counting all patients with periodontal disease in the same period—that is, if 50 of the 100 patients have periodontal disease, then the prevalence is 50%. Remember, incidence is a rate and requires a unit of time, whereas prevalence is a proportion and is expressed as a percentage of the population.

35. What is meant by test sensitivity and specificity? How are they calculated?

Frequently dentists wish to know if disease is present and may use some diagnostic test to arrive at an answer. In dentistry, the most frequent test is the radiograph. Dental radiographs are imperfect in that they do not distinguish all diseased from disease-free surfaces. Sensitivity and specificity are measures that describe how good the radiograph is in such differentiation.

Sensitivity measures the proportion of persons with the disease who are correctly identified by a positive test. That is the *true-positive rate*. **Specificity** measures the proportion of those without disease who are correctly identified by a negative test—the *true-negative rate*.

Sensitivity and specificity are inversely proportional, and as the specificity of a test increases, the sensitivity decreases. An ideal test would have both high specificity and sensitivity, yet tradeoffs can be made depending on the condition being tested. Sensitivity and specificity can be calculated from a 2 × 2 table as illustrated below. Sensitivity = TP/TP + FN; specificity = TN/FP + TN.

	With disease	Without disease
Test positive	True positive (TP)	False positive (FP)
Test negative	False negative (FN)	True negative (TN)

36. What is meant by positive predictive value (PPV)?

The PPV reflects the proportion of persons who have the disease, given that they test positive. This measures how well the test predicts the presence of a given disease. It can be calculated from a 2 × 2 table as PPV = TP/TP + FP. This takes into account the prevalence of disease.

37. What does the *p* value represent?

The probability that the observed result or something more extreme occurred by chance alone. Therefore, a *p* value of 0.05 indicates that there is only a 5% likelihood that the result observed was due to chance alone. Traditionally, a *p* value of 0.05 is considered statistically significant. If the *p* value is >0.05, chance cannot be ruled out as an explanation for the observed effect. It is important to remember that chance can never be ruled out as an explanation for the observed results. A statistically significant result indicates that chance is not likely.

38. What is relative risk? Odds ratio?

The **relative risk** measures the association between exposure and disease. It is expressed as a ratio of the disease rate among the exposed individuals to the rate among the unexposed. The rate measure estimates the strength or magnitude of an association. The calculation of relative risk requires incidence rates, provided by cohort studies.

The **odds ratio** provides an estimate of the relative risk in case-control studies; since disease has already occurred, the incidence of disease cannot be determined.

39. How do the mean, median, and mode differ?

These three terms are measures of central tendency and are used to provide a summary measure to characterize a group of individuals.

The **mean** represents the average. It is calculated by adding together all the observations and then dividing by the total number of measurements. The mean takes into account the magnitude of each observation and, as a result, is easily affected by extreme values. The **median** is defined as the middle-most measurement (the 50th percentile)—i.e., half the observations are below it and half are above. Therefore, the median is unaffected by extreme measures. The **mode** is the most frequently occurring observation.

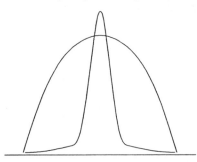

Two distributions with identical means, medians, and modes. (From Pagano M, Gauvreau K: Principles of Biostatistics. Boston, Harvard School of Public Health, 1991, with permission.)

40. Which of the following is most appropriate for testing differences between the means of two groups: ANOVA, *t*-test, chi-square?

A ***t*-test** is used to compare the means between two groups. ANOVA, or analysis of variance, compares the means in greater than two groups. The chi-square test is used to show differences in proportions.

41. Confidence intervals are frequently provided when data are reported. What do they indicate?

Confidence intervals (CI) are reported because they represent the range within which the true magnitude of the effect lies with a certain degree of certainty. For example, a relative risk of 2.1 may be reported with a 95% CI (1.5, 2.9). This indicates that the relative risk was determined to be 2.1 in this study, but we are 95% certain that the true relative risk is not <1.5 or >2.9. If the 95% CI includes the null value (1.0), then the result is not statistically significant.

42. Compare cross-sectional, case-control, and cohort studies.

Cross-sectional studies are a type of *descriptive* epidemiologic study in which the exposure and disease status of the population are determined at a given point in time. For example, the caries status of U.S. adults aged 45–65 in the year 1992 may be determined by a national dental survey and examination.

Case control and cohort studies are *analytical* epidemiologic studies. In a **case-control study** individuals are selected into the study on the basis of disease status. The "cases" are persons who have the disease of interest, and the control group comprises persons similar to the case group except they do not have the disease of interest. Information on exposure status is then obtained from each group to assess if an association exists between exposure and disease.

Cohort studies differ from case-control studies in that individuals are entered into the study on the basis of exposure status. Study participants must be free of the disease of interest at the time the study begins. A group of exposed and a group of nonexposed individuals are then followed over time to assess the association between exposure and specific diseases.

43. Which type of study—cohort, case-control, retrospective, or clinical trial—most closely resembles a true experiment?

In a clinical trial, the investigator allocates the subjects to the exposure groups of interest and then follows the groups over time to observe how they differ in outcome. This most closely resembles an experiment.

44. Discuss the importance of blinding and randomization in experimental studies.

Randomization and blinding are two methods of reducing bias in research studies. A **randomized study** is one in which all study participants have an equal likelihood of receiving the treatment of interest. For example, patients are randomly assigned into two groups, one of which receives a particular treatment and the other, placebo. Several techniques are available that help to ensure randomization of study participants.

In a **double-blind study,** the investigator who is observing the study results and the participant are both blinded—i.e., unaware—as to which study group the individual is assigned. One means of achieving a blinded study is with the use of placebos.

45. Distinguish between split-mouth and crossover designs.

In a split-mouth study, different treatments are applied to different sections of the mouth. It is important to remember that the effects of treatment must be localized to the region receiving the treatment. In crossover studies, patients serve as their own control and receive treatments in sequence—treatment A and then treatment B—and the disease course is compared between the two periods. The disease under investigation must be assumed to be stable over the period of time during which the treatments are administered.

46. What is the difference between inter-examiner and intra-examiner reliability?

The validity of an examination depends on the reliability of the examiner. Intra-examiner reliability refers to the ability of a single examiner to record the same findings the same way over a period of time. Inter-examiner refers to the ability of different examiners to record the same finding identically.

47. List and describe the most common dental indices used.

Measurements of dental caries are made with the **DMF index**. The DMF is an irreversible index and is used only with permanent teeth. *D* represents decayed teeth, *M* is for missing teeth, *F* is filled teeth. The DMF score for a person can range from 0 to 32. The DMF index can be applied to teeth (DMFT) or surfaces (DMFS).

The primary dentition uses the **def index**, where *d* is decayed teeth, *e* is for extracted teeth, and *f* is for filled teeth.

Gingivitis is most commonly scored with the **gingival index** of LOE and Silness. It grades the gingiva on the four surfaces of each tooth. Each area receives a score from 0 to 3, where 0 = normal gingiva; 1 = mild inflammation, no bleeding on probing; 2 = moderate inflammation; 3 = severe inflammation, ulceration, and spontaneous bleeding.

48. What is happening with the prevalence of caries in the U.S.?

The prevalence of caries has been declining in children during the 20th century. Results of the National Health and Nutrition Examination Surveys (NHANES) during the 1970s and 1980s show that the prevalence of caries has decreased significantly in the U.S. Elsewhere, the caries rate is also declining. A decline in adult caries is not as evident, as most adults grew up before the decline started. Fluoridation has received the most credit for the decline in the development of caries.

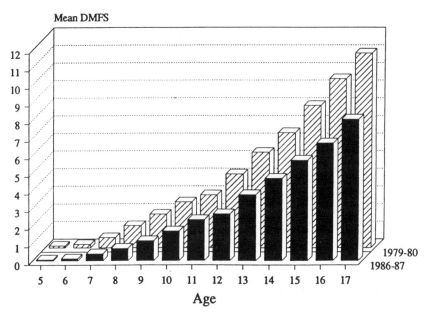

DMFS values for United States school children, aged 5 to 17, in 1979–1980 and 1986–1987. (From Burt BA, Eklund SA: Dentistry, Dental Practice and the Community. Philadelphia, W.B. Saunders, 1992, with permission).

49. What factors make a person susceptible to dental caries?
Three factors are essential for the development of caries:
- Host, a susceptible tooth
- Agent, acid-producing bacteria
- Environment, dental plaque

50. What did the Vipeholm study reveal about the effect of diet on dental decay?
This study, conducted in a mental institution in Vipeholm, Sweden, is considered unethical and will not be repeated. The study divided patients into groups who received different doses of sugars. The sugar differed as to the amount, form, frequency, and whether it was consumed between meals. The most significant finding of the study was that the form and frequency of sugar consumption were most related to the occurrence of dental caries—that is, frequent consumption of sticky sugars increased the occurrence of dental caries.

51. Root caries is seen predominantly in what patient population?
The elderly. The rising incidence of root caries can be attributed to the aging of populations in industrialized societies and the fact that most adults are retaining more teeth. In this population, there is increased gingival recession with exposure of root surfaces, leading to the development of root caries.

52. What is occurring with the prevalence of periodontal disease?
Gingivitis and periodontitis are universally prevalent, with more than 70% of all adults in most countries afflicted. Some data suggest that there is no difference in the prevalence of

periodontitis between developing and developed countries. More recent data obtained during the 1980s show that the prevalence of severe periodontitis ranges from 7 to 15% regardless of a country's economic state, oral hygiene, or availability of dental care.

53. What is a common factor in both caries and periodontal disease?
The presence of dental plaque is a causative agent in both these diseases.

54. How common are oral cancers?
Oral cancer accounts for 4 to 5% of all cancers diagnosed in the U.S. this year. Approximately one million new cancers are diagnosed in each year, and of these, about 40,000 will be cancers of the lips, tongue, floor of the mouth, palate, gingiva, alveolar mucosa, buccal mucosa, and oropharynx. Oral cancer is twice as prevalent in males as in females. The age-adjusted annual incidence of oral cancer in white patients aged 65 or older was 20/100,000 in 1980.

55. What are the risk factors?
Studies of oral cancer have identified smoking and other uses of tobacco as risk factors. In addition, alcohol consumption is a risk factor that may act as a promoter with tobacco.

HEALTH POLICY

56. Differentiate between licensure and registration.
Licensure is granted through a government agency to those who meet specified qualifications to perform given activities or to claim a particular title. Registration is when qualified individuals are listed by a governmental or nongovernmental organization.

57. What are the types of supervision for allied dental personnel as defined by the ADA?
1. **Indirect:** The dentist diagnoses a condition, then authorizes the allied dental personnel to carry out treatment while that dentist remains in the office as the treatment is being carried out.

2. **Direct:** The dentist diagnoses a condition, authorizes treatment, and evaluates the outcome.

3. **General:** General supervision is defined by practice acts within each state and may require that the dentist be available but not necessarily on the premise or site where care is delivered.

58. What are the basic components of the dental care delivery system?
A delivery system is a means by which health care is provided to a patient and consists of four main components: (1) the organizational structure in which doctors and patients come together; (2) how health care is financed and paid for; (3) the supply of health care personnel; and (4) the physical structures involved in the delivery of care.

59. What does "quality assurance" refer to?
Quality assurance is the process of examining the physical structures, procedures, and outcome as they affect the delivery of health care. It consists of assessment to identify any inadequacies, followed by the implementation of improvements to correct these inadequacies, followed by reassessment to determine if these improvements are effective.

60. Define the concepts of structure, process, and outcome as they relate to quality assurance.
Structure refers to the layout and equipment of a facility. Included are items such as the building, equipment, and record forms. **Process** involves the services the dentist and auxiliaries perform for the patients and how skillfully they accomplish these. **Outcome** is the change in health status that occurs as a result of the care delivered.

61. How do cost-benefit and cost-effectiveness analyses differ?

Cost-effectiveness and cost-benefit analyses are two similar yet distinct techniques to help allocate resources to maximize objectives. *Cost-benefit analysis* requires that all costs and benefits be expressed in dollar terms, to provide a measure of the net-benefit. *Cost-effectiveness analysis* allows alternative measures to value effectiveness. Objections to valuing life in terms of dollars lead to the use of cases of disease prevented, life-years gained, or of quality-adjusted life-years. The result is a cost-effectiveness ratio which expresses the cost per unit of effectiveness.

62. What is "adverse selection"?

Adverse selection occurs when individuals at high risk for an illness are the predominant purchasers of insurance, especially when the risk for illness and the premium are based on a low-risk population. Thus, high-risk individuals are attracted to the insurance by its low rates, which allow them to avoid payments for a likely illness.

63. What is "moral hazard"?

In the presence of insurance, patients demand more medical care than if they had to pay the cost themselves.

64. What is a "community rating"?

The premiums charged to all insurance subscribers are the same regardless of the individual risk. Regardless of who pays for medical care, the cost ultimately falls on the general public.

65. What are the different financing mechanisms for dental care?

Dentistry is financed mainly through fee-for-service self-pay; 56% of all dental expenses are paid out of pocket by the patient. Payment to the dentist by an organization other than the patient is called third-party payment. Third-party payers represented by private insurance pay about 33% of total dental expenses, followed by government-financed or public programs (i.e., Medicaid, Veterans Affairs).

66. What is capitation payment?

HMO premiums are usually made on a capitation basis. That is, HMO providers receive a given fee per enrollee, regardless of how much or little care is delivered.

67. Explain the differences between IPA, PPO, and HMO.

All three represent managed-care practices. Managed care refers to forms of insurance coverage in which utilization and service patterns are monitored by the insurer with the aim of containing costs. An HMO (health maintenance organization) is usually a self-contained staff-model practice where there is no distinction made between the providers of insurance and the providers of health care. HMO premiums are paid on a "capitation" basis; i.e., there is a given fee per enrollee. In contrast, IPA (independent practice association) and PPO (preferred provider organization) represent groups of doctors who practice in the community and are distinct from the insurance provider. However, the insurance agency contracts with these providers for discounted rates and may refer patients to these providers exclusively. If a patient elects to go to a different provider than one recommended by the insurance company, the patient may face a financial penalty such as an additional charge.

68. How do these managed-care arrangements differ from the traditional model of dental care?

Traditional medical and dental care has been paid fee-for-service. In this model, a patient chooses any provider in the community and the insurance company usually pays a certain percentage of the charge. In this era of cost-consciousness, many insurance companies are modifying or eliminating this model altogether. Fee-for-service usually provides no incentive for either the patient or provider to contain costs.

69. How do Medicaid and Medicare differ?

Medicare, an entitlement fund, was created to provide health insurance to individuals 65 years old and over, certain disabled groups, and individuals with certain kidney diseases. Medicare has two parts, an institutional or hospital portion (Part A), and a noninstitutional portion or physician-services (Part B). Part A has no premium, but Part B is supplemental and voluntarily purchased. Medicare does not provide for dental care.

Medicaid is a means-tested program to provide health insurance to poor individuals eligible for welfare assistance programs. Medicaid covers both hospital and physician costs without a premium or copayment. Medicaid is required by federal law to provide dental services to children. However, adult dental services are optional, and the decision whether to provide dental care is determined at a state level.

70. Which agency administers Medicare funds?

The Health Care Financing Administration (HCFA), a federal agency, is responsible for funding Medicare. It determines how much providers will be paid and what services are covered.

71. How are the funds for Medicaid provided?

Medicaid is a joint federal and state program with federal guidelines that allows states some flexibility in what services are provided and who is eligible. The federal government provides states with matching dollars.

72. What percentage of the gross national product (GNP) is spent on health care?

In 1992, 13.1% of the GNP was spent on health care. The GNP represents the total production in the USA.

73. What percentage of all US health care expenditures is for dental care?

In 1990, the HCFA estimated that 5% ($34 of $666 billion) of all U.S. health care expenditures was for dental services.

BIBLIOGRAPHY

1. American Dental Association: Principles of Ethics and Code of Professional Conduct. Chicago, American Dental Association, 1992.
2. Antczak-Bouckoms A, Tulloch JFC, Bouckoms AJ, et al: Diagnostic Decision Making. Anesth Prog 37:161–165, 1990.
3. A quality assurance primer for dentistry. J Am Dent Assoc 117:239–242, 1988.
4. Burt BA, Eklund SA: Dentistry, Dental Practice and the Community. Philadelphia, W.B. Saunders, 1992.
5. Dunning JM: Principles of Dental Public Health, 4th ed. Cambridge, MA, Harvard University Press, 1986.
6. Feldstein PJ: Health Care Economics. Albany, Delmar, 1988.
7. Hennekens CH, Buring JE: Epidemiology in Medicine. In Mayrent SL (ed). Boston, Little, Brown, 1987.
8. Jacobs P: The Economics of Health and Medical Care. Gaithersburg, MD, Aspen, 1991.
9. Jong A: Dental Public Health and Community Dentistry. St. Louis, Mosby, 1981.
10. Newburn E: Effectiveness of water fluoridation. J Public Health Dent 49:279–289, 1989.
11. Pagano M, Gauvreau K: Principles of Biostatistics. Boston, Harvard School of Public Health, 1991.
12. Public Health Focus: Fluoridation of community water systems. MMWR 1992; pp 372–375, 381.
13. Riordan PJ: Fluoride supplements in caries prevention: A literature review and proposal for a new dosage schedule. J Public Health Dent 53:174–189, 1993.
14. Ripa LW: A half century of community water fluoridation in the United States: Review and commentary. J Public Health Dent 53:17–44, 1993.
15. Rozier RG, Beck JD: Epidemiology of oral disease. Curr Opin Dent 1:308–315, 1991.
16. Silverman S: Oral Cancer. Atlanta, American Cancer Society, 1990.
17. Weinstein MC, Fineberg HV: Clinical Decision Analysis. Philadelphia, W.B. Saunders, 1980.
18. Weintraub JA, Douglass CW, Gillings DB: Biostatistics: Data Analysis for Dental Health Professionals. Chapel Hill, Cavco, 1985.

14. LEGAL ISSUES AND ETHICS IN DENTAL PRACTICE

Elliot V. Feldbau, D.M.D.

LEGAL ISSUES

1. What general principles of law apply to dental practice?
United States law is outlined under principles of criminal and civil law; the latter is divided as contract and tort law. Most legal issues related to dental practice involve civil wrongs or torts; that is, wrongful acts or injuries, not involving breach of contract, for which a court can bring a civil action for damages.

Negligence and malpractice are specific torts, requiring that the dentist's failure to employ the care and skill routinely practiced by other members of the profession is the "proximate cause" of a patient's injury. Both are considered unintentional torts and are normally covered by dental malpractice insurance.

Assault and battery are the unprivileged touching of another person's body. Both are termed intentional torts, and actions against dentists for battery usually center on issues of informed consent. Battery may include instances in which the patient consented to one procedure and the dentist performed another (e.g., working on the wrong tooth). The paramount question is whether the patient knew and agreed to what was done, not whether the dentist deviated from a certain standard of care.

Invasion of privacy, another intentional tort, results when a patient's image or name is used by a dentist for personal gain, such as in advertising. Discussing a patient by name without permission, with persons other than the clinical staff, also may be construed as a violation of the privacy implied by the doctor–patient relationship.

2. Under the law, how is the relationship between doctor and patient interpreted?
The law defines the doctor–patient relationship under the principles of contract law. The terms are usually implied but may be expressed. Upon accepting a patient for care, the dentist is obliged (1) to maintain confidentiality, (2) to complete care in a timely and professional manner, (3) to ensure that care is available in emergency situations or in the absence of the dentist, and (4) to be compensated for treatment by the patient. Of interest, the contract is termed binding at the earliest point of contact; that is, the moment of a telephone call to the dentist may be interpreted as the point of consummation of the contract, unless the dentist refuses to consider the caller for care or does not realize that the caller is a patient.

3. May a dentist dismiss a patient after beginning treatment?
Generally the dentist's liability for the patient's care continues even if treatment cannot be completed. Another competent practitioner must be found to take over care, and the dentist may be obliged to provide follow-up treatment. Abandonment is considered a breach of contract and grounds for a lawsuit.

4. What is considered adequate informed consent? What issues of law are considered when lack of informed consent is alleged?
A dentist must disclose to a patient in writing the procedure, the risks of the procedure, alternatives to the suggested treatment, and risks associated with the alternatives. A dentist may be liable for any resulting injury to the patient, even without negligence, if informed consent is not obtained. Furthermore, the patient must understand the disclosure, which should be phrased in simple and common terms. The disclosure is deemed adequate when it is measured by the standard of what a reasonable dental practitioner would disclose under similar circumstances.

Lack of informed consent is the fastest growing cause of action against dentists; therefore, it is often suggested that the document should be read and signed by the patient and witnessed by a dental assistant. The best defense for the practitioner is a proper document showing that he or she explained all material risks and alternatives and that the patient demonstrated understanding.

5. When may the issue of informed consent be bypassed?
In an emergency implied consent is recognized by good Samaritan statutes. Such an emergency exists when treatment cannot be postponed without jeopardizing the life or well-being of the patient and the patient is unable to grant consent because of physical impairment.

6. Who is responsible if a dental hygienist performs prophylactic treatment without proper premedication on a patient who develops subacute bacterial endocarditis after relating a history of rheumatic fever and heart valve replacement on their medical form?
Under the legal principle of "respondeat superior" ("let the master answer"), the employees of a dentist as well as the dentist may be sued for negligence (deviating from the standard of care) or other issues of malpractice or battery during the course of their employment.

7. Does a missed diagnosis or failure of treatment constitute negligence?
An incorrect diagnosis does not necessarily constitute negligence. Because of the many judgments involved in dental practice it is considered unrealistic to expect that a dentist be 100% correct. The plaintiff must demonstrate serious injury because of the dentist's failure to diagnose properly before there are grounds for negligence. Furthermore, it must be shown that the dentist failed to exercise the applicable standard of care. But injury alone is grounds to file a suit for negligence.

If the outcome of treatment is bad (e.g., a failed endodontic treatment due to a separated instrument), negligence is not necessarily supported if the appropriate standard of treatment is employed. However, if a dentist promises to effect a specific cure, to bring about a particular result, or to complete a procedure with no residual problems and he fails to fulfill the promise, a lawsuit may be filed on the basis of breach of contract rather than negligence.

8. When should a patient be referred?
A patient should be referred under the following circumstances:
1. When there is a question of appropriate treatment;
2. When periodontal treatment not routinely performed by the general dentist is indicated;
3. When periodontal disease is advanced with severe bone loss;
4. When shared responsibility is desirable for complex multidisciplinary cases;
5. When complex care is required for medically compromised patients; and
6. When the patient is refractory to treatment or unstable with a well-documented history of previous treatment failures.

9. What are common reasons for patients to sue?
1. Lack of informed consent: a patient does not know the specific nature and/or complications of treatment.
2. Failure to refer: for example, treating advanced periodontal disease with only scalings.
3. Failure to treat or diagnose adequately.
4. Abandonment: if the patient was dismissed for nonpayment of services, the dentist must show that other avenues were tried, such as small claims court or collection agencies. The dentist should document the reason for the dismissal and make available a referral source and any necessary emergency care for a period of 60 days. Communications to the patient should be through a registered letter.
5. Guarantees by doctor or staff.
6. Poor patient rapport.
7. Lack of communication.

8. Poor recordkeeping.
9. Issues related to fee collection.

10. What is necessary to prove negligence?
Two elements are necessary to prove negligence:
1. A relationship to the patient, which may begin with a telephone call, an examination, or a radiograph, and
2. The duty to render a standard of care and the breach of that duty with resultant injury to a patient.

11. What are gounds for revocation of a dental license?
Criminal convictions involving fraud and deception in prescribing drugs, gross immorality, or conviction of a felony under state law are grounds for revocation, usually by decision of the state licensing board.

12. What issues may constitute a defense against malpractice?
In a claim of malpractice or negligence, the patient must show that his or her injuries are directly associated with the dentist's wrongful acts or that standards of care were not followed. Failure to achieve successful treatment or to satisfy a patient with esthetic results does not necessarily constitute negligence.

"Contributory negligence" is a special phrase used in the law to describe what the plaintiff may have done to contribute to his or her own injury. Contributory negligence may occur if the patient does not comply with specific instructions regarding medications or home care and summarily dismisses any claims of negligence.

13. What elements are contained in a complete dental record?
Identification data

Medical history, including updated antibiotic regimens for prophylaxis of subacute bacterial endocarditis, effects of medication on birth control pills, and medical consultations when needed

Dental history

Clinical examination

Diagnosis and interpretation of radiographs

Treatment plans

Progress notes

Consent forms for surgical procedures

Completion notes

14. How should records be written and corrections be made?
All entries require ink or typed notes, not pencil, and errors must be lined out with a single line and initialed, with the substitute entry correcting the error. This procedure guards against any challenge to the reliability of record entries.

ETHICS

15. How is the practice of dentistry broadly governed?
The ethical rules and principles of professional conduct for the practice of dentistry are set fourth in the American Dental Association's publication, *Principles of Ethics and Code of Professional Conduct,* which describes the role of the professional in the practice of dentistry.

16. What three ethical principles are outlined in the code?
1. Beneficence: being kind and/or doing good
2. Autonomy: respect of the patient's right of self-decision
3. Justice: the quality of being impartial and fair

17. How does the code define beneficence in the practice of dentistry?
The dentist is obliged:

    1. To give the highest quality of service of which he or she is capable. This implies that professionals will maintain their level of knowledge by continued skill development.

    2. To preserve healthy dentition unless it compromises the well-being of other teeth; and

    3. To participate in legal and public health–related matters.

18. Who is expected to be responsible for practices of preventive health maintenance?
The patient is expected to be responsible for his or her own preventive practices. The dentist is responsible for providing information and supportive care (e.g., recall and prophylaxis), but the patient has the ultimate responsibility to maintain oral health.

19. Outline the essential elements implied in the principle of autonomy.
The principle of autonomy requires a respect for the patient's rights in the areas of confidentiality, informed consent for diagnostic and therapeutic services, and truthfulness to the patient. The dentist should work with patients to allow them to make autonomous decisions about their care. The dentist is obliged to provide services for which the patient contracts.

20. How does the profession serve justice, according to the code?
The individual dentist and the profession as a whole are obligated to be just and fair in the delivery of dental services. Self-regulation is a basic tenet of this obligation as well as calling attention to any social injustices in the allocation of societal resources to the delivery of dental health services.

21. Discuss the ethical principles that apply to decision making in each of the following examples.

    1. A 29-year-old patient with poor oral hygiene and multiple caries requests full-mouth extractions and dentures. A complete examination reveals a basically sound periodontium and carious lesions that can be restored conservatively. How does one best serve this basic case of neglect without advanced disease?

    Respect for the patient's autonomy and requests is evaluated and judged against the duty of the dentist to provide the highest type of service of which he or she is capable. After full disclosure about long-term effects of edentulism, as well as the costs and benefits of saving teeth, the assessment of the patient's motivation is most important. Saving teeth that will only fall into disrepair through neglect and the patient's lack of commitment to maintain oral health have to be considered carefully before a final treatment is elected or rejected.

    2. A patient rejects the use of radiographs for examination of his teeth. How should this situation be handled, according to the code?

    The dentist's only recourse is to use informed consent about the risks and benefits of an incomplete examination and the possible consequences of such a decision. The respect of the patient's right to choose (autonomy) prevails, even if it generates a negative obligation not to interfere with a patient's choice.

    3. An adolescent presents with a suspected lesion of a sexually transmitted disease (STD) and asks that no one, especially his parents, be told. What are the ethical considerations?

    The right of autonomy and respect for privacy is overturned by the public health law that requires the reporting of STDs to the health department. Public law is often the determinant in such situations.

    4. A patient requests that all her amalgam restorations be replaced. Is this an ethical issue?

    It is not unethical to replace amalgams on request. It is considered untruthful, and hence unethical, to make any claim that a patient's general health will be improved or that the patient will rid her body of toxins by replacing amalgam restorations. It would be unethical to ascribe any disease to the use of dental amalgam, because no causal relationship has been proved, or to attempt to treat any systemic disease by the removal of dental amalgams.

22. What disciplinary penalties may be imposed on a dentist found guilty of unethical conduct?

1. Censure: a disciplinary sentence written to express severe criticism or disapproval for a particular type of conduct or act.

2. Suspension: a loss of membership privileges for a period of time with automatic reinstatement.

3. Probation: a specified period without the loss of rights in lieu of a suspended disciplinary penalty.

4. Expulsion: absolute severance from the profession.

23. For what acts may a dentist be charged with unethical conduct?

1. A guilty verdict for a criminal felony.

2. A guilty verdict for violating the bylaws or principles of the Code of Ethics.

24. To what guiding principle does the ADA's Principles of Conduct and Code of Professional Ethics ascribe?

Service to the public and quality of care are the two aspects of the dental profession's obligation to society elaborated in the code.

25. May a dentist refuse to care for certain patients?

It is unethical for a dentist to refuse to accept patients because of race, creed, color, sex, or national origin or because the patient has acquired immunodeficiency syndrome (AIDS) or is infected with the human immunodeficiency virus (HIV). Treatment decisions and referrals should be made on the same basis as they are made for any patient that the dentist treats. Such decisions should be based only on the need of a dentist for another dentist's skills, knowledge, equipment, or experience to serve best the patient's health needs.

26. May a dentist relate information about a patient's seropositivity for HIV to another dentist to whom he or she is referring the patient?

The laws that safeguard the confidentiality of a patient's record are not uniform throughout the United States with regard to HIV status. It may be prohibited to transfer this information without the written permission of the patient. As a rule, the treating dentist is advised to seek written permission from the patient before releasing any information to the consulting practitioner.

27. May a dentist accept a copayment from a dental insurance company as payment in full for services and not request the patient's portion?

It is considered "overbilling" and hence unethical to collect only the third-party payment without full disclosure to the insurance company.

28. What is overbilling?

Overbilling is the misrepresentation of a fee as higher than in fact it is; for example, when a patient is charged one fee and an insurance company is billed a higher fee to benefit the patient's copayment.

29. May a dentist charge different fees to different patients for the same services?

It is considered unethical to increase a fee to a patient because the patient has insurance. However, different treatment scenarios and conditions may prevail and dictate different fees, regardless of the form of payment.

30. Is it appropriate to advance treatment dates on insurance claims for a patient who otherwise would not be eligible for dental benefits?

It is considered false and misleading representation to the third-party payer to advance treatment dates for services not undertaken within the benefit period.

31. What are the standards for advertising by dentists?

Advertising is permitted as long as it is not false or misleading in any manner. Infringements of the standards involve statements that include inferences of specialty by a general dentist, use of unearned degrees as titles or nonhealth degrees to enhance prestige, or use of "HIV-negative health results" to attract patients without conveying information that clarifies the scientific significance of the statement.

32. How may specialization be expressed? What are the standard guidelines?
To allow the public to make an informed selection between the dentist who has completed accredited training beyond the dental degree and the dentist who has not, an announcement of specialization is permitted. The areas of ethical specialty recognized by the American Dental Association are dental public health, endodontics, oral pathology, oral surgery, orthodontics, pediatric dentistry, periodontics, and prosthodontics. Any announcement should read "specialist in" or practice "limited to" the respective field. Dentists making such announcements must have met the educational requirements of the ADA for the specialty.

33. What are the stated guidelines for the name of a dental practice?
Because the name of a practice may be a selection factor on the patient's part, it must not be misleading in any manner. The name of a dentist no longer associated with the practice may be continued for a period of 1 year.

34. What does the code state about chemical dependency of dentists?
It is unethical for a dentist to practice while abusing alcohol or other chemical substances that impair ability. All dentists are obligated to urge impaired colleagues to seek treatment and to report firsthand evidence of abuse by a colleague to the professional assistance committee of a dental society. The professional assistance committee is obligated to report noncompliers to the appropriate regulatory boards for licensing review.

35. How are problems of interpretation of the "Principles of Ethics and Code of Professional Conduct" to be resolved?
Problems involving questions of ethics should be resolved by the local dental society. If resolutions cannot be achieved, an appeal to the ADA's Council on Ethics, Bylaws and Judicial Affairs is the next step.

BIBLIOGRAPHY

Law and Dental Practice

1. Barsley RE, Herschaft EE: Dental malpractice. In Hardin JF (ed): Clark's Clinical Dentistry, vol. 5. Philadelphia, J.B. Lippincott, 1992, ch 23A, pp 1–26.
2. Brackett RC, Poulsom RC: The law and the dental health practitioner. In Hardin JF (ed): Clark's Clinical Dentistry, vol. 5. Philadelphia, J.B. Lippincott, 1992, ch 37, pp 1–42.
3. Pollack B: Risk management in dental office practice. In Hardin JF (ed): Clark's Clinical Dentistry, vol. 5. Philadelphia, J.B. Lippincott, 1992, ch 23A, pp 1–26
4. Pollack B: Legal risks associated with implant dentistry. In Hardin JF (ed): Clark's Clinical Dentistry, vol. 5. Philadelphia, J.B. Lippincott, 1992, ch 45A, pp 1–8.
5. Pollack B: Legal risks associated with management of the temporomandibular joint. In Hardin JF (ed): Clark's Clinical Dentistry, vol. 5. Philadelphia, J.B. Lippincott, 1992, ch 35, pp 1–11.
6. Risk Management Foundation of the Harvard Medical Institutions. Claims Management and the Legal Process. Cambridge, MA, 1994.

Ethics and Dentistry

7. American Dental Association: Principles of Ethics and Code of Professional conduct, with official advisory opinions revised to May 1992. Chicago, American Dental Association, 1992.
8 Massachusetts Dental Society. Code of Ethics. Natick, MA, 1986.
9. McCullough LB: Ethical issues in dentistry. In Hardin JF (ed): Clark's Clinical Dentistry, vol. 1. Philadelphia, J.B. Lippincott, 1992, ch. 36, pp 1–17.
10. Ozar DT: AIDS, ethics, and dental care. In Hardin JF (ed): Clark's Clinical Dentistry, vol. 1. Philadelphia, J.B. Lippincott, 1992, ch. 36, 1–17.

INDEX

Page numbers in **boldface** type indicate complete chapters.